Hypertension in Pregnancy

Hypertension in Pregnancy

edited by

Michael A. Belfort
University of Utah Health Sciences Center
Salt Lake City
and Utah Valley Regional Medical Center
Provo, Utah, U.S.A.

Steven Thornton
University of Warwick
Coventry, England

George R. Saade
University of Texas Medical Branch
Galveston, Texas, U.S.A.

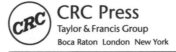
CRC Press
Taylor & Francis Group
Boca Raton London New York

CRC Press is an imprint of the
Taylor & Francis Group, an **informa** business

CRC Press
Taylor & Francis Group
6000 Broken Sound Parkway NW, Suite 300
Boca Raton, FL 33487-2742

© 2003 by Taylor & Francis Group, LLC
CRC Press is an imprint of Taylor & Francis Group, an Informa business

No claim to original U.S. Government works

Visit the Taylor & Francis Web site at
http://www.taylorandfrancis.com

and the CRC Press Web site at
http://www.crcpress.com

For my wife, Joanne; my children, Sarah and Benjamin; and my late grandfather, Meyer Michael Belfort, who would have been so happy to see a Belfort edit a book.

Michael A. Belfort

To my parents, Harry and Connie; wife, George; and children, Joe and Sarah.

Steven Thornton

To my parents, Robert and Malak.

George R. Saade

Preface

Preeclampsia and the hypertensive disorders of pregnancy remain significant problems in modern obstetrics. Although there have been huge advances in basic science over the past two decades, we still have no defined etiology for preeclampsia/eclampsia. Despite this obvious void in our knowledge, there have been significant clinical advances in the management of preeclampsia and its severe complications, and the care of women affected by these conditions continues to be refined.

The format and scope of this book are such that it is not intended to be an exhaustive reference text but rather a focused spotlight on the latest additions to our literature. Our intention is to inform the reader about important new developments in the classification, etiology, differential diagnosis, and management of preeclampsia, related hypertensive diseases during pregnancy, and their complications. This volume was conceptualized to achieve a number of rather specific aims. The first and most pressing of these was to focus attention on recent findings that may not yet be reflected in the most recent editions of general obstetric textbooks. This was achieved by having a rapid turnaround from writing to publication. Even so, a number of the chapters required extensive rewriting due to significant new findings. We appreciate the efforts of our contributors who were affected by this and who responded so magnificently by rewriting and updating their material.

Another aim was to decrease the differences between standards of practice on different continents. To this end we asked leading experts from around the world to use an evidence-based approach to the writing of their chapters, rather than describe their local or regional techniques. Where appropriate we have had to accept slight differences in practice that may exist but, in general, these are few and far between and represent drug availability in the different countries more than anything else. One of the more glaring of the practice differences has recently been addressed by the publication of the MAGPIE Study findings, and Chapter 9, on the use of magnesium sulfate in preeclampsia, highlights this.

The final major aim was to address aspects of management as they specifically apply to the patient with preeclampsia. We have therefore included chapters on new methods of noninvasive evaluation of cardiac function and hemodynamics in preeclampsia, fetal monitoring, anesthesia, and on specific drug therapy for preeclampsia and its complications.

Michael A. Belfort
Steven Thornton
George R. Saade

Contents

Contributors

John Anthony, M.B.Ch.B., F.C.O.G.(S.A.) Professor, Department of Obstetrics and Gynaecology, University of Cape Town, Cape Town, South Africa

Philip N. Baker, M.R.C.O.G., D.M. Professor, Maternal and Fetal Health Research Centre, The University of Manchester, Manchester, England

Michael A. Belfort, M.B.B.C.H., D.A.(S.A.), M.R.C.O.G., F.A.C.O.G., M.D., Ph.D. Professor, Department of Obstetrics/Gynecology, University of Utah Health Sciences Center, Salt Lake City, and Utah Valley Regional Medical Center, Provo, Utah, U.S.A.

Mark A. Brown, M.D. Professor, Departments of Renal Medicine and Medicine, St. George Hospital and University of New South Wales, Sydney, New South Wales, Australia

Rosie Burton, M.D. University of Cape Town, Cape Town, South Africa

John M. Davison, M.D., M.Sc., F.R.C.O.G. Professor, Department of Obstetrics and Gynaecology, Royal Victoria Infirmary, University of Newcastle Upon Tyne, Newcastle Upon Tyne, England

Gustaaf Albert Dekker, M.D., Ph.D. Professor, Department of Obstetrics and Gynaecology, Lyell McEwin Health Service, University of Adelaide, Adelaide, South Australia, Australia

Gary A. Dildy III, M.D.   Professor, Department of Obstetrics and Gynecology, Louisiana State University School of Medicine, New Orleans, Louisiana, U.S.A.

Pragasan Dean Gopalan, M.B.Ch.B., F.C.A.(S.A.), CritCare(S.A.)   Senior Specialist and Lecturer, Department of Anaesthetics, Nelson R. Mandela School of Medicine, University of Natal, Durban, South Africa

Michael D. Hnat, D.O., F.A.C.O.G.   Fellow, Division of Maternal-Fetal Medicine, Department of Obstetrics and Gynecology, University of Cincinnati College of Medicine, Cincinnati, Ohio, U.S.A.

Christy M. Isler, M.D.   Assistant Professor, Department of Obstetrics and Gynecology, Brody School of Medicine, East Carolina University, Greenville, North Carolina, U.S.A.

Louise C. Kenny, M.B.Ch.B.(Hons), M.R.C.O.G.   Clinical Lecturer, Maternal and Fetal Health Research Centre, The University of Manchester, Manchester, England

Garrett K. Lam, M.D.   Clinical Instructor and Fellow, Division of Maternal-Fetal Medicine, Department of Obstetrics and Gynecology, University of North Carolina, Chapel Hill, North Carolina, U.S.A.

Everett F. Magann, M.D., F.A.C.O.G., F.R.A.N.Z.C.O.G.   Professor, Department of Obstetrics and Gynecology, University of Western Australia, Perth, Australia

James Martin, Jr., M.D.   Professor, Department of Obstetrics and Gynecology, Director, Division of Maternal-Fetal Medicine, and Chief of Obstetrics, University of Mississippi Medical Center, Jackson, Mississippi, U.S.A.

Kenneth J. Moise, Jr., M.D.   Professor, Division of Maternal-Fetal Medicine, Department of Obstetrics and Gynecology, University of North Carolina, Chapel Hill, North Carolina, U.S.A.

Justine C. Norman, M.D., Ch.B.   Fellow, Department of Obstetrics and Gynaecology, Royal Victoria Infirmary, University of Newcastle Upon Tyne, Newcastle Upon Tyne, England

Robyn A. North, M.B.Ch.B., Ph.D.   Associate Professor, Department of Obstretrics and Gynaecology, University of Auckland, Auckland, New Zealand

D. A. Rocke, M.R.C.P., F.C.A.(S.A.), F.R.C.P. Professor and Head, Nelson R. Mandela School of Medicine, University of Natal, Durban, South Africa

Roxann Rokey, M.D., F.A.C.C. Clinical Professor of Medicine, University of Wisconsin, Madison, and Co-Director of Echocardiography and Director, Adult Congenital Heart Disease Clinic, Department of Cardiology, Marshfield Clinic, Marshfield, Wisconsin, U.S.A.

Baha M. Sibai, M.D. Professor and Chairman, Department of Obstetrics and Gynecology, University of Cincinnati College of Medicine, Cincinnati, Ohio, U.S.A.

Usha Singh, D.A.(S.A.), F.C.A.(S.A.) Department of Anaesthesiology, Nelson R. Mandela School of Medicine, University of Natal, Durban, South Africa

Michael W. Varner, M.D. Professor, Department of Obstetrics and Gynecology, University of Utah, Salt Lake City, Utah, U.S.A.

Andrea G. Witlin, D.O., Ph.D. Assistant Professor, Women's Reproductive Health Research Scholar, Department of Obstetrics and Gynecology, University of Texas Medical Branch, Galveston, Texas, U.S.A.

Hypertension in Pregnancy

1

Diagnosis and Classification of Preeclampsia and Other Hypertensive Disorders of Pregnancy

Mark A. Brown
St. George Hospital and University of New South Wales, Sydney, New South Wales, Australia

I. INTRODUCTION

The diagnostic criteria for disorders of hypertension in pregnancy are not currently uniform and there are a number of different systems promulgated by major working groups and international societies. There has been some progress toward unifying the classification and the major consensus statements now agree on most of the terminology. As for preeclampsia, the two extremes of the diagnostic spectrum take either a "restrictive" or an "inclusive" approach. The former requires both de novo hypertension after 20 weeks and the presence of proteinuria > 300 mg/24 hours, while the latter assumes that preeclampsia is a multisystem disorder and a diagnosis of preeclampsia is based upon symptoms and signs in the organs commonly affected in this condition. Proponents of the restrictive concept argue that broadening the definition includes women who may not have true preeclampsia and this may influence the interpretation of research data. Others argue that since maternal and fetal outcomes are similar regardless of the specificity of the classification, it is safer to use the inclusive definition. A second controversial issue is the definition of hypertension in pregnancy.

A blood pressure of ≥ 140/90 mmHg has traditionally been used to make the diagnosis. Further studies are required to determine whether this cutoff provides the optimal balance between sensitivity and specificity. On a positive note, until recently, the method of measurement has been debated, but it is now accepted that the Korotkoff V sound should be used to determine diastolic pressure. While the most recent guidelines of the American College of Obstetricians and Gynecologists (ACOG) have excluded any comparison with early-trimester/nonpregnant blood pressure as part of the diagnostic criteria, many investigators still believe that adherence to an absolute blood pressure limit may miss a subgroup of women with preeclampsia. Moreover, this change in the ACOG guidelines may temper some of the conclusions derived from studies that included such women.

As for proteinuria, the diagnosis is far more inaccurate and subjective than that of hypertension. Recent studies confirm that dipstick urinalysis in hypertensive pregnancy is at best a rough screen for the presence or absence of true proteinuria.

The diagnosis and classification of the hypertensive disorders of pregnancy has been reviewed recently (1). This chapter attempts to update some of these issues, including the variability in diagnoses, the detection of proteinuria, and the difficulty of making the distinction between gestational hypertension and preeclampsia.

II. THE EXTENT OF THE PROBLEM

The authors of two recent reviews have analyzed manuscripts relating to preeclampsia published between 1997 and 1998 (2,3). These reviews demonstrated that the various methods for defining hypertension and proteinuria were so diverse that data could rarely be considered comparable. In an analysis of 135 articles from nine major journals, Harlow and Brown (3) found that there were major variations in the terminology and diagnostic criteria. In up to 30% of papers, no adequate definition of preeclampsia was given. When preeclampsia was defined, 80% of the papers required that both hypertension and proteinuria be present, while other papers required evidence of hypertension and multisystem organ dysfunction (e.g., renal, liver, cerebral involvement, thrombocytopenia) or only hypertension and edema. The methods for defining proteinuria varied. Up to one-fifth of papers relied on dipstick urinalysis despite its high false-positive and false-negative rates (discussed below). Seven percent of articles used urinary protein concentration (rather than excretion rate), which may be inaccurate due to the fact that it is influenced by the state of hydration and the urine flow rate. The definition of hypertension was generally around 140/90 mmHg. We noted that in about three-quarters of the papers, the authors included either systolic or diastolic pressure for their diagnosis. Chappell (2) found that about half relied on diastolic pressure alone. In two-thirds of the studies, hypertension was diagnosed on the basis of a single blood pressure reading despite the fact that "white-coat hypertension" has been shown to account for at least 25% of cases of elevated blood pressure in the clinic (4).

The three main variables affecting the accuracy of a blood pressure measurement are the device employed, the Korotkoff sound used to record the diastolic blood pressure, and the size of the blood pressure cuff. These details were not documented at all in 70 to 90% of the articles reviewed. In other words, even though there seems to be reasonable agreement in the literature as to what constitutes hypertension in pregnancy, there is still great variability in the way in which we arrive at such a blood pressure measurement. These two reviews are important in that they agree in their analyses and show that the diversity of definitions and diagnostic criteria for preeclampsia are such that the groups of women reported in these international journals could rarely be considered truly comparable.

III. COMPARISON OF AVAILABLE CLASSIFICATION SYSTEMS

Classifying the hypertensive disorders stimulates opposing opinions. The "inclusive" system is based on a pathophysiological description of preeclampsia as a multisystem disorder (5) and has been adopted by the Australasian Society for the Study of Hypertension in Pregnancy (ASSHP) (6). The "restrictive" classification, adopted by the (USA) National High Blood Pressure Education Program (NHBPEP) (8), limits the criteria of the diagnosis of preeclampsia to that of hypertension and proteinuria and provides differential guidance for clinical and research purposes.

It could be argued that a classification system for hypertension in pregnancy is not necessary. Increased blood pressure, whether associated with proteinuria or not, is a sign that deserves attention. On one hand, artificial classification may falsely reassure the clinician and lead to inadequate investigation and treatment of hypertension. On the other hand, an inclusive and generalized classification may lead to expensive and unnecessary intervention. The majority of care providers still find a classification system useful in order to translate research findings and management guidelines into clinical practice.

A. Requirements of a Good Classification System

The first major requirement of a classification system for hypertension in pregnancy should be the ability to stratify patients according to risk for adverse maternal and perinatal outcome, so that appropriate intervention and management can be instituted. An important discriminator is whether the hypertension arose de novo during the pregnancy or predated it. A system that can differentiate between de novo preeclampsia and underlying chronic hypertension would identify women at higher risk for adverse pregnancy outcomes but lower long-term risk. At a time when outpatient management is becoming popular, the ability to classify patients according to risk has become paramount.

B. Terminology of the Currently Available Systems

Chronic hypertension is perhaps the least debated term in current usage. Within this group, differentiation between women with essential hypertension and those with secondary hypertension is important, particularly since the latter may be reversible. This distinction is clearly made in the ASSHP and the Canadian (8) systems.

De novo hypertension in pregnancy is given a wide range of terms, including *preeclampsia* and *gestational hypertension*. The fact that preeclampsia does not include the word *hypertension* is a distinct advantage, as preeclampsia should be thought of as a multisystem disorder with elevated blood pressure as one component. *Gestational hypertension* describes high blood pressure pertaining to pregnancy with no other features of preeclampsia. This term seems appropriate, as blood pressure returns to normal after delivery. The inclusion of the word *hypertension* in this terminology is appropriate, because elevation of blood pressure is the only abnormality. Preeclampsia has been classified as mild or severe in some classification systems (9,10), but the definition of mild preeclampsia is inconsistent. This may lead to confusion between mild preeclampsia and gestational hypertension, and for this reason the latest ASSHP classification does not stratify preeclampsia (6). Gestational hypertension should not be confused with mild preeclampsia, since the two conditions are distinct.

C. Current Classification Systems

The currently used classification systems are summarized in Tables 1 through 4. The International Society for the Study of Hypertension in Pregnancy (ISSHP) has a detailed classification system, adopted from Davey and MacGillivray (11) (Table 1). This has not been revised for more than a decade, while at least four other systems have been proposed in that time. The merit of this ISSHP system is that it attempts to cover all possible presentations of the hypertensive disorders of pregnancy, but it is too unwieldy for routine clinical use. In essence, the system makes the diagnosis of preeclampsia when de novo hypertension in pregnancy is accompanied by proteinuria.

The NHBPEP published its first classification system in 1990 (12) and has slightly modified it in its current iteration (Table 2). This is a clinically focused classification. A diagnosis of preeclampsia is made when de novo hypertension in pregnancy is accompanied by proteinuria. Edema, a feature of the earlier NHBPEP classification, has now been discarded as a diagnostic criterion. Isolated hypertension is now referred to as gestational hypertension of pregnancy.

The Australasian Society of the Study of Hypertension in Pregnancy published its first consensus statement in 1993 (9). In this, it defined all de novo hypertension as preeclampsia, subclassifying it as mild preeclampsia when hypertension was the only feature and severe preeclampsia when there was any evidence of multisystem disorder in the mother. While this was an easy classification

Table 1 International Society for the Study of Hypertension in Pregnancy
Classification of Hypertension in Pregnancy

A. New-onset hypertension and/or proteinuria in pregnancy[a]
   1. Gestational hypertension (without proteinuria)
   2. Gestational proteinuria (without hypertension)
   3. Preeclampsia (hypertension with proteinuria)
B. Chronic hypertension and renal disease
   1. Chronic hypertension and renal disease
   2. Chronic renal disease (proteinuria with or without hypertension)[b]
   3. Chronic hypertension with superimposed preeclampsia (i.e., with new-onset
       proteinuria in pregnancy)[c]
C. Unclassified
   1. Hypertension and/or proteinuria noted *when first presentation* is after 20 weeks.
   2. As above, when noted for the first time during pregnancy, labor, or puerperium
       and there are insufficient background data to permit a diagnosis from category A
       or B above.
D. Eclampsia

---

[a]Presenting antenatally, in labor, or the puerperium.
[b]Many renal disorders will not include proteinuria, particularly in their early stages.
[c]In many cases, the distinction between progressive renal disease and superimposed preeclampsia may
be impossible on clinical grounds.
Source: Ref. 11.

system to follow, the inclusion of the term *mild preeclampsia* was misleading
when the only abnormality was elevated blood pressure. This approach does not
equate with our current understanding of the pathogenesis of preeclampsia as a
multisystem disorder (5,13).

The ISSHP and the early NHBPEP and ASSHP classifications created different reporting systems for preeclampsia. In order to compare these systems, we
prospectively audited 1183 consecutive women diagnosed with hypertension in
pregnancy in our unit, representing 6.7% of all deliveries during a 6-year period
(14). For the purpose of this analysis, we considered the NHBPEP and ISSHP
systems as one, both systems requiring proteinuria for a diagnosis of preeclampsia. We compared this system (proteinuric preeclampsia versus gestational/
transient hypertension) with the classification system then proposed by the
ASSHP [mild (nonproteinuric) versus severe (proteinuric) preeclampsia] (15).
Significant differences in the reporting of outcomes of these pregnancies were
apparent using these two classification methods. Preeclampsia was diagnosed in
only 16% of our patients using the former classification (NHBPEP) but in 77%
using the ASSHP classification (14). It should be noted that the apparent low
prevalence of preeclampsia using the NHBPEP classification probably resulted
from our very strict requirements for proteinuria. This required that the 24-hour
urine protein be $\geq$300 mg/day, persistently $\geq$2+ dipstick testing, or a spot urine

Table 2 National High Blood Pressure Education Program Classification of
Hypertension in Pregnancy

A. Chronic hypertension[a]
   Hypertension present before pregnancy, diagnosed before 20 weeks' gestation, or
   failing to resolve within 12 weeks postpartum
B. Preeclampsia—eclampsia[b]
   Usually occurring after 20 weeks, defined by hypertension and proteinuria
C. Preeclampsia superimposed upon chronic hypertension[c]
   New-onset proteinuria in those without proteinuria at start of pregnancy
   An increase in proteinuria, blood pressure levels, or thrombocytopenia or abnormal
   liver enzymes in those who already had proteinuria at the start of pregnancy
D. Gestational hypertension
   De novo hypertension during pregnancy without proteinuria
   Include women with features of preeclampsia who have not manifested proteinuria
   Reclassified 3 months postpartum as "transient hypertension" if blood pressure
   returned to normal

---

[a]Does not clearly divide essential and secondary forms of hypertension.
[b]Preeclampsia is suspected if proteinuria is absent, but de novo hypertension is accompanied by
features such as headache, blurred vision, abdominal pain, thrombocytopenia, or abnormal liver
function.
[c]A diagnosis of superimposed preeclampsia in a patient with primary renal disease can be suspect if it
relies only on an increase in protein excretion or blood pressure.
Source: Ref. 7.

protein:creatinine ratio ⩾30 mg protein per millimole of creatinine. Women
classified as having preeclampsia in the ISSHP/NHBPEP system were at much
greater risk for complications than those identified by the ASSHP system, with a
significantly higher prevalence of all maternal complications, perinatal mortality,
and earlier gestation at delivery.

The two classification systems were also compared to determine which
system better stratified women with de novo hypertension in pregnancy at *low* risk
for complications. Women classified as having mild preeclampsia according to the
old ASSHP system (isolated hypertension, now referred to as gestational hypertension in the revised ASSHP 2000 document) were compared with those categorized as having gestational/transient hypertension in the NHBPEP/ISSHP classifications (nonproteinuric hypertension). Maternal complication rates were all
significantly higher (except for renal insufficiency) in low-risk patients classified
using the NHBPEP/ISSHP system, although perinatal mortality rates did not
differ significantly (Table 5, Figure 1).

The ASSHP system was revised in 2000 (6) and has taken the broad
"inclusive" approach of defining preeclampsia as de novo hypertension after 20
weeks gestation in a patient who has any of the features known to occur in
preeclampsia (Table 3). It does not confine the diagnosis to those with proteinuria.

Table 3 The Australasian Society for the Study of Hypertension in Pregnancy 2000 Classification System for Hypertensive Pregnancies

1. Gestational hypertension: De novo hypertension after 20 weeks' gestation, without any other features of preeclampsia, returning to normal within 3 months postpartum
2. Preeclampsia: De novo hypertension[a] arising after 20 weeks' gestation returning to normal within 3 months postpartum and one or more of the following:
   Proteinuria—$\geq$ 300 mg/day or spot urine protein: creatinine $\geq$ 30 mg/mmol
   Renal insufficiency—plasma creatinine $\geq$ 0.09 mmol/L or oliguria
   Liver disease—raised serum transaminases and/or severe epigastric/right upper-quadrant pain
   Neurological problems—convulsions (eclampsia), hyperreflexia with clonus, severe headaches with hyperreflexia, persistent visual disturbances (scotomata)
   Hematological disturbances—thrombocytopenia, hemolysis, disseminated intravascular coagulation
   Fetal growth restriction
3. Chronic hypertension
   (a) Essential hypertension: Blood pressure $\geq$ 140 mmHg systolic and/or $\geq$ 90 mmHg diastolic preconception or in the first half of pregnancy without an apparent secondary cause or evidence of "white-coat" hypertension.
   (b) Secondary hypertension
4. Preeclampsia superimposed on chronic hypertension

[a]Hypertension in pregnancy is defined as an absolute BP $\geq$ 140 mmHg systolic and/or $\geq$ 90 mmHg diastolic. Edema is not included in any part of this classification system. Proteinuria is not mandatory for a diagnosis of preeclampsia.
Source: Ref. 6.

Table 4 Canadian Hypertension Society Classification System for Hypertensive Pregnancies

A. Preexisting hypertension
   1. Essential
   2. Secondary
B. Gestational hypertension
   1. Without proteinuria[a]
   2. With proteinuria[b]
C. Preexisting hypertension plus superimposed gestational hypertension with proteinuria
D. Unclassifiable antenatally[c]

[a]Equates to NHBPEP definition of gestational hypertension.
[b]Equates to NHBPEP definition of preeclampsia. Both groups of "gestational hypertensives" may have "adverse conditions" that involve problems such as eclampsia, thrombocytopenia, pulmonary edema, or elevated liver enzymes.
[c]Refers to women in whom blood pressure was not measured until after 20 weeks' gestation. Only allows 6 weeks for blood pressure to normalize postpartum before applying a retrospective label of "preexisting hypertension."
Source: Ref. 8.

Table 5 Maternal and Fetal Outcomes and Laboratory Data in Women with Nonproteinuric de Novo Hypertension in Pregnancy According to Classification System Used

	Gestational hypertension (ASSHP)	Gestational/transient hypertension (NHBPEP/ISSHP)	p Value
Number of women	502	665	
Age (years)	28 (5)	28 (5)	0.30
Nulliparas (%)	59	60	0.73
Gestation—presentation (weeks)	36 (5)	36 (5)	0.87
Gestation—delivery (weeks)	38 (2)	38 (2)	0.92
Hyperuricemia (%)	47	53	0.03
Maternal complications (%)			
Severe hypertension	2	13	<0.0001*
Thrombocytopenia	1	8	<0.0001*
Renal insufficiency	0	1	0.009
Liver disease	1	7	<0.0001*
Neurological	1	7	<0.0001*
Laboratory data			
Plasma creatinine (mmol/L)	0.07 (0.02)	0.07 (0.02)	0.09
Plasma uric acid (mmol/L)	0.37 (0.12)	0.38 (0.18)	0.35
Plasma albumin (g/L)	35 (3)	34 (4)	0.06
Hemoglobin (g/L)	122 (14)	122 (16)	0.41
Hematocrit (%)	36.1 (4.2)	35.8 (5.1)	0.50
Platelets ($\times 10^9$/L)	245 (77)	234 (81)	0.03
Fetal complications			
Small for gestational age (%)	14	17	0.11
Perinatal mortality rate (per 1000)	6	6	1.0
Birth weight (g)	3194 (541)	3097 (601)	0.004*

Data are percentages or mean (standard deviation). * = Statistically significant after correction for multiple comparisons.

The document states that this is largely a clinical classification and that for research purposes a more restrictive diagnosis, such as that of the NHBPEP, is more appropriate.

The American College of Obstetricians and Gynecologists published a technical bulletin in 1996 which was at odds with their national body's NHBPEP publication (10). The ACOG bulletin uses the term *pregnancy-induced hypertension* and defines this as mild and severe in much the same way as the original ASSHP document defined mild and severe preeclampsia.

A further classification has been proposed by Redman and Jefferies (16) in which the diagnosis of preeclampsia depends on an initial diastolic blood pressure less than 90 mm Hg with a subsequent rise of at least 25 mmHg to more than 90

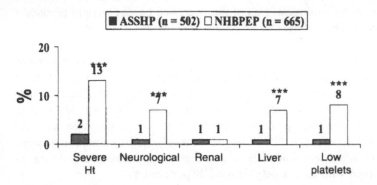

Figure 1 Comparison of maternal outcomes in low-risk hypertensive pregnant women with gestational hypertension as diagnosed by the ASSHP (n = 502) versus NHBPEP (n = 665) classification systems. The *** denotes a significant difference. (Adapted from Ref. 14.)

mmHg. No mention is made in this classification of the other pathophysiologic features of preeclampsia.

North et al. (17) recently studied 1496 nulliparous women. They defined gestational hypertension as a systolic blood pressure $\geq$ 140 mmHg with a rise of at least 30 mmHg from early pregnancy, or as a diastolic blood pressure $\geq$ 90 mmHg, with a rise of at least 15 mmHg. Preeclampsia was defined as hypertension with proteinuria $\geq$ 300 mg/day or $\geq$ 1 g/L (2+) on dipstick testing. Those with hypertension but lower degrees of proteinuria, including 0.3 g/L (1+) on dipstick testing, were considered to have gestational hypertension. Five percent of this cohort developed preeclampsia and 8% developed gestational hypertension; 40% of the women who developed preeclampsia had one or more features of multi-system dysfunction (e.g., abnormal liver function, thrombocytopenia), and 56% had episodes of severe hypertension. About 10% of women with gestational hypertension had features of multisystem dysfunction and 22% had episodes of severe hypertension. Further analysis of the gestational hypertension patients showed that those with 1+ proteinuria had a higher incidence of severe maternal disease or severe hypertensive episodes. This may be expected, since these women would have been classified as preeclamptic in most other systems.

The final significant contribution to classification systems is that of the Canadian Hypertension Society (8), published in 1997, which is very similar to the current NHBPEP document.

D. Consolidation of the Classification Systems

The most recently published statements on this topic are remarkably consistent (NHBPEP 2000, ASSHP 2000) and use virtually identical terminology. It would alleviate some of the confusion if all of the interested parties were to produce a unified document. There is general agreement that hypertension before 20 weeks of gestation is not preeclampsia (unless associated with gestational trophoblastic disease) or gestational hypertension but is either essential or secondary chronic hypertension. There is agreement (though with differing terminology) that de novo hypertension after 20 weeks associated with proteinuria defines preeclampsia. There is still a difference of opinion regarding: (a) whether women with de novo hypertension who do not have proteinuria but do have one or more features of preeclampsia should be classified as preeclamptic or gestational hypertensive and (b) whether a diagnosis of gestational hypertension should be restricted to women who have solely de novo hypertension.

E. How Should We Approach These Different Viewpoints?

We have previously analyzed the outcomes of women with preeclampsia defined by the "inclusive" ASSHP classification (14). In this category we defined women as having preeclampsia on the basis of hypertension as well as one or more of proteinuria, neurological, renal, hepatic, or thrombocytopenic abnormalities. This description accounts for the systemic nature of preeclampsia but does not insist on proteinuria for a diagnosis; in fact, 49% of this group had proteinuria (rigorously defined as either $\geq 2+$ proteinuria and/or ≥ 300 mg/day). When this system of classifying preeclamptics was compared with the NHBPEP/ISSHP system (which requires proteinuria) there was no significant difference in maternal or fetal outcomes between the groups (Table 6, Fig. 2). In other words, this category of the ASSHP classification system takes account of what we understand to be the pathophysiology of preeclampsia, does not insist upon proteinuria for a diagnosis as long as other evidence of the pathophysiology is present, but gives a similar stratification of risk as does the diagnosis of "proteinuric preeclampsia."

The disadvantages are that this remains a relatively small sample for analysis and that in this system of classification the signs are "soft," e.g., what one clinician calls hyperreflexia another might not. Further, laboratory abnormalities are hard to categorize, e.g., because the platelet count may fall without consequence in up to 8% of otherwise normal pregnancies (18), at what level should thrombocytopenia be defined in a hypertensive pregnant woman? Liver transaminase levels generally remain unchanged in pregnancy (19) and serum creatinine falls as part of the increase in glomerular filtration rate in normal pregnancy so any elevation of AST or ALT ≥ 40 IU/L or serum creatinine ≥ 0.09 mmol/L should be considered abnormal. Other symptoms and signs also remain difficult to standardize, e.g., epigastric pain in a hypertensive pregnant woman should be considered extremely serious as it may represent subcapsular hematoma of the liver, but it might equally turn out to be no more than indigestion!

Therefore, the ASSHP system of defining preeclampsia is an "inclusive"

Table 6 Maternal and Fetal Outcomes and Laboratory Data in Women with de Novo Hypertension in Pregnancy According to Classification System Used

	Preeclampsia (NHBPEP/ISSHP)	Preeclampsia (ASSHP)	p Value
Number of women	160	323	
Age (years)	28 (5)	29 (5)	0.33
Nulliparas (%)	68	65	0.64
Gestation—presentation (weeks)	34 (6)	35 (5)	0.17
Gestation—delivery (weeks)	36 (4)	37 (3)	0.5
Hyperuricemia (%)	79	76	0.52
Maternal complications (%)			
Severe hypertension	53	50	0.50
Thrombocytopenia	19	24	0.21
Proteinuria	100	49	0.0001*
Renal insufficiency	21	17	0.38
Liver disease	21	23	0.52
Neurological	33	29	0.49
Laboratory data			
Plasma creatinine (mmol/L)	0.08 (0.07)	0.08 (0.05)	0.74
Plasma uric acid (mmol/L)	0.42 (0.09)	0.42 (0.08)	0.40
Plasma albumin (g/L)	30 (7)	32 (7)	0.02
Hemoglobin (g/L)	115 (32)	117 (27)	0.50
Hematocrit (%)	33.9 (6.8)	34.6 (7.0)	0.40
Platelets ($\times 10^9$/L)	196 (79)	198 (81)	0.80
Fetal complications			
Small for gestational age (%)	24	26	0.65
Perinatal mortality rate (per 1000)	38	22	0.31
Birth weight (g)	2498 (866)	2646 (788)	

Data are percentages or mean (standard deviation). * = Statistically significant after correction for maternal comparisons.

and sensitive system, which should drive good clinical practice by alerting clinicians to look for the multisystem features of preeclampsia but is likely to be much less specific than the "restrictive" NHBPEP, ISSHP, and Canadian systems. Accordingly, for basic research studies, when we want to study only women who truly have preeclampsia, the latter systems are more functional.

A further point to note is that gestational hypertensives as defined by the ASSHP system constitute a very low risk group of women who can be managed as outpatients. It should not be forgotten however that 15–25% of these women will develop features of the systemic disorder of preeclampsia at some stage and this transition is more likely with early onset of gestational hypertension (20).

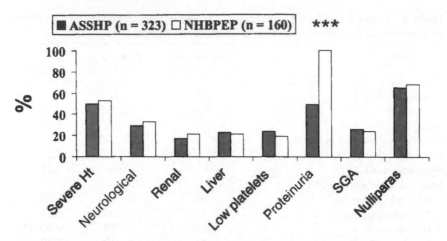

Figure 2 Comparison of maternal outcomes in high-risk hypertensive pregnant women with preeclampsia diagnosed by the ASSHP (*n* = 323) versus NHBPEP (*n* = 160). The *** denotes a significant difference. (Adapted from Ref. 14.)

IV. THE "CLASSIC" DIAGNOSIS OF PREECLAMPSIA

Unfortunately, little attention has been paid to the accuracy with which hypertension, proteinuria and edema have been evaluated, and many feel that the medical literature is now replete with an overdiagnosis of preeclampsia.

A. Hypertension

Hypertension in pregnancy is most typically diagnosed by the presence of an absolute blood pressure ⩾140 mmHg systolic and/or ⩾ 90mmHg diastolic. Previously the definition included a rise in blood pressure from preconception or first-trimester values of more than 25–30 mmHg systolic and/or 15 mmHg diastolic. It is uncertain how these discriminant levels of blood pressure were chosen. It is known that a diastolic blood pressure ⩾ 90 mmHg is associated with a higher incidence of proteinuria (21) and that systolic blood pressure is more predictive of adverse fetal outcome than diastolic blood pressure (22). Surveys have shown differences in the way clinicians record blood pressure during pregnancy. In the same patient, discrepancies in blood pressure as great as 20 mmHg can be ascribed simply to differences in the technique of measurement (23–25).

One particular controversy has surrounded the use of phase 4 (K4) or phase 5 (K5) Korotkoff sounds to record diastolic pressure. The Canadian Society, ISSHP, and ASSHP originally recommended K4. Recent studies have clearly shown that the K5 is recorded with greater accuracy and reliability than K4 during pregnancy (26). Furthermore, this sound corresponds more closely to true intra-arterial diastolic blood pressure in pregnant women (27). A prospective, randomized, open study compared maternal and fetal outcomes amongst hypertensive pregnant women when blood pressure was recorded using either K4 or K5. No clinically significant differences in outcome were apparent. Episodes of severe elevation of the diastolic blood pressure ($\geqslant$110 mmHg) were detected in 16% less women when the K5 was used (28). Use of the K5 was associated with a more reliable measurement, and changing from K4 to K5 did not appear to have an adverse impact on maternal or fetal outcome (28). For these reasons the ISSHP has now recommended universal adoption of K5 (29), and the most recent ASSHP and NHBPEP documents have followed suit.

The recognition of problems inherent in the use of the traditional stethoscope-and-sphygmomanometer method of determination of blood pressure in pregnancy has led to demands for the use of automatted devices. Automated devices may not necessarily be as accurate as mercury sphygmomanometry, and proper validation of each device is required (30,31). Use of such devices may remove interobserver variability, but it is imperative that their accuracy be checked on a regular basis. Irrespective of their accuracy, mercury sphygmomanometers are unlikely to enjoy continued use in most industrialized countries because of issues associated with mercury toxicity (32).

The use of an incremental increase in BP (25–30/15 mmHg from "booking" or preconception blood pressure) is no longer considered part of the classification systems of ASSHP and NHBPEP. This decision was made because pregnancy outcomes are similar irrespective of the magnitude of the incremental increase (17,33). The NHBPEP and ASSHP statements emphasize that a marked incremental increase in blood pressure should not be ignored, although it is not used for diagnosis.

B. Edema

Edema is not helpful for the diagnosis of preeclampsia. It occurs with similar frequency in both preeclamptic and normal pregnant women. While the rapid appearance of edema (particularly when it involves the face and hands) may herald the advent of preeclampsia, there is little reason to use this sign as a diagnostic criterion in a classification scheme for preeclampsia. The pathophysiological processes producing edema in preeclampsia and normal pregnancy may well be different, but there is no way of distinguishing them on clinical grounds. Accordingly, the use of edema has been abandoned as part of the diagnostic process for preeclampsia.

C. Proteinuria

The diagnosis of proteinuria in pregnancy is fraught with difficulty. The standard method of semiquantitative analysis, using a dipstick technique, may overestimate proteinuric preeclampsia by as much as 50% when 1+ is used as the cutoff value

(34–36). The reliability may be improved by automated devices and by the use of a midstream urine specimen. We and others (36,37) have found that a spot urine protein:creatinine ratio of ≥30 mg protein per millimole of creatinine reflects more than 300 mg/day proteinuria. The protein-to-creatinine ratio may offer a faster alternative to the current gold standard of a 24-hour urine collection.

Two studies have shown a high false-negative rate with dipstick testing for predicting a 24-hour urinary protein excretion of more than 300 mg (38,39). For this reason, women may be put at risk if it is assumed that proteinuria is present only when dipstick urinalysis is positive (40). Reasons for such high false-negative rates in these studies but not in others may be that dipsticks differ in their chemical sensitivity to proteinuria according to the manufacturer, or that, at lower levels of protein concentration, which are not detected by dipstick, significant total proteinuria (>300 mg/day) may be present if urine volume is high enough (e.g., a urine protein concentration of 0.2 g/L will not be detected as more than a "trace" by dipstick but could equate to 400 mg/day if urine volume were at least 2 L/24 hours). Furthermore, the laboratory method of measuring proteinuria is not always standardized, though most often the benzethonium chloride protein assay is used. In addition, the most widely quoted and accepted definition of proteinuria, ≥300 mg/day, is based on some less-than-rigorous studies that were not specifically designed to address this issue (described in Ref. 41); the only recent study on this issue concluded that a 24-hour urine protein ≥200 mg/day is abnormal (35). Finally, a 24-hour urine protein remains the gold standard for measuring proteinuria in hypertensive pregnancy, but this process of urine collection is fraught with error due to over- or undercollection by the patient. Even in the most motivated and diligent patient, the dilated ureters and renal pelves may themselves interfere with collection of a complete urine volume. What should be obvious is that reliance on dipstick alone is completely inadequate—a disturbing point, given that about one in five papers on the subject of preeclampsia do just this (2,3).

V. CONCLUSIONS

The classification of hypertension in pregnancy has been confusing, but a number of respected authorities have recently produced similar well-thought-out schema. The differences in these systems are fundamental and revolve around the inclusion of proteinuria as a defining criterion. There is also difficulty associated with the clinical measurement of hypertension and the appropriate cutoff. The K5 sound should be used to define the diastolic blood pressure. The adoption of this practice has been accepted by all of the major governing bodies in hypertension in pregnancy. There is still some work to be done in this evolving field, and we look forward to a time when all agree on a single classification system for hypertension in pregnancy.

REFERENCES

1. Brown MA, de Swiet M. Classification of hypertension in pregnancy. In: Brown MA, ed. Pregnancy and Hypertension. Baillière's Best Practice and Research. Clinical Obstetrics and Gynaecology. London: Baillière Tindall, London 1999:13:27–39.
2. Chappell L, Poulton L, Halligan A, Shennan AH. Lack of consistancy in research papers over the definition of pre-eclampsia. Br J Obstet Gynecol 1999; 106:983–985.
3. Harlow FH, Brown MA. The diversity of diagnosis of pre-eclampsia. Hypertens Pregnancy 2001; 20:57–67.
4. Brown MA, Robinson A, Jones M. The white coat effect in hypertensive pregnancy: much ado about nothing? Br J Obstet Gynaecol 1999; 106:474–480.
5. Roberts JM, Redman CWG. Pre-eclampsia: more than pregnancy-induced hypertension. Lancet 1993; 341:1447–1450.
6. Brown MA, Hague WM, Higgins J, Lowe S, McCowan L, Oats J, Peek MJ, Rowan JA, Walters BNJ. The detection, investigation and management of hypertension in pregnancy: full consensus statement. Aust NZ J Obstet Gynaecol 2000; 40:139–156.
7. National High Blood Pressure Education Program working group report on high blood pressure in pregnancy. Am J Obstet Gynecol 2000; 183:1–22.
8. Helewa ME, Burrows RF, Smith J, Williams K, Brain P, Rabkin SW. Report of the Canadian Hypertension Society consensus conference: definitions, evaluation and classifications of hypertensive disorders in pregnancy. Can Med Assoc J 1997; 157: 715–725.
9. Australasian Society for the Study of Hypertension in Pregnancy. Management of hypertension in pregnancy: consensus summary. Med J Aust 1993; 15:700–702.
10. Hypertension in Pregnancy. ACOG Technical Bulletin. Washington, DC: American College of Obstetrics and Gynecology, 1996.
11. Davey DA, MacGillivray I. The classification and definition of the hypertensive disorders of pregnancy. Am J Obstet Gynecol 1988; 158:892–898.
12. National High Blood Pressure Education Program Working Group: Report on high blood pressure in pregnancy. Am J Obstet Gynecol 1990; 163:1691–1712.
13. Brown MA. The physiology of pre-eclampsia. Clin Exp Pharmacol Physiol 1995; 22: 781–791.
14. Brown MA, Buddle ML. What's in a name? Problems with the classification of hypertension in pregnancy. J Hyperten 1997; 15:1049–1054.
15. Brown MA, Buddle ML. Hypertension in pregnancy: material and fetal outcomes according to laboratory and clinical features. Med J Aust 1996; 165:360–365.
16. Redman CWG, Jeffries M. Revised definition of pre-eclampsia. Lancet 1988; 1:809–812.
17. North RA, Taylor RS, Schellenberg JC. Evaluation of a definition of pre-eclampsia. Br J Obstet Gynaecol 1999; 106:767–773.
18. Letsky E. Hematologic disorders. In: Barron WM, Lindheimer MD, eds. Medical Disorders During Pregnancy. St. Louis: Mosby, 1991:272–322.
19. Freund G, Arvan DA. Clinical biochemistry of pre-eclampsia and related liver diseases of pre-eclampsia: a review. Clin Chim Acta 1990; 191:123–152.
20. Saudan P, Brown MA, Buddle ML, Jones M. Does gestational hypertension become pre-eclampsia? Br J Obstet Gynaecol 1998; 105:1177–1184.

21. MacGillivray I. Pre-eclampsia. London: Saunders, 1983:1–12.
22. Seligman S. Which blood pressure? Br J Obstet Gynaecol 1987; 94:497–498.
23. Bisson DL, Golding J, MacGillivray I, Thomas P, Stirrat GM. Blood pressure lability. Contemp Rev Obstet Gynaecol 1990; 2:11–16.
24. Brown MA, Simpson JM. Diversity of blood pressure recording during pregnancy: implications for the hypertensive disorders. Med J Aust 1992; 156:306–308.
25. Perry IJ, Wilkinson LE, Shinton RA, Beevers DG. Conflicting views on the measurement of blood pressure in pregnancy. Br J Obstet Gynaecol 1991; 98:241–243.
26. Shennan A, Gupta M, Halligan A, Taylor D, De Swiet M. Lack of reproducibility in pregnancy of Korotkoff phase IV as measured by mercury sphygmomanometry. Lancet 1996; 347:139–142.
27. Brown MA, Reiter L, Smith B, Buddle ML, Morris R, Whitworth JA. Measuring blood pressure in pregnant women: a comparison of direct and indirect methods. Am J Obstet Gynecol 1994; 171:661–667.
28. Brown MA, Buddle ML, Farrell TJ, Davis G, Jones M. The impact of choice of Korotkoff sounds on the outcomes of hypertensive pregnancies. Lancet 1998; 352:777–781.
29. de Swiet M. K5 rather than K4 for diastolic blood pressure measurement in pregnancy. Hypertens Pregnancy 1999; 18:3–5.
30. Shennan A, Kissane J, De Swiet M. Validation of the Spacelabs 90207 ambulatory blood pressure monitor for use in pregnancy. Br J Obstet Gynaecol 1993; 100:904–908.
31. Gupta M, Shennan A, Halligan A, Taylor D, De Swiet M. Accuracy of oscillometric blood pressure monitoring in pregnancy and pre-eclampsia. Br J Obstet Gynaecol 1997; 104:350–355.
32. O'Brien E. Replacing the mercury sphygmometer. Br Med J 2000; 320:815–816.
33. Levine RJ. Should the definition of preeclampsia include a rise in diastolic blood pressure ≥15 mmHg? (Abstract.) Am J Obstet Gynecol 2000;182:225.
34. Brown MA, Buddle ML. Inadequacy of dipstick proteinuria in hypertensive pregnancy. Aust NZ J Obstet Gynaecol 1995; 35:366–369.
35. Kuo VS, Koumantakis G, Gallery EDM. Proteinuria and its assessment in normal and hypertensive pregnancy. Am J Obstet Gynecol 1992; 167:723–728.
36. Saudan PJ, Brown MA, Farrell T, Shaw L. Improved methods of assessing proteinuria in hypertensive pregnancy. Br J Obstet Gynaecol 1997; 104:1159–1164.
37. Ramos JGL, Martins-Costa SH, Mathias MM, Guerin YLS, Barros EG. Urinary protein/creatinine ratio in hypertensive pregnant women. Hypertens Pregnancy 1999; 18:209–218.
38. Meyer NL, Mercer BM, Friedman SA, Sibai BM. Urinary dipstick protein: a poor predictor of absent or severe proteinuria. Am J Obstet Gynecol 1994; 170:137–141.
39. Bell S, Halligan AWF, Martin A, Ashmore J, Shennan AH, Lambert PC, Taylor DJ. The role of observer error in antenatal dipstick proteinuria analysis. Br J Obstet Gynaecol 1999; 106:1177–1180.
40. Halligan AWF, Bell SC, Taylor DJ. Dipstick proteinuria: caveat emptor. Br J Obstet Gynaecol 1999; 106:1113–1115.
41. Lindheimer MD, Katz AI. Kidney Function and Disease in Pregnancy. Philadelphia: Lea & Febiger. 1977:78.
42. Douglas K, Redman C. Eclampsia in the United Kingdom. Br Med J 1994; 309:1395–1399.

2

The Etiology of Preeclampsia

Louise C. Kenny and Philip N. Baker
Maternal and Fetal Health Research Centre, The University of
Manchester, Manchester, England

I. INTRODUCTION

The precise etiology of preeclampsia, the "disease of theories" (1), has eluded physicians since the time of Hippocrates. At the turn of the last century, the presence of a circulating toxin of fetal origin was postulated as the cause of eclampsia, and hence the disease became known as "toxemia of pregnancy." More than a century later, the toxemic theory remains the favored hypothesis. It is now widely accepted that preeclampsia is associated with abnormal placental implantation, which is believed to result in relative placental ischemia. Furthermore, as yet unidentified maternal or fetal genes may confer susceptibility. The syndrome of preeclampsia, which normally presents in the third trimester, possibly results from an immunologically based maternal response to abnormal placental implantation. This response, which can affect almost every major system of the body, reflects the involvement of the maternal vascular endothelium, now widely regarded as the target cell of the disease process. These observations have led to the development of a two-stage etiological model of preeclampsia (see Figure 1). This model, and in particular the link between the two stages, has been the subject of intense research and debate in recent years and is the principal focus of this chapter.

II. THE GENETICS OF PREECLAMPSIA

A familial factor has been recognized in the pathogenesis of preeclampsia for many years. Epidemiological studies have demonstrated a three- to fourfold

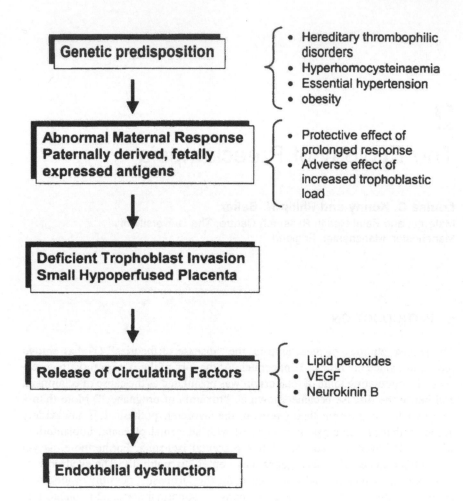

Figure 1 The proposed pathogenesis of preeclampsia.

increase in the incidence of preeclampsia in first-degree relatives of affected women (2,3). Pedigree data have been reported to support models of maternal inheritance due to a recessive gene with a population frequency of 0.16 to 0.31 (2,3) or a dominant gene with a population frequency of 0.14 to 48% penetrance (3). However, data on the incidence of preeclampsia in identical twin sisters, although limited, indicate that discordance is more common than concordance, implicating factors other than the maternal genotype (4).

One possible factor is the contribution of the fetal genotype. Epidemiological data have been reported consistent with fetal recessive inheritance (5) or maternal-fetal sharing of a recessive gene (6). Genetic studies of preeclampsia are beset with difficulties. Extended pedigrees are relatively uncommon. In part this is due to the fact that males cannot be tested for susceptibility and that females can be tested only if they become pregnant. Furthermore, preeclampsia is predominantly a disease of the first pregnancy; therefore the interaction between maternal and fetal genotypes can be tested only once. Finally, the definition and diagnosis of preeclampsia, even in the recent past, have been variable and imprecise. Hence, retrospective analysis of hospital records, when they are available, is often frustrating and unreliable.

There are presently several projects attempting to address the complex issues surrounding genetic studies in preeclampsia. One such study, the Genetics of Pre-eclampsia Collaborative Study (GOPEC), is a multicenter UK project. The aim is to utilize transmission disequilibrium testing (TDT) in order to examine distortions in the transmission of marker alleles from heterozygous (informative) parents to affected individuals. In the first instance, the GOPEC study will investigate various candidate genes that have been implicated in previous studies. The genes under investigation are as follows:

1. Angiotensinogen. Affected pedigree member analysis of Scottish and Icelandic families with preeclampsia has demonstrated significant distortion of allele sharing at the angiotensinogen locus (7). An angiotensinogen variant T235 was associated with preeclampsia in a study from the USA (8), although a study from the UK did not confirm this (9). There is also some preliminary evidence for increased transmission of an angiotensinogen dinucleotide allele repeat from mother to fetus in pre-eclampsia (9).

2. Angiotensin II type I receptor. Women with preeclampsia are exquisitely sensitive to the vasopressor effects of angiotensin II and demonstrate increased expression of angiotensin II type I receptors on platelets. There is preliminary evidence for increased maternal-fetal transmission of an angiotensin II receptor dinucleotide repeat allele in preeclampsia (10).

3. Factor V Leiden. A point mutation in the factor V gene, which results in substitution of glutamine for arginine, renders factor V resistant to inactivation by protein C and is believed to account for the sevenfold increase in the risk of venous thrombosis in carriers of the mutation. A population-based study has demonstrated an increased risk of developing preeclampsia in women heterozygous for factor V Leiden (11).

4. Tumor necrosis factor α (TNFα). A billalelic polymorphism in the promoter region of the TNFα gene has been reported to be associated with increased expression of TNFα mRNA levels and preeclampsia (12).

The genetic inheritance of preeclampsia is undoubtedly complex. However it is highly likely that the advent of complete disclosure of the human genome and rapidly evolving genotyping technology will make genomewide screening by TDT a realistic possibility within the next few years.

III. IMMUNOLOGICAL ASPECTS

The underlying reason for the failure of trophoblast invasion in preeclampsia is unknown. It has been suggested that disordered placentation reflects an abnormal maternal immunological response to fetal antigens derived from the father. The increased prevalence of preeclampsia in multiple pregnancies, molar pregnancies, and those associated with increased placental mass suggests that fetal antigen load and trophoblast volume have a pathological role in this disorder (13).

There is extensive epidemiological evidence to implicate immunological factors in the etiology of preeclampsia. A strong association between the disease and parity was recognized over 300 years ago by Mauriceau, who wrote "primigravidas are at far greater risk of convulsions than multiparas." Several large studies have confirmed this observation and furthermore have demonstrated that the association does not hold for nulliparity and nonproteinuric hypertension (14,15). This clearly suggests that preeclampsia and nonproteinuric gestational hypertension are different disorders and further emphasizes the need for care when analyzing data from studies where no attempt has been made to distinguish between the two.

Epidemiological data have revealed that the incidence of preeclampsia in multigravid women is associated with a change in partner. Li and Wi (16) conducted a cohort study based on 140,147 women with two consecutive births during 1989–1991. Among women without preeclampsia in the first birth, changing partners resulted in a 30% increase in the risk of preeclampsia in the subsequent pregnancy compared with those who did not change partners. However, among women with preeclampsia in the first birth, changing partners resulted in a 30% reduction in the risk of preeclampsia in the subsequent pregnancy. These findings demonstrate that preeclampsia is a disease of primipaternity rather than primigravidity and are consistent with the hypothesis that normal pregnancy reflects a state of tolerance to the foreign paternally derived antigens of the fetus, whereas in women with preeclampsia, this immunological tolerance is impaired.

In line with this hypothesis, several studies have demonstrated that the incidence of preeclampsia may be related to the duration of prior exposure to paternal antigens in sperm. It has been suggested (17) but not confirmed (18) that the use of barrier methods of contraception that prevent exposure to sperm and seminal fluid are associated with an increased risk of developing preeclampsia during the subsequent pregnancy. Furthermore, oral sex and the swallowing of seminal fluid is correlated with a diminished occurrence of preeclampsia (19). Epidemiological studies have demonstrated that the duration of sexual cohabitation before conception is inversely related to the incidence of preeclampsia (20). This suggests that during a protracted sexual relationship, women develop an immune response against paternal antigens expressed on spermatozoa or in seminal fluid, which is possibly impaired in women using barrier methods of contraception and enhanced by oral exposure. This induces an allogeneic tolerance that immunologically protects against exposure to paternally derived fetal antigens in a subsequent pregnancy.

IV. THE ROLE OF THE ENDOTHELIUM

The vascular endothelium is no longer thought to be simply an inert lining of the vasculature but is now recognized as a highly specialized, metabolically interactive interface between blood and the underlying tissues. In recent years it has been increasingly appreciated that an intact endothelium plays an obligatory role in mediating vascular tone and maintaining thromboresistance as well as participating in the inflammatory response.

As our understanding of the role of the endothelium has evolved, a concept has formed that the endothelial cell is the target of the disease process in preeclampsia. This hypothesis is attractive as the ubiquitous nature and diverse functions of the vascular endothelium would account for the complex multisystem nature of the clinical manifestations of the disease process.

Evidence for endothelial involvement in preeclampsia abounds. The best-characterized morphological abnormality of this syndrome, once assumed to be pathognomonic of the condition, glomerular endotheliosis, involves endothelial cells (21). Preeclampsia is also associated with a loss of endothelial cell integrity and a consequent increase in vascular permeability (22). There is also a plethora of evidence from the study of circulating endothelial cell markers in preeclampsia. Levels of fibronectin, factor VIII antigen, von Willebrand factor, tissue plasminogen activator, and plasminogen activator inhibitor-1 have been found to be elevated in the circulation of women with preeclampsia (23,24). Although these substances are synthesized by several cell types, they are all produced in the vascular endothelium. Furthermore, several studies have reported increased levels of circulating endothelin-1 in preeclampsia (25,26), which may reflect increased synthesis by activated endothelial cells (27,28).

An intact endothelium is a vital component of the coagulation system (29). Widespread deposition of fibrin, associated with diffuse vascular damage suggesting activation of the coagulation system, has long been recognized as a pathological feature of preeclampsia. However, unless preeclampsia is complicated by disseminated intravascular coagulation, routine coagulation tests are normal. More sensitive indicators of coagulation abnormalities are present in a high proportion of women with this disorder and include an altered ratio of factor VIII–related antigen to coagulation activity (30), a reduction in the platelet count (31) and an increase in the levels of plasma β-thromboglobulin. Significantly, these changes antedate the onset of clinical manifestations of the disease by several weeks.

One of the most striking and consistent pathophysiological abnormalities of women with preeclampsia is an increased sensitivity to pressor agents such as angiotensin II (32). The mechanism underlying both the suppressed response to pressor agents in normal pregnancy, and the increased sensitivity observed in preeclampsia is yet to be fully elucidated. However, there is well-documented evidence that endothelium-dependent relaxation of resistance arteries is impaired in preeclampsia. McCarthy et al. used the technique of wire myography to examine subcutaneous vessels from nonpregnant, normal pregnant women and women with preeclampsia (33). The authors reported comparable responses to the endothelium-dependent vasodilator acetylcholine (ACh) in vessels isolated from nonpregnant and normal pregnant women. However, they found significantly impaired ACh-mediated relaxation in the arteries of women with preeclampsia. Similarly, impaired responses to other endothelium-dependent vasodilators in a variety of vascular preparations have been described by other investigators (34,35). There are now known to be at least three endothelium-derived agents responsible for mediating endothelium-dependent relaxation in resistance arteries and thereby modulating vascular tone; nitric oxide, prostacyclin, and endothelium-derived hyperpolarizing factor (EDHF). Furchgott and Zawadski first described the obligatory role of the endothelium in the relaxation of isolated arteries in ACh in 1980 (36). They demonstrated that relaxation did not occur if the endothelium was removed completely and hypothesized that it was mediated by an endothelium-derived relaxing factor, identified in 1987 as nitric oxide (37). However, as knowledge of endothelium-dependent responses has advanced, it has become clear that the endothelial release of nitric oxide cannot account for all endothelium-dependent relaxation. Long before nitric oxide was described it was known that ACh caused hyperpolarization of smooth muscle (38), the endothelial dependence of this response was first described in the mesenteric artery of the guinea pig by Bolton et al. (39). This initial observation has now been repeated in various blood vessels from many species including a limited number of human vessels (40). In many of these models, the hyperpolarization and the relaxation that accompany it are resistant to inhibitors of nitric oxide and prostacylin. This suggests the presence of an additional endothelium-derived factor. This factor, EDHF, has yet to be identified and its pharmacological nature remains the topic of much controversy. Candidates include, derivates of the cytochrome P450 pathway, potassium ions, endogenous cannabinoids, and communication via gap junctions (41).

Intriguingly, several studies have suggested that endothelium-dependent responses in vessels isolated from normal pregnant women are not significantly affected by inhibition of nitric oxide and prostacylin, implicating a role for EDHF. A study investigating endothelium-dependent responses in myometrial resistance vessels demonstrated that in vessels isolated from nonpregnant women, responses to bradykinin were significantly attenuated by combined inhibition of nitric oxide. In contrast, in vessels isolated from normal pregnant women, endothelium-dependent relaxation was largely independent of nitric oxide but was almost abolished by partial depolarization, implicating a role for EDHF (42). This suggests that in normal pregnancy there is a change in the mechanism of endothelium-dependent relaxation from one involving nitric oxide to one predominantly mediated by EDHF. Furthermore, in vessels isolated from women with preeclampsia, response to bradykinin was almost entirely mediated by nitric oxide. This implies that EDHF mediates endothelium-dependent responses in pregnancy and that the release of, or sensitivity to, EDHF is diminished in preeclampsia (43).

In summary, the vascular endothelial cell appears to be the target of the disease process in preeclampsia. A variety of studies have reported evidence of widespread endothelial cell activation and impaired endothelial-dependent responses. Many of the clinical manifestations of preeclampsia can be accounted for by activation of this cell type. However, the exact nature of the activation and subsequent function of the endothelial cell in vivo has not been fully elucidated.

V. THE ROLE OF THE PLACENTA

Relative placental ischemia is thought to play a pivotal role in the pathogenesis of preeclampsia. This hypothesis is supported by the observation that the incidence of preeclampsia is increased in situations where placental oxygen demand is increased. This occurs in the presence of multiple pregnancies, hydatidiform moles and hydropic placentas. Cytotrophoblast cells reside in chorionic villi of two types; floating and anchoring villi. Floating villi, which represent the vast majority of chorionic villi, are bathed in maternal blood and primarily perform gas and nutrient exchange for the developing embryo. During early placentation, cytotrophoblast cells in the floating villi proliferate and differentiate by fusing to form the multinucleate syncytiotrophoblast layer. Cytotrophoblast cells in anchoring villi either fuse to form the syncytiotrophoblast layer, or break through the syncytium at selected sites and form multilayered columns of nonpolarized extravillous trophoblast cells, which physically connect the embryo to the uterine wall. The extravillous trophoblast cells consist of two populations:

1. Interstitial cytotrophoblasts invade the decidual stroma and reach the superficial myometrium by the eighth week of gestation. Subsequently,

they invade deeper into the myometrium, especially in the center of the placental bed. Trophoblast cells cluster around spiral arteries; these perivascular trophoblasts are seen in around 20% of myometrial spiral arteries at 8 weeks and around 60% at 16 to 18 weeks (44). At the end of their invasion path, cytotrophoblast cells fuse to form multinuclear giant cells, and this probably accounts for the reduced number of cytotrophoblasts cells in the deeper myometrium after 11 weeks of gestation.

2. Endovascular cytotrophoblasts invade into the lumina of the spiral arteries and then migrate in a retrograde fashion. This process probably starts as early as 4 to 6 weeks of gestation and reaches the lumen in less than 5% of myometrial arteries at 10 weeks but in about 32% at 16 to 18 weeks. It has been proposed that the endovascular invasion occurs in two waves; the initial decidual phase being completed by around 10 weeks, and the later myometrial phase starting 4 to 5 weeks later (45). The exact morphological basis and the physiological significance of this "two-wave" hypothesis is unclear.

This process of trophoblast invasion leads to the transformation of the spiral arteries supplying the intervillous space. These small, narrow-caliber arteries are gradually converted into large sinusoidal vessels, as the endothelium and the internal elastic lamina are replaced by trophoblasts. These changes transform the vascular supply to a low pressure, high flow system, allowing an adequate blood flow to the placenta and fetus.

There is histological evidence that in women who later develop pre-eclampsia there has been defective penetration by the cytotrophoblast, so that these maternally derived arteries retain the musculoelastic elements of their walls (46). In placental bed biopsies from preeclamptic pregnancies in the third trimester, the endothelial lining of these arteries appears to be focally disrupted by attached intraluminal endovascular trophoblasts (47). However, it should be noted that endovascular trophoblast invasion is not an all or nothing phenomenon in normal and pre-eclamptic pregnancies and that probably a spectrum of invasion and spiral artery morphological change occur (48).

The cause of this impaired placentation is not fully understood but may in part be due to poor invasive properties of the trophoblastic cells or changes in the maternal dicidual tissues, which regulate trophoblast behaviour, perhaps mediated via multifunctional cytokine pathways. The cytotrophoblastic expression of adhesion molecules, which influence invasion, is altered in women with preeclampsia (49). In vivo studies have shown lower attachment of trophoblasts from pre-eclamptic placentas on fibronectin and vitronectin compared to normotensive controls, which may reflect differences in expression of matrix receptors (49). Maternal factors leading to inhibition of trophoblast invasion include reduced expression of the histocompatibility antigen HLA-G (50), local inflammatory cell behavior (51) and cytokine regulation of integrin expression (52).

Endothelial disruption within the placenta will predispose to platelet aggregation, vasospasm and thrombosis. The balance between endothelial release of vasoconstrictors such as endothelin and thromboxane, and vasodilators such as prostacyclin, is altered in preeclampsia in favor of vasoconstriction. The combined effect of the above changes is a reduction in uteroplacental perfusion, particularly later in pregnancy. This is presumed to trigger the release of a factor into the maternal circulation.

VI. CIRCULATING FACTORS

The link between deficient trophoblastic invasion early in pregnancy and the widespread endothelial dysfunction manifesting much later has eluded researchers for many years. The observation that terminating the pregnancy and, more specifically, delivery of the placenta, results in resolution of the disease suggest that the placenta is the focus of production of the putative factor(s) that attack the endothelial cell. This hypothesis and the nature of the circulating factor(s) has been investigated in a wide variety of both in vivo and ex vivo studies. One of the first studies to investigate the potential of circulating factors was reported over a decade ago and is widely credited with reviving the concept of toxemia (53). This much-cited study demonstrated that serum from women with preeclampsia was cytotoxic to cultured human umbilical vein endothelial cells (HUVECS) when compared with control sera from normal pregnant women. The cytotoxic effect of serum collected prior to delivery was greater than that collected postpartum; this rapid disappearance of cytotoxic activity suggested that the putative factor(s) had a short half-life and provided evidence that they were related to products of conception. Interestingly, the cytotoxic effect persisted when a combination of antenatal sera from normal pregnant women and women with preeclampsia was utilized, providing further evidence of an active circulating factor as opposed to a relative deficiency of a protective factor. This landmark study has subsequently been extended by other investigators in a wide variety of cultured cell types. It now appears that the circulating factor(s) induce an alteration in endothelial function rather than gross morphological injury and cell death, as was initially suggested (54,55). This assumption is further supported by the observation that when seeded in the presence of sera from women with preeclampsia, endothelial cells proliferate, attach, and spread in a manner similar to those seeded in sera from normal pregnant women. Moreover, endothelial cells continue to grow well during incubation with serum from women with preeclampsia, and any metabolic changes can be reversed by replacing the serum from women with preeclampsia with standard culture medium (56).

Serum from women with preeclampsia has been reported to stimulate greater mitogenic activity and increase production of platelet-derived growth factor (PDGF) and also to stimulate greater expression of endothelial cell PDGF-B-chain mRNA in cultured HUVECS than serum isolated from normotensive pregnant women (57). Plasma from women with preeclampsia has been demonstrated to increase cellular permeability, an effect mediated through the protein kinase C (PKC) pathway (58). Lorentzen et al. reported that cultured endothelial cells incubated with sera from women with preeclampsia acquired a large number of sudanophilic granules that had lipid appearance on electron microscopy. The triglyceride content of these cells was also increased in comparison with control cells (56). Paradoxically, endothelial cell production of prostacyclin and nitric oxide is increased by exposure to plasma and sera from women with preeclampsia (59,60).

There are a number of caveats applying to cell culture studies that make interpretation and extrapolation of the results problematic. Endothelial production of nitric oxide and prostacyclin is dependent upon the cell type utilized (61). Moreover, the effects of plasma and sera differ according to the duration of the experiment: plasma from women with preeclampsia has been found to stimulate initially (at 24 hours) then inhibit (at 72 hours) endothelial cell prostacyclin production (62). It is therefore illogical to extrapolate these findings, or compare them, to a disease process which develops over months. Finally, endothelial cells in culture exist in isolation from the vascular smooth muscle and not in the context of a dynamic organ that is a resistance artery.

In an attempt to overcome some of these cell culture limitations, several investigators have used the technique of small vessel myography to study endothelial behavior in isolated whole vessels in vitro.

Using this technique, Ashworth et al. observed that incubation of vessels isolated from normal pregnant women, with plasma from women with preeclampsia, induced an alteration in endothelium-dependent responses. The response to bradykinin was markedly impaired and mimicked the behavior of vessels isolated from women with preeclampsia (63). Further investigation of this phenomenon has revealed that the effect is independent of the parity of the patient from whom the vessel is isolated, but is specific to vessels from pregnant women. Preliminary characterization of the plasma effect has revealed that it is dose dependent and of rapid onset, with alterations in endothelial function occurring within one hour. The one or more plasma factors responsible for inducing this change appear to be heat labile at 60°C and retain their activity after reconstitution following precipitation with a 70% ammonium sulfate solution. Although the activity of plasma from women with preeclampsia is partially removed by charcoal precipitation, suggesting a possible lipid component, the observations more readily support the conclusion that a protein/glycoprotein may be responsible (64).

In summary, there is an abundance of evidence to implicate the presence of a placentally derived circulating factor that targets the endothelial cell in preeclampsia and induces widespread activation. Evidence suggests that there are a number of characteristics any putative factor must possess. These include the ability to pass freely into the maternal circulation, increase cellular permeability and possibly cell turnover, alter prostacyclin and nitric oxide production and lead to a functional change in the response to endothelium-dependent agonists. A number of factors have been advanced as potential candidates for this role.

A. Vascular Endothelial Growth Factors (VEGFs)

VEGFs comprise a family of glycoproteins that includes five VEGF isoforms and the homologous placental growth factor. They express their biological activity of promoting blood vessel permeability, endothelial cell growth, and angiogenesis by binding to one of two receptors: fetal liver tyrosine-like (flt-1) receptor and a kinase domain receptor (65,66). VEGF contains a hydrophobic secretary signal sequence and exerts in vitro effects specific to vascular endothelial cells at concentrations similar to circulating levels found in vivo (67). VEGF has been shown to induce an increase in vascular permeability through the protein kinase C pathway, an ability shared by plasma from women with pre-eclampsia (58).

There is some controversy surrounding the concentration of circulating VEGF levels in women with pre-eclampsia. Several groups have reported that serum VEGF levels are significantly elevated in patients with preeclampsia (68,69). However, Lyall et al. measured serum VEGF concentrations in women with preeclampsia, normal pregnant women and nonpregnant controls and reported that levels were significantly lower in normal pregnant women than in nonpregnant women and further reduced in preeclampsia (70). An explanation for the apparent discrepancy was provided by the demonstration that quantification of VEGF in pregnancy is affected by interference from binding proteins. When VEGF levels were measured using the commercially available enzyme-linked immunosorbent assay (ELISA) used by Lyall et al., spiking of pregnant serum with VEGF did not alter the ELISA result (71). This promoted speculation that the binding protein might be the soluble form of the VEGF receptor flt-1, and the presence of such a receptor in the plasma has been confirmed (72).

The source of the elevated circulating levels of VEGF in pregnancies complicated by preeclampsia is unclear. VEGF is expressed in placental tissue and when trophoblast cells are cultured in hypoxic conditions, VEGF production is increased. However, studies of placental tissue are equivocal; some have demonstrated that the expression of VEGF mRNA is decreased in pregnancies complicated by preeclampsia (73), whereas others, using immunohistochemical analysis have reported that staining for VEGF is increased in pregnancies complicated by preeclampsia (74). In addition, several alternative explanations have been advanced to account for the increase in circulating levels of VEGF observed in preeclampsia. It has been postulated that VEGF may increase secondary to impaired renal function and diminished excretion. Alternatively, VEGF production may increase in response to vascular endothelial cell injury as it has recently been demonstrated that VEGF produced in vascular smooth muscle may contribute the initiation of endothelial repair (75). As endothelial cell damage is widespread in preeclampsia, this would lead to an increase in both local and circulating concentrations of VEGF.

The effect of VEGF on the vascular endothelium has been investigated by a variety of cell culture studies. VEGF increases microvascular endothelial cell prostacylin production in a dose-dependent manner analogous to the acute effects of plasma from women with preeclampsia (76). Furthermore, the addition of an antibody to plasma derived from women with preeclampsia inhibits the release of prostacyclin from cultured endothelial cells. Fractionation of plasma from women with preeclampsia has demonstrated that the fraction within the plasma responsible for stimulating prostacylin production has a molecular weight between 40 and 55kDa (77). This is a similar molecular weight to that of VEGF and lends further support to the hypothesis that VEGF is one of the factors associated with endothelial dysfunction in preeclampsia.

VEGF has also been demonstrated to induce a functional change in the response of myometrial resistance arteries to the endothelium-dependent vasodilator bradykinin. Incubation with VEGF induces a dose and time-dependent diminution in endothelium-dependent relaxation in these arteries which mirrors that found following incubation with plasma from patients with preeclampsia. Intriguingly, pre-treatment of both VEGF and plasma from women with preeclampsia with an antibody to VEGF protects against loss of endothelium-dependent relaxation (78). This suggests that the elevated levels of VEGF observed in preeclampsia may play a role in the pathogenesis of vascular damage, rather than merely being an epiphenomenon.

B. Neurokinin B

Neurokinin B is a neuropeptide and one of three known mammalian tachykinins; the others being substance P and neurokinin A. The tachykinins are normally restricted to the nervous tissue and exert their effects peripherally by release from nerve endings and activation of the neurokinin receptors, NK1, NK2, and NK3. Neurokinin B preferentially binds to the NK3 receptor, activation of which has been demonstrated to induce hypertension by contraction of the rat portal vein and mesenteric vasculature (79) and increase canine heart rate (80). Neurokinin B was previously thought to be restricted to the brain. However, Page et al. have recently reported that the syncytiotrophoblast of the human placenta expresses neurokinin B mRNA (81). Moreover, they found that plasma levels of the peptide were significantly elevated in women with preeclampsia as compared with the levels in normal pregnant women. They speculated that, in response to placental ischemia consequent upon defective trophoblastic invasion, placental production of neurokinin B increases, in order to increase blood pressure and correct the hypoperfusion of the fetoplacental unit. The subsequent stimulation of the neurokinin B receptors is hypothesized to cause constriction of the mesenteric vascular bed and the portal veins, leading to an increase in blood pressure, damage to the liver and kidneys and the symptoms of abdominal pain. Reduction in blood flow to the liver is speculated to lead to an accumulation of undetoxified metabolites, such as lipid peroxides, which may contribute to endothelial cell damage and dysfunction. The authors also suggest that in severe cases of pre-eclampsia, concentrations of neurokinin B may be sufficient to stimulate peripheral NK 1 receptors on platelets and neutrophils and hence contribute to the other symptoms of preeclampsia associated with activation of these cells. Finally, the authors suggest that increased secretion of neurokinin B may predate the development of clinical signs and symptoms of preeclampsia and therefore increased levels of neurokinin B in early pregnancy may identify pregnancies destined to develop preeclampsia. The neurokinin B hypothesis is attractive, particularly as there are several potent and commercially available selective antagonists for NK receptors, allowing for the implementation of a much-needed pharmacological intervention early in the disease process. However, the findings of this small study await confirmation. In particular, the localization of NK receptors in the human vasculature and the effect of neurokinin B on human vascular tone await elucidation. Quantitative analysis of the placental production of neurokinin B in normal and compromised human pregnancy and circulating maternal plasma levels in all three trimesters of pregnancy await clarification in a longitudinal study. Undoubtedly this area will be the focus of intense research in the immediate future.

C. The Role of Oxidative Stress and Lipid Peroxides

Oxidative stress is a pathological state, implicated in the etiology of many disorders including atherosclerosis, in which pro-oxidants dominate over antioxidants. The resultant increase in the formation of reactive oxygen species can damage cell membranes, proteins and DNA. Epidemiological studies have revealed that many of the risk factors associated with the development of preeclampsia such as obesity, black race, lipid abnormalities, insulin resistance, and raised serum homocysteine are also associated with the risk of developing atherosclerosis in later life. These observations have led to the emerging hypothesis suggesting that reduced placental perfusion generates oxidative stress and leads to widespread endothelial dysfunction in preeclampsia. Wang and Walsh (82) demonstrated that enzyme activities and mRNA expression of the placental antioxidant enzymes superoxide dismutase and glutathione peroxidase were significantly decreased in placentas from women with pregnancies complicated by preeclampsia as compared to those from normal pregnant women. This is thought to lead to an abnormal increase in placental production of lipid peroxides in preeclampsia. In support of this, markers of lipid peroxidation, including malondialdehyde (83) and 8-epiprostaglandin-F2α (84) are increased in the plasma of women with preeclampsia. Furthermore, it has been reported that both the water-soluble antioxidant, ascorbic acid and the lipid-soluble antioxidants alpha-tocopherol and beta-carotene levels are decreased in the plasma of women with preeclampsia compared with those of normal pregnant women. This suggests that antioxidant nutrients may be utilized to a greater extent in preeclampsia to counteract free radical–mediated cell disturbances, resulting in a reduction in antioxidant plasma levels in this disease (85). The increase in lipid peroxide formation by the placenta in preeclampsia may account for many of the pathological changes seen in this disease. With half-lives extending up to minutes, lipid peroxides formed at a primary site may accumulate in lipoproteins and be transferred throughout the circulation. Elevated lipid peroxide levels in plasma inhibit the enzyme prostaglandin synthase, with a consequent fall in the production of prostacylin. However, platelet thromboxane A2 synthesis is unaffected by such compounds. This could potentially lead to an alteration in the ratio of prostacylin to thromboxane production comparable to that observed in preeclampsia (86). Lipid peroxides have also been noted to induce smooth muscle contractions in a variety of isolated arterial preparations. Furthermore, elevation of circulating levels of lipid peroxide products induced by deprivation of vitamin E in rats produced an increased pressor responsiveness to angiotensin II and a decreased isolated mesenteric artery relaxation to acetylcholine (87).

Recently, the results of a prospective randomized placebo-controlled trial suggested that supplementation with vitamins C and E in women at increased risk of preeclampsia was associated with a significant decrease in plasma markers of vascular endothelial cell activation and placental insufficiency. This study also demonstrated a significant reduction in the occurrence of preeclampsia in the treated group. Confirmation of this encouraging finding by a larger trial is awaited.

D. Syncytiotrophoblast Microvillous Membranes (STBMs)

STBMs have been proposed to be the factor linking the defective placentation to the endothelial dysfunction (88). Morphological evaluation of placentas from women with preeclampsia shows abnormally shaped syncytiotrophoblast microvilli and areas of focal necrosis, associated with a reduced number of microvilli. These changes are similar to those seen in placental villi, cultured under hypoxic conditions. In vitro experiments have demonstrated that STBMs can interfere with endothelial cell growth in cultured endothelial cells by suppressing proliferation and disrupting the cell monolayer (88). Furthermore, perfusion of isolated subcutaneous arteries with a high concentration of STBM abolishes ACh-induced vasodilatation (89).

STBMs prepared from placentas of normal women and women with preeclampsia had similar effects on endothelial cells, indicating the effect of STBMs in preeclampsia to be quantitative rather than qualitative (88). Knight et al. studied the presence of STBMs in pregnant women and reported the concentrations of STBMs to be significantly increased in the maternal circulation of women with preeclampsia. The concentrations in the uterine vein exceeded those in the peripheral venous circulation, indicating the placental origin of the STBMs (91). The mechanism by which STBMs exert effects on endothelial cells is unclear, but recent evidence has suggested a link to oxidative stress. It has been reported that incubation of cultured endothelial cells with STBM produced a substance that activates peripheral leukocytes and primes peripheral monocytes to give greater responses after activation (91).

VII. CONCLUSION

In 1939, Johnstone (92) concluded that "no completely satisfactory explanation of the disease or of the nature or source of the toxin can as yet be offered," and this conclusion is no further advanced today. It is difficult to construct a unifying hypothesis. However, the primary event in preeclampsia appears to be abnormal trophoblastic invasion early in pregnancy. Maternal genotype and fetal phenotype may confer susceptibility and as a result the maternal immunological response to fetal antigen is abnormal. The resulting hypoperfused placenta secretes a factor(s) into the maternal circulation, which targets the vascular endothelium and gives rise to the clinical sequelae of the disease. The nature of this factor(s) remains uncertain and the effect on endothelial function at cellular level has not been fully elucidated.

REFERENCES

1. Zwiefel P. Eklampsie. In: Dodelein A, ed. Handbuch der Geburtshilfe, Vol II. Wiesbaden, Germany, Bergmann, 1916:672–723.
2. Chesley LC, Cooper DW. Genetics of hypertension in pregnancy: possible single gene control of pre-eclampsia and eclampsia in the descendants of eclamptic women. Br J Obstet Gynaecol 1986; 93(9):898–908.
3. Arngrimsson R, Bjornsson S, et al. Genetic and familial predisposition to eclampsia and pre-eclampsia in a defined population. Br J Obstet Gynaecol 1990; 97(9):762–769.
4. Thornton JG, Macdonald AM. Twin mothers, pregnancy hypertension and pre-eclampsia. Br J Obstet Gynaecol 1999; 106(6):570–575.

5. Cooper DW, Liston WA. Genetic control of severe pre-eclampsia. J Med Genet 1979;
    16(6):409–416.
6. Liston WA, Kilpatrick DC. "Is genetic susceptibility to pre-eclampsia conferred by
    homozygosity for the same single recessive gene in mother and fetus?" Br J Obstet
    Gynaecol 1991; 98(11):1079–1086.
7. Arngrimsson R, Purandare S, et al. Angiotensinogen: a candidate gene involved in
    preeclampsia? Nat Genet 1993; 4(2):114–115.
8. Ward K, Hata A, et al. A molecular variant of angiotensinogen associated with
    preeclampsia. Nat Genet 1993; 4(1):59–61.
9. Morgan L, Crawshaw S, et al. Maternal and fetal angiotensinogen gene allele sharing
    in pre-eclampsia. Br J Obstet Gynaecol 1999; 106(3):244–251.
10. Morgan L, Crawshaw S, et al. Distortion of maternal-fetal angiotensin II type I
    receptor allele transmission in pre-eclampsia. J Med Genet 1998; 35(8):632–636.
11. Dizon-Townson DS, Nelson LM, et al. The factor V Leiden mutation may predispose
    women to severe preeclampsia. Am J Obstet Gynecol 1996; 175(4 Pt 1):902–905.
12. Chen G, Wilson R, et al. Tumour necrosis factor-alpha (TNF-alpha) gene polymor-
    phism and expression in pre-eclampsia. Clin Exp Immunol 1996; 104(1):154–159.
13. Taylor RN. Review: immunobiology of preeclampsia. Am J Reprod Immunol 1997;
    37(1):79–86.
14. Campbell DM, Carr-Hill R, et al. Pre-eclampsia in a second pregnancy. Clin Exp
    Hypertens [B] 1983; 2(2):303–306.
15. Misra DP, Kiely JL. The association between nulliparity and gestational hypertension.
    J Clin Epidemiol 1997; 50(7):851–855.
16. Li DK, Wi S. "Changing paternity and the risk of preeclampsia/eclampsia in the
    subsequent pregnancy." Am J Epidemiol 2000; 151(1):57–62.
17. Klonoff-Cohen HS, Savitz DA, et al. An epidemiologic study of contraception and
    preeclampsia. JAMA 1989; 262(22):3143–3147.
18. Mills JL, Klebanoff MA, et al. Barrier contraceptive methods and preeclampsia.
    JAMA 1991; 265(1):70–73.
19. Koelman CA, Coumans AB, et al. Correlation between oral sex and a low incidence of
    preeclampsia: a role for soluble HLA in seminal fluid? J Reprod Immunol 2000;
    46(2):155–166.
20. Robillard PY, Hulsey TC. Association of pregnancy-induced-hypertension, pre-
    eclampsia, and eclampsia with duration of sexual cohabitation before conception.
    Lancet 1996; 347(9001):619.
21. Spargo B, McCartney C, et al. Glomerular capillary endotheliosis in toxaemia of
    pregnancy. Arch Pathol 1959; 68:593–599.
22. Campbell DM, Campbell AJ. Evans blue disappearance rate in normal and pre-
    eclamptic pregnancy. Clin Exp Hypertens [B] 1983; 2(1):163–169.
23. Roberts JM, Taylor RN, et al. Preeclampsia: an endothelial cell disorder. Am J Obstet
    Gynecol 1989; 161(5):1200–1204.
24. Friedman SA, Schiff E, et al. Biochemical corroboration of endothelial involvement
    in severe preeclampsia. Am J Obstet Gynecol 1995; 172(1 Pt 1):202–203.
25. Taylor RN, Varma M, et al. Women with preeclampsia have higher plasma endothelin
    levels than women with normal pregnancies. J Clin Endocrinol Metab 1990; 71(6):
    1675–1677.

26. Mastrogiannis DS, O'Brien WF, et al. Potential role of endothelin-1 in normal and hypertensive pregnancies. Am J Obstet Gynecol 1991; 165(6 Pt 1):1711–1716.

27. MacCumber MW, Ross CA, et al. Endothelin: visualization of mRNAs by in situ hybridization provides evidence for local action. Proc Natl Acad Sci USA 1989; 86 (18):7285–7289.

28. Yoshimoto S, Ishizaki Y, et al. Cerebral microvessel endothelium is producing endothelin. Brain Res 1990; 508(2):283–285.

29. Roberts JM, Redman CW. Pre-eclampsia: more than pregnancy-induced hypertension. Lancet 1993; 341(8858):1447–1451.

30. Redman CW, Denson KW, et al. Factor-VIII consumption in pre-eclampsia. Lancet 1977; 2(8051):1249–1252.

31. Redman CW, Bonnar J, et al. Early platelet consumption in pre-eclampsia. Br Med J 1978; 1(6111):467–469.

32. Gant NF, Daley GL, et al. A study of angiotensin II pressor response throughout primigravid pregnancy. J Clin Invest 1973; 52(11):2682–2689.

33. McCarthy AL, Woolfson RG, et al. Abnormal endothelial cell function of resistance arteries from women with preeclampsia. Am J Obstet Gynecol 1993; 168(4):1323–1330.

34. Knock GA, Poston L. Bradykinin-mediated relaxation of isolated maternal resistance arteries in normal pregnancy and preeclampsia. Am J Obstet Gynecol 1996; 175(6): 1668–1674.

35. Ashworth JR, Warren AY, et al. Loss of endothelium-dependent relaxation in myometrial resistance arteries in preeclampsia. Br J Obstet Gynaecol 1997; 104(10):1152–1158.

36. Furchgott RF, Zawadzki JV. The obligatory role of endothelial cells in the relaxation of arterial smooth muscle by acetycholine. Nature 1980; 288(5789):373–376.

37. Palmer RM, Ferrige AG, et al. Nitric oxide release accounts for the biological activity of endothelium-derived relaxing factor. Nature 1987; 327(6122):524–526.

38. Kuriyama H, Suzuki H. The effects of acetylcholine on the membrane and contractile properties of smooth muscle cells of the rabbit superior mesenteric artery. Br J Pharmacol 1978; 64(4):493–501.

39. Bolton TB, Lang RJ, et al. Mechanisms of action of noradrenaline and carbachol on smooth muscle of guinea-pig anterior mesenteric artery. J Physiol (Lond) 1984; 351: 549–572.

40. Nakashima M, Mombouli JV, et al. Endothelium-dependent hyperpolarization caused by bradykinin in human coronary arteries. J Clin Invest 1993; 92(6):2867–2871.

41. Randall MD, Kendall DA. Endocannabinoids: a new class of vasoactive substances. Trends Pharmacol Sci 1998; 19(2):55–58.

42. Kenny LC, Dunn WR, et al. Endothelium-dependent relaxation of myometrial resistance arteries in normal pregnancy is mediated by EDHF. J Soc Gynecol Invest 1999; 6(1 suppl):717A.

43. Kenny LC, Baker PN, et al. Differences in endothelial function in pregnancy and pre-eclampsia. Br J Pharmacol 1999; 128:44P.

44. Pijnenborg R, Bland JM, et al. Uteroplacental arterial changes related to interstitial trophoblast migration in early pregnancy. Placenta 4(4):397–413.

45. Robertson WB, Khong TY, et al. The placental bed biopsy: review from three European centers. Am J Obstet Gynecol 1986; 155(2):401–412.

46. Brosens IA. Morphological changes in the utero-placental bed in pregnancy hypertension. Clin Obstet Gynaecol 1977; 4(3):573–593.

47. Khong TY, Sawyer IH, et al. An immunohistologic study of endothelialization of uteroplacental vessels in human pregnancy—evidence that endothelium is focally disrupted by trophoblast in preeclampsia. Am J Obstet Gynecol 1992; 167(3):751–756.

48. Meekins JW, Pijnenborg R, et al. A study of placental bed spiral arteries and trophoblast invasion in normal and severe pre-eclamptic pregnancies. Br J Obstet Gynaecol 1994; 101(8):669–674.

49. Pijnenborg R, Luyten C, et al. Attachment and differentiation in vitro of trophoblast from normal and preeclamptic human placentas. Am J Obstet Gynecol 1996; 175(1): 30–36.

50. Colbern GT, Chiang MH, et al. Expression of the nonclassic histocompatibility antigen HLA-G by preeclamptic placenta. Am J Obstet Gynecol 1994; 170(5 Pt 1): 1244–1250.

51. Butterworth BH, Greer IA, et al. Immunocytochemical localization of neutrophil elastase in term placenta decidua and myometrium in pregnancy-induced hypertension. Br J Obstet Gynaecol 1991; 98(9):929–933.

52. Vinatier D, Monnier JC. Pre-eclampsia: physiology and immunological aspects. Eur J Obstet Gynecol Reprod Biol 1995; 61(2):85–97.

53. Rodgers GM, Taylor RN, et al. Preeclampsia is associated with a serum factor cytotoxic to human endothelial cells. Am J Obstet Gynecol 1988; 159(4):908–914.

54. Tsukimori K, Maeda H, et al. The possible role of endothelial cells in hypertensive disorders during pregnancy. Obstet Gynecol 1992; 80(2):229–233.

55. Roberts JM, Edep ME, et al. Sera from preeclamptic women specifically activate human umbilical vein endothelial cells in vitro: morphological and biochemical evidence. Am J Reprod Immunol 1992; 27(3–4):101–108.

56. Lorentzen B, Endresen MJ, et al. Sera from preeclamptic women increase the content of triglycerides and reduce the release of prostacyclin in cultured endothelial cells. Thromb Res 1991; 63(3):363–372.

57. Taylor RN, Musci TJ, et al. Preeclamptic sera stimulate increased platelet-derived growth factor mRNA and protein expression by cultured human endothelial cells. Am J Reprod Immunol 1991; 25(3):105–108.

58. Haller H, Hempel A, et al. Endothelial-cell permeability and protein kinase C in pre-eclampsia. Lancet 1998; 351(9107):945–949.

59. Baker PN, Davidge ST, et al. Plasma from women with preeclampsia increases endothelial cell nitric oxide production. Hypertension 1995; 26(2):244–248.

60. de Groot CJ, Davidge ST, et al. Plasma from preeclamptic women increases human endothelial cell prostacyclin production without changes in cellular enzyme activity or mass. Am J Obstet Gynecol 1995; 172(3):976–985.

61. Wellings RP, Brockelsby JC, et al. Activation of endothelial cells by plasma from women with preeclampsia: differential effects on four endothelial cell types. J Soc Gynecol Invest 1998; 5(1):31–37.

62. Baker PN, Davidge ST, et al. Plasma of preeclamptic women stimulates and then inhibits endothelial prostacyclin. Hypertension 1996; 27(1):56–61.

63. Ashworth JR, Warren AY, et al. Plasma from pre-eclamptic women and functional change in myometrial resistance arteries. Br J Obstet Gynaecol 1998; 105(4):459–461.

64. Hayman R, Brockelsby J, et al. Preeclampsia: the endothelium, circulating factor(s) and vascular endothelial growth factor. J Soc Gynecol Invest 1999; 6(1):3–10.
65. Vaisman N, Gospodarowicz D, et al. Characterization of the receptors for vascular endothelial growth factor. J Biol Chem 1990; 265(32):19461–19466.
66. Terman BI, Dougher-Vermazen M, et al. Identification of the KDR tyrosine kinase as a receptor for vascular endothelial cell growth factor. Biochem Biophys Res Commun 1992; 187(3):1579–1586.
67. Ferrara N, Houck K, et al. Molecular and biological properties of the vascular endothelial growth factor family of proteins. Endocr Rev 1992; 13(1):18–32.
68. Baker PN, Krasnow J, et al. Elevated serum levels of vascular endothelial growth factor in patients with preeclampsia. Obstet Gynecol 1995; 86(5):815–821.
69. Sharkey AM, Cooper JC, et al. Maternal plasma levels of vascular endothelial growth factor in normotensive pregnancies and in pregnancies complicated by pre-eclampsia. Eur J Clin Invest 1996; 26(12):1182–1185.
70. Lyall F, Greer IA, et al. Suppression of serum vascular endothelial growth factor immunoreactivity in normal pregnancy and in pre-eclampsia. Br J Obstet Gynaecol 1997; 104(2):223–228.
71. Anthony FW, Evans PW, et al. Variation in detection of VEGF in maternal serum by immunoassay and the possible influence of binding proteins. Ann Clin Biochem 1997; 34(Pt 3):276–280.
72. Banks RE, Forbes MA, et al. Evidence for the existence of a novel pregnancy-associated soluble variant of the vascular endothelial growth factor receptor, Flt-1. Mol Hum Reprod 1998; 4(4):377–386.
73. Lyall FA, Young A, et al. Placental expression of vascular endothelial growth factor in placentae from pregnancies complicated by pre-eclampsia and intrauterine growth restriction does not support placental hypoxia at delivery. Placenta 1997; 18(4): 269–276.
74. Simmons LA, Hennessy A, et al. Uteroplacental blood flow and placental vascular endothelial growth factor in normotensive and pre-eclamptic pregnancy. Br J Obstet Gynaecol 2000; 107(5):678–685.
75. Tsurumi Y, Murohara T, et al. Reciprocal relation between VEGF and NO in the regulation of endothelial integrity. Nat Med 1997; 3(8):879–86.
76. Brockelsby JC, Anthony FW, et al. The effects of vascular endothelial growth factor on endothelial cells: a potential role in preeclampsia. Am J Obstet Gynecol 2000 182(1 Pt 1):176–183.
77. Davidge ST, Signorella AP, et al. Distinct factors in plasma of preeclamptic women increase endothelial nitric oxide or prostacyclin. Hypertension 1996; 28(5):758–764.
78. Brockelsby J, Hayman R, et al. VEGF via VEGF receptor-1 (Flt-1) mimics preeclamptic plasma in inhibiting uterine blood vessel relaxation in pregnancy: implications in the pathogenesis of preeclampsia. Lab Invest 1999; 79(9):1101–1111.
79. D'Orleans-Juste P, Claing A, et al. Neurokinins produce selective venoconstriction via NK-3 receptors in the rat mesenteric vascular bed. Eur J Pharmacol 1991; 204(3): 329–334.
80. Thompson GW, Hoover DB, et al. Canine intrinsic cardiac neurons involved in cardiac regulation possess NK1, NK2, and NK3 receptors. Am J Physiol 1998; 275(5 Pt 2):R1683–R1689.

81. Page N, Woods RJ, et al. Excessive placental secretion of neurokinin B during the third trimester causes pre-eclampsia. Nature 2000; 405(6788):797–800.

82. Wang Y, Walsh SW. Antioxidant activities and mRNA expression of superoxide dismutase, catalase, and glutathione peroxidase in normal and preeclamptic placentas. J Soc Gynecol Invest 1996; 3(4):179–184.

83. Hubel CA, McLaughlin MK, et al. Fasting serum triglycerides, free fatty acids, and malondialdehyde are increased in preeclampsia, are positively correlated, and decrease within 48 hours post partum. Am J Obstet Gynecol 1996; 174(3):975–982.

84. Barden A, Beilin LJ, et al. Plasma and urinary 8-iso-prostane as an indicator of lipid peroxidation in pre-eclampsia and normal pregnancy. Clin Sci 1996; 91(6):7111–718.

85. Mikhail MS, Anyaegbunam A, et al. Preeclampsia and antioxidant nutrients: decreased plasma levels of reduced ascorbic acid, alpha-tocopherol, and beta-carotene in women with preeclampsia. Am J Obstet Gynecol 1994; 171(1):150–157.

86. Wang YP, Walsh SW, et al. The imbalance between thromboxane and prostacyclin in preeclampsia is associated with an imbalance between lipid peroxides and vitamin E in maternal blood. Am J Obstet Gynecol 1991; 165(6 Pt 1):1695–1700.

87. Hubel CA, Griggs KC, et al. Lipid peroxidation and altered vascular function in vitamin E–deficient rats. Am J Physiol 1989; 256(6 Pt 2):H1539–H1545.

88. Smarason AK, Sargent IL, et al. The effect of placental syncytiotrophoblast microvillous membranes from normal and pre-eclamptic women on the growth of endothelial cells in vitro. Br J Obstet Gynaecol 1993; 100(10):943–949.

89. Cockell AP, Learmont JG, et al. Human placental syncytiotrophoblast microvillous membranes impair maternal vascular endothelial function. Br J Obstet Gynaecol 1997; 104(2):235–240.

90. Knight M, Redman CW, et al. Shedding of syncytiotrophoblast microvilli into the maternal circulation in pre-eclamptic pregnancies. Br J Obstet Gynaecol 1998; 105(6): 632–640.

91. von Dadelszen P, Hurst G, et al. Supernatants from co-cultured endothelial cells and syncytiotrophoblast microvillous membranes activate peripheral blood leukocytes in vitro. Hum Reprod 1999; 14(4):919–924.

92. Johnstone R. Toxaemias in pregnancy. In: Comrie JD, ed. A Textbook of Midwifery. Edinburgh: 1939:252.

3

The Immunological Aspects of Preeclampsia: Links with Current Concepts on Etiology and Pathogenesis

Gustaaf Albert Dekker
Lyell McEwin Health Service, University of Adelaide, Adelaide, South Australia, Australia

I. INTRODUCTION

Preeclampsia occurs in 3 to 5% of pregnancies and is a major cause (15–20%) of maternal mortality in developed countries. It is also a leading cause of (iatrogenic) preterm birth and intrauterine growth restriction (IUGR). Shallow, endovascular cytotrophoblast invasion in the spiral arteries, inappropriate endothelial cell activation, and an exaggerated inflammatory response are features in the pathogenesis (see Chapter 2). In the late 1980s, generalized endothelial dysfunction was considered to be one of the triggering steps (1). More recent evidence suggests that inappropriate endothelial activation is part of a more generalized inflammatory reaction involving intravascular leukocytes as well as the coagulation and complement systems. Redman et al. (2) demonstrated that normal pregnancy in and of itself is characterized by a marked inflammatory response and that the differences between preeclampsia and normal pregnancy are less striking than those between the pregnant and nonpregnant states. A number of hypotheses on the etiology and early pathogenesis of preeclampsia are currently popular (3):

1. The placental ischemia hypothesis: Increased trophoblast deportation, as a consequence of placental ischemia, may result in endothelial cell dysfunction. In more recent publications, poor placentation is consid-

ered to be a separate pathologic mechanism, not the cause of preeclampsia but rather a powerful predisposing factor. Poor placentation
is a separate disorder that, once established, usually but not always
leads to the maternal syndrome. This depends on the extent to which the
placental ischemia initiates inflammatory signals (modulated by fetal
genes) and the nature of the maternal response to those signals (regulated by maternal genes).

2. The very low density lipoprotein (VLDL) versus toxicity-preventing
   activity (TxPA) hypothesis: In preeclampsia, circulating free fatty acids
   (FFAs) have been shown to be increased 15 to 20 weeks before the onset
   of disease. These FFAs may have a variety of adverse effects on
   endothelial physiology. Plasma albumin exists as several isoelectric
   species, which range from isoelectric point (pI) 4.8 to pI 5.6. The
   greater the binding of FFAs to albumin, the lower the pI. Plasma
   albumin in the pI 5.6 form exhibits toxicity-preventing activity (TxPA).
   Since higher ratios of FFA to albumin cause a shift in plasma albumin
   from the pI 5.6 to the pI 4.8 form, preeclamptic patients (who have
   elevated VLDL levels) will have lower amounts of protective TxPA (pI
   5.6) than normotensive pregnant women. A low ratio of TxPA to VLDL
   results in cytotoxicity and triglyceride accumulation in endothelial
   cells. In some pregnant women (possibly those with lower albumin
   concentrations), the burden of transporting extra FFAs from adipose
   tissue to the liver (in response to the increased energy demands), is
   likely to reduce the concentration of TxPA to a point where VLDL
   toxicity is expressed, leading to endothelial injury (4,5).

3. The hyperdynamic disease model: This hypothesis is based on the
   finding that in early pregnancy, some women destined to develop
   preeclampsia have an elevated cardiac output with compensatory vasodilatation. Dilated systemic terminal arterioles and renal afferent arterioles expose downstream capillary beds to systemic pressures and
   increased flow rates, eventually leading to shear stress and the endothelial cell injury characteristic of preeclampsia (6).

4. The immune/immunogenetic maladaptation hypothesis: It is known
   that the interaction between decidual leukocytes and invading cytotrophoblast cells is essential for normal trophoblast invasion and development. Immune maladaptation may cause the shallow invasion of the
   spiral arteries by endovascular cytotrophoblast cells, and endothelial
   cell dysfunction mediated by an increased decidual release of Thl
   cytokines, proteolytic enzymes, and free radical species (3).

5. The genetic hypothesis: the development of preeclampsia-eclampsia
   may be based on a single recessive gene or a dominant gene with
   incomplete penetrance. Penetrance may be dependent on the fetal genotype.

6. The genetic-conflict hypothesis. The maternal and fetal genomes perform different roles during development. Inheritable paternal, rather than maternal, imprinting of the genome is necessary for normal trophoblast development.

Preeclampsia may relate to a "hefty" genetic conflict, or a mother unable to cope with a "physiologic" genetic conflict. It should be stressed that these hypotheses are certainly not mutually exclusive, but most likely interactive to some extent. Although the etiology of preeclampsia is still unknown, many risk factors (7) have been identified (Table 1). Knowledge of these may allow the clinician to target groups of patients at high risk of preeclampsia. However, understanding the pathogenetic background of these risk factors could be of even

Table 1 Risk Factors for Preeclampsia

Preconceptional and/or Chronic Risk Factors
  Partner-related risk factors
    Nulliparity/primipaternity/teenage pregnancy
    Limited sperm exposure, donor insemination, oocyte donation
    Oral sex (risk reduction)
    Partner who fathered a preeclamptic pregnancy in another woman
  Non–partner-related risk factors
    History of previous preeclampsia
    Age, interval between pregnancies
    Family history
  Presence of specific underlying disorders
    Chronic hypertension and renal disease
    Obesity, insulin resistance, low birth weight
    Gestational diabetes, type I diabetes mellitus
    Activated protein C resistance (factor V mutation), protein S deficiency
    Antiphospholipid antibodies
    Hyperhomocysteinemia
    Sickle cell disease, sickle cell trait (?)
  Exogenous factors
    Smoking (risk reduction)
    Stress, work-related psychosocial strain
    In utero diethylstilbestrol exposure
Pregnancy-Associated Risk Factors
  Multiple pregnancy
  Structural congenital anomalies
  Hydrops fetalis
  Chromosomal anomalies (trisomy 13, triploidy)
  Hydatidiform moles
  Urinary tract infection

greater importance in our search for the obstetric "holy grail" (i.e., understanding the etiology and pathogenesis of preeclampsia).

II. THE IMMUNOLOGY OF PREECLAMPSIA: SPERM EXPOSURE, PRIMIPATERNITY, AND THE PATERNAL FACTOR

Generally, preeclampsia is thought of as a disease of first pregnancies (1). Indeed, a previous normal pregnancy is associated with a markedly lowered incidence of preeclampsia, and even a previous abortion provides some protection in this respect (8). The protective effect of multiparity, is however lost with a change in partner. The term *primipaternity* was introduced by Robillard et al. (9,10) to define the relationship between severe preeclampsia and changes in paternity patterns among multigravidae. In 61.7% of multiparous women with preeclampsia, the father of the current pregnancy was different to that of the former pregnancy, compared to 16.6% in the control group ($p < 0.0001$). Therefore these authors suggested the preeclampsia may be a problem of primipaternity rather than primigravidity. Robillard's study (9) was criticized because preeclampsia in these multiparous women was not defined by the classic combination of pregnancy-induced hypertension plus proteinuria. Tubbergen et al. (11) repeated this study in a Dutch population of 392 hypertensive multiparous patients and showed that multiparous women with strictly defined preeclampsia and/or hemolysis, elevated liver function tests, low platelets (HELLP) syndrome had a new partner in 22 to 25% of cases versus 3.4% in a control group of 182 normotensive multiparous patients. Trupin et al. (12), in a prospective study of 5,068 nulliparas and 5800 multiparas, of whom 573 had new partners, found that the incidence of pre-eclampsia in nulliparas (3.2%) and multiparas with changed paternity (3%) is similar, and much higher than the 1.9% incidence in multiparas with no change in partner. Li and Wi (13) showed that the effect of changing partners depends on the history of preeclampsia. They studied a cohort of 140,147 Californian women with two consecutive births during 1989–1991. Among women without preeclampsia in the first pregnancy, changing partners resulted in a 30% increase in the risk of preeclampsia in the subsequent pregnancy compared with those who did not change partners (95% CI 1.1–1.6). On the other hand, among women with pre-eclampsia in the first pregnancy, changing partners resulted in a 30% reduction in the risk of preeclampsia in the subsequent pregnancy (95% CI 0.4–1.2).

The duration of sexual cohabitation is also an important determining risk factor. Marti and Herrman (14) were the first to describe that the number of sexual cohabitations preceding pregnancy is about three times higher in normal pregnant women than in preeclamptic women, and concluded that their findings might also provide an explanation for the high incidence of preeclampsia in teenage pregnant girls. Klonoff et al. (15) subsequently conducted a case-control study, comparing the contraceptive histories of 110 primiparous women with preeclampsia with 115 pregnant women without preeclampsia. Their data indicated a 2.4-fold increased risk of preeclampsia for users of contraceptives that prevent exposure to sperm. Robillard et al. (16) were the first to launch a prospective study on the relationship between sperm exposure and preeclampsia; 1011 consecutive women delivering in one obstetric unit were interviewed about paternity and duration of sexual cohabitation before conception. The incidence of pregnancy-induced hypertension was 11.9% among primigravidae, 4.7% among same-paternity multigravidae, and 24.0% among new-paternity multigravidae. For both primigravidae and multigravidae, length of sexual cohabitation before conception was inversely related to the incidence of pregnancy-induced hypertension ($p < 0.0001$). Taking women cohabiting for more than 12 months as reference, a cohabitation period of 0 to 4 months was shown to be associated with a typical odds ratio (OR) of 11.6, a period of 5 to 8 months with a typical OR of 5.9, and a period of 9 to 12 months with a typical OR of 4.2. The very high incidence (24.0%) of pregnancy-induced hypertension among new-paternity multiparous women was shown to be related to a remarkably short period of sperm exposure preceding conception. In contrast to Robillard's study, a recent retrospective case-control study (17) in a group of 68 women of mixed parity with pregnancy-induced hypertensive disorders found that for primiparous women, a shorter duration of sexual cohabitation was associated with only a small and nonsignificant reduction in the risk of pregnancy-induced hypertensive disorders. For multiparous women, the greater the duration between stopping barrier contraceptives and pregnancy, the greater the risk of pregnancy-induced hypertensive disorders. However, this study has been criticized because a relatively high percentage (20–40% of cases) had a history of a previous abortion and the cases and the controls appear to have had some significant fertility issues. The mean duration of unprotected sexual activity was 13.2 months and 10.9 months respectively in the primiparous hypertensive cases and controls, and 49.4 and 27.1 months respectively in the multiparous hypertensive cases and controls.

Oral tolerance of antigens is quite easy to establish because the gut is a powerful tolerance induction site (18) and oral tolerance induction to MHC molecules has been shown in the rat model. In humans, Koelman et al. (19,20) assessed the effects of oral sex and found that, when comparing strictly defined primiparous preeclamptic women with primiparous control women, 18/41 preeclamptic women (44%) had oral sex with their partner before the index pregnancy versus 36/44 (82%) in the control group ($p = 0.0003$). In addition, significantly fewer (17% of 41) preeclamptic patients than control patients (48% of 44) confirmed that they swallowed the seminal fluid and sperm ($p = 0.003$).

Analogous to altered paternity and/or a short period of sperm exposure, Need (21) was the first to report the higher incidence (about twofold) of preeclampsia in pregnancies after artificial donor insemination. This has since been reported by several investigators [reviewed by Dekker et al. (20)]. Hoy et al. (22) compared a cohort of 152 donor-insemination pregnancies with 7717 normally conceived pregnancies. This study provided solid evidence that donor insemination is a risk factor for preeclampsia. Oocyte donation is also associated with an increased incidence of preeclampsia (20). In a retrospective analysis (23) of 232 ovum donation pregnancies, it was noted that 23% were complicated by hypertension. Salha et al. (24) compared the incidence of preeclamptic pregnancies conceived after donor insemination versus partner insemination and also after egg donation and embryo donation. In this study, 72 infertility patients who had conceived as a result of sperm, ovum, or embryo donation were compared with 72 age- and parity-matched controls who became pregnant with their own gametes, either spontaneously or following intrauterine insemination with their partners' spermatozoa. The overall incidence of preeclampsia in the donated-gamete study group was 18.1%, versus 1.4% in the age- and parity-matched controls. The incidence of preeclampsia in pregnancies resulting from donated spermatozoa was 18.2%, compared with 0% in the age- and parity-matched partner-insemination group. The incidence of preeclampsia resulting from ovum donation was also significantly higher (16% in the study group versus 3.7% in the age- and parity-matched control group). Four of the 12 (33.3%) women who conceived with donated embryos developed hypertension compared with none of their age- and parity-matched controls.

Recent data also provide evidence for the existence of the so-called dangerous father. Lie et al. (25) recently published data based on a Norwegian population analysis (1967–1992; about 60,000 births a year). There were 363,758 pairs of first and second pregnancies when the children had the same parents; 14,266 pairs of pregnancies when the children had the same mother but different fathers; and 26,152 pairs where the children had the same father but different mothers. One of the major findings was that men who fathered one preeclamptic pregnancy were nearly twice as likely to father a preeclamptic pregnancy in a different woman (OR 1.8; 95% CI 1.2–2.6; after adjustment for parity), regardless of whether or not she had already had a preeclamptic pregnancy. Thus women having a second pregnancy with a man who had previously fathered a preeclamptic first pregnancy in another woman had a substantially increased risk of preeclampsia in their second pregnancy (2.9%). This risk was nearly as high as the average risk among first pregnancies.

All these findings on the effect of change in partner, the protective effect of sperm exposure, and the "preeclampsia" partner are consistent with the immune/immunogenetic maladaptation hypothesis. Medawar (26) first noted the immunologically privileged nature of the fetal allograft in 1953. According to the laws of tissue transplantation, fetal alloantigens encoded by polymorphic genes inherited from the father ought to provoke maternal immune responses leading to fetal rejection soon after blastocyst implantation in the uterine wall. The expression of MHC molecules is an important factor in determining the antigenicity of the conceptus, and its capacity to invoke a specific maternal immune response. All mammals possess the MHC, a cluster of genes referred to as the HLA complex in humans. MHC molecules expressed on the cell surface are principally involved in the discrimination between self and nonself. The diversity of the MHC molecules within a species is enormous. This is due to polymorphism, which is the presence of multiple alleles at a given locus that confers the MHC uniqueness of an individual. MHC class I molecules, the major transplantation antigens, are ubiquitously expressed by the majority of somatic cells and are associated with tissue rejection through T lymphocyte–mediated immune responses. MHC class II is expressed by antigen presenting cells (APCs) and is classically involved in the induction of immune response through the presentation of foreign peptides to effector cells of the immune system (27). Immunologically, the trophoblast plays the most important role in the maternal response to the fetus at implantation. RT-PCR techniques have been used to demonstrate that both maternal and paternal MHC antigens are present in the murine embryo before its first cleavage division (28). However, the syncytiotrophoblast does not express class I MHC mRNA. While all of the classic class I HLA antigens are absent (apart from low-grade expression of HLA-C), the invading cytotrophoblast does express the nonclassical HLA-G (20) and HLA-G alternate transcripts. The presence of this nonpolymorphic MHC class I molecule probably plays an important role in the afferent arm of maternal tolerance of the fetus by failing to be perceived as "foreign" while still protecting the trophoblast from natural killer (NK) cell–mediated cytotoxicity. HLA-G–positive trophoblast cells express the transporter protein TAP1, which is essential in peptide presentation and MHC assembly. This suggests that the HLA-G molecule may also function by presenting peptide to target leukocytes (30). NK cells express killer-inhibitory and killer-activatory receptors capable of recognizing HLA class I molecules. Interestingly, the repertoire of the above receptors expressed by the large granular lymphocytes (LGL cells ≈ decidual NK cells) differs between women. HLA-C appears to be the most pertinent in influencing NK-cell function. The two killer inhibitory receptors that are specific for all HLA-C alleles also recognize HLA-G suggesting that HLA-G is the universal inhibitor of cytolysis by NK cells. Interestingly, analogous MHC-like molecules and their receptors have not yet been found in rodents. This suggests that HLA-G/C may have evolved after rodent and primate ancestors diverged. It might be that these processes evolved due to the need to protect a greater fetal mass for longer periods of time in larger mammalian species (27). MHC class II alloantigens are not expressed at the maternal-fetal interfaces. This removes a critical factor eliciting CD4+ T cell responses—significant components of effector and helper T-cell responses that target tissue allografts, leading to rejection (27). Trophoblast invasion is actually dependent on appropriate cytokines being produced by uterine LGLs in response to HLA-G expressed on cytotrophoblast. This phenomenon is called immunotrophism. Several cytokines, in a close and complex interaction with steroids and prostaglandins, are essential to early pregnancy development. For instance TNF, IFN-α, IFN-β, IFN-γ, and TGF-1β inhibit trophoblast growth. Conversely IL-1, VEGF, GM-CSF, and IL-6 stimulate trophoblast growth. Lack of HLA-G expression in extravillous trophoblast is associated with preeclampsia (31). However, no association between a polymorphism associated with reduced expression of HLA-G and preeclampsia could be demonstrated (32).

    Overall T-lymphocyte activity is downregulated in normal pregnancy (33). In 1986, two distinct and mutually inhibitory types of T-helper cells were described. The first type of cell, termed Th1, secretes IL-2, IFN-γ, and lymphotoxin. This contrasts with Th2 cells, which secrete Il-4, IL-6, Il-10 (34). Th1 cytokines are associated with cell-mediated immunity and delayed hypersensitivity reactions, whereas Th2 cytokines foster antibody response and allergic reactions. A Th2 switch characterizes pregnancy. During pregnancy, expression of both CD4 and CD8 is transiently downregulated on αβ TcR+ splenic T cells specific for a paternal HLA class I antigen, which represents a reduced Th response (35). Cytotrophoblast HLA-G induces a Th2 response in decidual leukocytes (36). Several substances such as progesterone, PGE2, TGF-β2, GM-CSF, and especially IL-10 play a part in the immunoendocrine network that is pivotal in maintaining pregnancy. IL-10 acts as a cytokine-synthesis-inhibitory factor and as an inducer of ACTH. Placental and decidual cells both produce Th2 cytokines (37). The importance of the Th2 switch is supported by the finding that decidual CD4 and CD8 T-cell clones of recurrent spontaneous miscarriage patient show reduced IL-4 and IL-10 production. Also, when measured in peripheral leukocytes, normal pregnancy is characterized by a Th2 cytokine pattern, whereas spontaneous miscarriages are characterized by a Th1 cytokine profile (38). The majority of studies on preeclampsia have found increased TNF-α and IL-1 levels, and increased levels of soluble TNF-α receptors and IL-1 receptor antagonists (39). Serum levels of IL-2, an important cytokine in the T-cell pathway, are also increased in preeclampsia. Both the placenta and the decidua are important sources of these Th1 cytokines. A deficiency of placental IL-10 has been identified in preeclampsia (37). In addition, decidual production of IL-2 is increased, which may lead to increased proliferative and cytotoxic activities of the U-LGL and conversion to lymphokine-activated killer (LAK) cells (40). Hamai et al. (41) provided data that the increase in IL-2 and TNFα levels in women who go on to develop preeclampsia is already detectable at the end of the first trimester. Saito et al. (42) demonstrated that the Th1–Th2 imbalance in preeclampsia is recognizable (by flow cytometry methodology) at the cellular level.

    Sacks et al. (43) proposed that suppression of the specific arm of the maternal response is accompanied, and perhaps compensated for, by activation of the nonspecific innate immune system. Furthermore, they propose that there is a unique dysregulation between the innate and specific arms of the maternal immune system in which the monocyte rather than the lymphocyte assumes a central role in the maternal immunological adaptation. The normal function of the innate immune system is to instigate an immune response by processing and presenting antigens, in association with MHC class I and II molecules, to lymphocytes, the so-called signal 1. Full responses also require adjuvants such as endotoxin, which, through interaction with the innate immune system, produce signal 2, in the form of costimulatory surface molecules or cytokines. Signal 2 appears to determine the biological significance of antigens and communicates this information to the adaptive immune system. In effect, it instructs the adaptive system to either respond or not, although it is debated whether the instruction distinguishes between self and nonself, infection and noninfection, or danger versus no danger. Marked activation of the innate immune system is a characteristic of normal pregnancy. There are increased numbers of monocyte and granulocytes with activated phenotypes. Monocyte phagocytosis and the respiratory burst activity are increased. Monocyte surface expression of the endotoxin receptor CD 14 is increased, and, in response to endotoxin, monocytes from normal pregnant women produce more of the proinflammatory type 1 cytokine IL-12. Many studies have demonstrated granulocyte activation and changes in plasma levels of soluble innate factors in pregnancy, and these findings are typical of an acute-phase response. Not all components of the innate system are activated in the maternal circulation. Most notably, cytotoxic activity and IFN-γ production by NK cells are suppressed, perhaps by specific inhibitory factors such as soluble HLA-G.

Delayed neutrophil programmed cell death, or apoptosis may explain the previously idiopathic neutrophilia of pregnancy (44). Inhibition of spontaneous neutrophil apoptosis is a marker of systemic inflammation and is consistent with normal pregnancy being a (pro) inflammatory state. Neutrophil apoptosis was found to be further delayed in preeclampsia, but not in normotensive IUGR. This is support for the hypothesis that although preeclampsia and normotensive IUGR share a common placental abnormality, it is the aberrant maternal response that eventually causes the maternal syndrome of preeclampsia. Von Dadelszen et al. (44) hypothesized that women who acquire preeclampsia may have a genetic tendency to delayed neutrophil apoptosis. According to Sacks et al. (43), placental particulate and/or soluble products can act as adjuvants, stimulating signal 2 of the classical immune response, but a relative absence of specific antigen presentation (signal 1) prevents a T cell–mediated rejection response. In this model, the immune response to normal pregnancy is thus signal 2 in the absence of signal 1.

This induction of signal 2 is potentially dangerous, as it primes the adaptive immune responses to fetal, foreign, or autoimmune antigens. According to Sacks et al. (43), the signal 2 is generated primarily in the blood, where sustained contact between APCs and lymphocytes is unlikely. Even in the event of such antigen presentation, placental factors such as progesterone, PGE2, and Th2 cytokines (e.g., IL-10) would bias the response to a Th2 pattern. An alternative explanation might be that a specific paternal factor, a unique maternal-paternal immunogenetic interaction, and/or the (partial) absence of a partner-specific immune tolerance induced by prolonged and repeated sperm exposure translates into degrees of signal 1 expression/suppression (45). One problem is that it is not obvious whether cytokine imbalances are caused by inappropriate T-cell responses or vice versa (27). Animal models have shown that maternal T cells specific for paternally inherited antigens could be induced to participate in immune responses leading to fetal rejection. According to Mellor and Dunn (72), there are compelling reasons for assuming that some, perhaps many, human pregnancy failures are caused by an immune dysfunction that upsets the delicate balance between maternal tolerance and fetal nurturing. Given the largely and necessarily descriptive nature of the evidence available from studies on human pregnancies, it is difficult to assess definitely whether maternal T cells are participants, facilitators, or merely by-standers in processes that lead to postimplantation loss of human fetuses. Maternal T cells are aware of fetal alloantigens during pregnancy (35). HLA allosensitiza-tion has also been demonstrated in human pregnancy, as evidenced by detectable IgG antibodies to fetal HLA alloantigens in the blood of 20 to 30% of primigravid and 50 to 65% of multiparous women (46). In pregnancy, maternal T-cell toler-ance must be induced and maintained either by trophoblast cells or by fetal cells that enter the maternal circulation and establish a reservoir. This reservoir of cells is either stable or continuously replenished. Studies on pregnant women show that fetal cells appear in the maternal circulation at an early stage in gestation and that genetic microchimerism may persist for many years after parturition (27). It has been assumed that fetal cells migrating into maternal tissues excite a T-cell response that results in T-cell tolerance and destruction of the fetal cells. This scenario might also explain why maternal tolerance disappeared shortly after parturition in the study of Tafuri et al. (35), since a continuous supply of fetal cells may be necessary to maintain T-cell tolerance. T-cell tolerance did, however, persist after parturition in another model reported by Jiang and Vacchio (47).

The adaptive immune system is a marvel of flexibility and precision. How-ever, immunization with foreign antigens requires a crude proinflammatory adju-vant (signal 2) in order to elicit an adaptive response. According to Janeway, costimulatory signals from the innate immune system indicating that "infection" is present are necessary in order to give "permission" to the adaptive immune system to activate. By extension, tissues that were not infected or inflamed would not support lymphocyte activation and would thus operationally be considered "self" regardless of the antigens they displayed. Janeway's hypothesis has been extended to include any signals that indicate microenvironmental tissue injury, not just infection. Bonney and Matzinger (48) proposed that any condition that the immune system recognizes as connoting danger to the host could be permissive for lymphocyte activation. Thus the innate immune system is not a primitive line of first defense but actually acquires critically important information regarding the nature of the threat to the host via its array of specialized receptors that detect microbial products, tissue damage, complement activation, clotting factors, etc. According to Mellor and Dunn (27), it makes sense that the highly specialized recognition and memory functions of the adaptive system should be regulated by the "older and wiser" innate immune system. In the context of reproductive biology, it is important to emphasize the paradigm that the adaptive immune response is regulated by the innate immune system. Lymphocyte responses are not simply driven by encounter with antigen but rather are strongly influenced by the context in which this encounter occurs. The Th cytokine milieu at the maternal-fetal interface is likely to be of immense importance in this respect. In normal pregnancy, the innate immune system is activated, local and systemic inflammation occurs, and the adaptive immune system is fully aware of paternal alloantigens. However, unlike the case of an organ allograft, the nature of the inflammatory response is immunosuppressive (27). The T-cell repertoire capable of responding to fetal antigens is made aware of the presence of these antigens during pregnancy and rendered unresponsive to them in an antigen-specific manner. Thus the key difference between the fetal allograft and a solid-organ transplant lies not in the ability of the adaptive system to see and respond to fetal alloantigens, but rather in the way in which the innate immune system threats the presence of the fetus. The innate system is alerted and responds actively to the fetal invasion, but the type of inflammation jointly created by fetally derived cells and the maternal innate immune system is not a milieu in which rejecting T-cell responses are produced. However, far from being hidden from the maternal adaptive immune system, fetal alloantigens are actively involved in establishing a condition of antigen-specific tolerance during pregnancy (27). According to Schuiling et al. (49), it is in the interest of the fetus to regulate the cytokine network in such a way that the fetus is not directly attacked. Theyproposed that only healthy zygotes are able to regulate the local inflammatory response so that they are not harmed by it. As such, postimplantation pregnancy loss may be part of the human reproductive strategy and be the necessary consequence of adequate selection and subsequent elimination of unfit zygotes.

The mechanism by which sperm exposure protects and the way the paternal factor exerts its effects are still unclear. It is possible that previous regular sperm exposure is important in creating a nondanger signal for the innate immune system. Deposition of semen in the female genital tract provokes a cascade of cellular and molecular events that resemble a classic inflammatory response. The trafficking of leukocytes within the endometrium and their phenotypic behavior appear to be under the control of steroid hormones and seminal factors acting through cytokines emanating from the uterine epithelium. The production of one of these cytokines, GM-CSF, is increased 20-fold following mating and is believed to play a central role in the recruitment of endometrial leukocytes. The critical seminal factor appears to be seminal-vesicle derived TGFβ1. Interestingly, seminal vesicle-derived TGFβ1 is secreted predominantly in a latent form. Seminal, plasma, and uterine factors transform the latent form in bioactive TGFβ1. Intrauterine insemination of TGFβ1 in vivo results in an increase in GM-CSF production that is sufficient to initiate an endometrial leukocytosis comparable with that seen following mating. In addition to initiating a GM-CSF production, TGFβ1 may also directly mediate an endometrial inflammatory response through its own chemotactic activity for macrophages and neutrophils. The introduction of TGFβ1 into the uterus in combination with paternal ejaculate antigens may favor the growth and survival of the semiallogeneic fetus in two ways. Firstly, by initiating a postinflammatory reaction, TGFβ1 increases the ability to sample and process paternal antigens contained within the ejaculate. Animal studies have shown that intrauterine insemination with sperm in combination with rTGFβ1 results in a significant increase in fetal and placental weight compared to immunization with sperm alone. Another important role of TGFβ1 and the subsequent postcoital inflammatory response is the initiation of a strong Th2 immune deviation. The processing of an antigen by APCs in an environment containing TGFβ1 is likely to initiate a Th2 phenotype within these responding T cells. By initiating a Th2 immune response toward paternal ejaculate antigens, seminal TGFβ1 may inhibit the induction of Th1 responses against the semiallogeneic conceptus that are thought to be associated with poor placental development and fetal loss (50). Decidual macrophages, present in an immunosuppressive phenotype from the moment of implantation, may inhibit NK-cell lytic activity through their release of molecules such as TGFβ, IL-10, and PGE2. Furthermore, the generation of non-complement-fixing antibodies following mating may help mask paternal trophoblast antigens, thereby preventing their recognition by more destructive components of the maternal immune system. Under the influence of the local cytokine environment, APCs such as macrophages, dendritic cells, and possibly even uterine epithelial cells may take up, process, and present ejaculate antigens (sperm, somatic cells, and soluble antigens) to T cells in the draining lymph nodes. The exact way by which the female organism is exposed to the paternal HLA message is uncertain. Koelman et al. (19) demonstrated the presence of soluble class I HLA molecules which might represent a straightforward way of exposing the endometrium to "the foreign antigen." Interestingly, soluble HLA molecules have also been demonstrated to induce apoptosis in human cytotoxic T cells (51), and induction of apoptosis may be a mechanism of inducing specific tolerance against HLA molecules of the male partner. According to Clark (52), the genital tract has unusual T cells with δ rather than α,β type receptors for antigen, and one possibility is that these T cells respond to antigens in the vagina and uterus. If such recognition were exempt from the usual requirement for simultaneous binding to an HLA-A, -B, -C, or -D type antigen on the antigen-presenting cell, that would pave the way to recognition of human trophoblasts lacking classical HLA surface antigens. Quantitative aspects [i.e., frequency of exposure (vaginally and orally)] and the level of soluble HLA may be important for the induction and sustaining of a state of tolerance. The induction of alloantibodies by pregnancy indicates that the maternal immune system is confronted with paternal HLA-A and -B antigens of the child. It might well be that the tolerance originally induced by soluble HLA-A and -B antigens or translated sperm mRNA spreads to epitopes of nonclassical HLA antigens expressed on the trophoblast (53). A generally accepted phenomenon in inflammation, a pregnancy characteristic, is an increased expression of classical HLA-antigens. For this reason, immune responses to classical HLA class I molecules cannot be excluded in the etiology of preeclampsia. Data from Smith et al. (54) suggest that the protective factor is on the spermatozoa and not in the seminal fluid. Sperm cells do not express HLA. In mice, uptake of sperm mRNA encoding for paternal HLA by decidual APCs has been shown to occur with subsequent translation of sperm mRNA encoding paternal MHC class I molecules within these maternal APCs. These APCs traffic from the uterus to the draining lymph nodes during the postcoital inflammatory response. It is unknown whether or not this fascinating mechanism is operative in humankind. HLA-G is certainly not involved here, since human sperm cells do not have mRNA for HLA-G (55,56).

The observation of an inverse relationship between the duration of sexual cohabitation and the incidence of preeclampsia suggests the long-term sperm exposure may be more important for the success of human implantation than acute exposure. This makes physiological sense since the human female is one of the few mammals exposed to her partner's semen on multiple occasions prior to conception. From an evolutionary perspective, it can be argued that induction of paternal antigen tolerance through repeated sperm exposure may have reproductive advantages, perhaps by promoting implantation and survival of embryos conceived in long-term relationships, where it could be argued that the male parent may be more committed to the well-being of the resultant child. In terms of evolution, the relatively high incidence of preeclampsia represents a significant reproductive disadvantage in humans as compared with other mammals. In most developing countries today, and until the 1950s in developed countries, approximately 1% of human births were complicated by eclampsia. Many authors think that because of its high incidence, the disease might mask an adaptive advantage somewhere. This may be true for the increase in blood pressure per se, since the increased maternal systemic blood pressure will increase uterine perfusion pressure (57). However, overall, the presence of preeclampsia means that humanity has had to adapt to a tremendous reproductive burden. The major difference between the human embryo and its mammal counterparts is the size of the brain. The human fetus has a brain which requires about 60% of its total nutritional needs during the extraordinary phase of brain development in the second and third trimesters of pregnancy. The large size of the human fetal brain requires deep endovascular trophoblast invasion, and this can only occur as a result of major immunogenetic compromise in terms of maternal-paternal tissue tolerance. According to Robillard (personal communication), the price that humankind had to pay for its large brain is the low fecundity rate (25%) and loss of estrus. In mathematical population models, demographers use a mean interval of 7 to 8 months after constitution of a couple (without contraception) in the calculation of fecundity. Being very fertile in a first pregnancy can be considered a disadvantage because of the high risk of preeclampsia. According to Robillard, a fecundity rate of 25% (as observed in the human species) is the best compromise between the risk of preeclampsia and the threat of reduced fertility in additional pregnancies (multiparity) with the same partner. In most human societies, babies from multigravidae represent 60 to 80% of total births. To remove the preeclampsia risk, the human female would need a fecundity rate of approximately 10%. Such a low rate would be disadvantageous to multiparous women and to the reproductive success of the human species. Loss of estrus in the human female remains partially unexplained in terms of biological necessity. There are several theories as to why this occurred. First, an estrus reproduction process is synonymous with a high fecundity rate. Second, an obligatory low fecundity rate induced a "repetition of trials" too hazardous with estrus reproduction once or twice a year. Third, the protective effect of semen exposure with a specific partner (lost with the absence of constant sexual cohabitation) made it necessary for the human female to be constantly sexually attractive.

An important discovery in reproductive immunology was the finding that parental sharing of human leukocyte antigens (HLAs) may be associated with adverse pregnancy outcome (46). This finding is consistent with the knowledge that inbred mating is associated with deleterious reproductive outcomes. Although still not well understood, maternal immune tolerance is probably initiated by fetal (paternal) immunologic stimulation. Parental HLA sharing may result in a lack of adequate antigenic stimulation and a failure to establish immune tolerance. This could lead to a series of adverse pregnancy outcomes including infertility, recurrent spontaneous abortions, and IUGR. The strongest evidence derives from the association between paternal HLA sharing and recurrent spontaneous abortion. IUGR pregnancies are also associated with a greater-than-expected degree of parental HLA sharing. HLA-incompatible fetuses are known to be at an advantage in human pregnancy (46). Parental HLA sharing has also been hypothesized to be a potential underlying mechanism for preeclampsia. However, only a limited number of studies have examined this hypothesis, and results are not consistent. At the moment the allegedly stronger relationship with HLA-DR4 sharing between mother and fetus has neither been confirmed nor refuted (58,59). The tumor necrosis factor allele, TNF1, may be associated with preeclampsia and certainly elevated concentrations of the cytokine are a feature of preeclampsia. The inducibility of TNF-α is HLA-class II–dependent, and the relevance of HLA-class

II genes might be entirely in relation to TNF-α synthesis and secretion (60). Li and Wi's study (13) was also based on the assumption that women with preeclampsia have a high likelihood of sharing HLA antigens with their partners. Thus those who changed partners were postulated to reduce the likelihood of HLA sharing. Their data suggest it is not the new set of paternal antigens per se that increases the risk of preeclampsia. Parental HLA sharing could impair the establishment of maternal immune tolerance needed to sustain a successful pregnancy. In a couple without HLA sharing, a prior successful pregnancy should provide enough protection against the risk of preeclampsia in a future pregnancy fathered by the same partner. Therefore, when a parous women changes partners, the protective effect offered by the previous pregnancies no longer exists; thus her risk of preeclampsia in a pregnancy fathered by a new partner is higher than that of a woman who remains with the same partner. The reported increased risk of preeclampsia associated with changing partners in many other studies may have reflected this phenomenon among women without parental HLA sharing because they comprised the majority of those study populations. On the contrary, if a woman had prior preeclampsia, thus indicating her sharing of HLA antigens with her current partner, her ability to establish the protective immune tolerance would be limited due to lack of immunologic stimulation resulting from HLA sharing. Changing a partner, which likely results in less HLA sharing, would reduce the risk of preeclampsia because of the enhanced immunologic stimulation from the fetus fathered by the new partner. Similar findings were reported by Lie et al. (25). In this Norwegian study, the risk of preeclampsia was 1.7% in second pregnancies in mothers with a history of a normotensive first pregnancy and who had their second pregnancy with the same partner. A woman who had preeclampsia in her first pregnancy had a risk of 13.1% if she had her second pregnancy with the same partner. This risk dropped to 11.8% if she changed partners (25). An alternative and/or additional explanation for this observed effect may be paternally related factors, genetic or otherwise. In other words, a relatively small percentage of men in the general population may carry a higher risk of fathering a pregnancy with preeclampsia. The Norwegian data clearly show the impact of the partner, since men who fathered one preeclamptic pregnancy were nearly twice as likely to father a preeclamptic pregnancy in a different woman (OR 1.8; 95% CI 1.2–2.6 after adjustment for parity), regardless of whether she had already had a preeclamptic pregnancy or not. So the paternal factor could be the degree of HLA sharing, specific genetic risk factors, and/or some sustained male sexual preference such as oral sex. Seminal factors such as the level of soluble HLA, TGFβ1, and plasmin might well be characteristics completely under genetic control. For example some HLA class I types are associated with low or high levels of soluble HLA levels in seminal plasma (19). Haig (61) has proposed a completely alternative hypothesis. According to Haig, the evolutionary theory of a parent offspring conflict hypothesizes that sperm cells are differently imprinted in the testes of males in short- and long-term relationships. In the evolutionary theory, by a mechanism to prevent propagation of their own genetic bloodline, males would imprint their sperm more "aggressively" when they do not expect to have offspring with that female or if a mother already has existing children by another man. In this view, the sperm exposure theory to habituate the female to paternal antigens becomes irrelevant. It is important to keep in mind that the paternal factor is not the only determinant of preeclampsia. Also Li and Wi's (13) data show that maternal factors are definitely strongly involved. If a paternal factor were the sole determinant of preeclampsia, one would have expected the risk to be similar among women who changed partners (assuming random mating), regardless of their history of preeclampsia. However, after changing partners, the risk of pre-eclampsia was still much higher (6.4%) among women with a history of pre-eclampsia in Li and Wi's (13) study than among women without such a history (0.9%). One of the potential mechanisms for this maternal importance could be that a history of preeclampsia is a marker for women who do not respond to fetal (paternal) immune stimulation as strongly as do women without such a history. Thus such women are less likely, under the same fetal stimulation, to establish the immune tolerance needed for a successful pregnancy. The failure in establishing immune tolerance to protect pregnancy could make women more susceptible to various adverse pregnancy outcomes, including preeclampsia. Poor response to paternal immune stimulation has been reported among women with recurrent spontaneous abortions. Therefore, a history of preeclampsia may be a marker for women with reduced capacity for mounting a reproductive immune response, and who are thus at a higher risk for preeclampsia. Other maternal reasons for a poor immune response might be a sustained maternal sexual preference—e.g., having a limited length of sexual cohabitation with new partner before conceiving. The latter phenomenon was demonstrated to be present in Robillard's (16) study in multiparous preeclamptic patients.

In summary, the protective effect of sperm exposure, the higher incidence after donor insemination and oocyte donation and the paternal factor strongly support the immune/immunogenetic maladaptation hypothesis. Further research in this field should focus on identifying the mechanism that allows for non–danger recognition by the maternal innate immune system in successful pregnancy. Elucidating these mechanisms is likely to pave the way to a more complete understanding of not only preeclampsia but also of the variety of human reproductive disorders linked to failed implantation.

REFERENCES

1. Roberts JM, Redman CWG. Pre-eclampsia: more than pregnancy-induced hypertension. Lancet 1993; 341:1447–1451.

2. Redman CWG, Sacks GP, Sargent IL. Preeclampsia: An excessive maternal inflammatory response to pregnancy. Am J Obstet Gynecol 1999; 180:499–506.
3. Dekker GA, Sibai BM. Etiology and pathogenesis of preeclampsia: current concepts. Am J Obstet Gynecol 1998; 179:1359–1375.
4. Lorentzen B, Endresen MJ, Clausen T, Henriksen T. Fasting serum free fatty acids and triglycerides are increased before 20 weeks of gestation in women who later develop preeclampsia. Hypertens Pregnancy 1994; 13:103–109.
5. Arbogast BW, Leeper SC, Merrick RD, Olive KE, Taylor RN. Hypothesis: which plasma factors bring about disturbance of endothelial function in pre-eclampsia? Lancet 1994; 343:340–341.
6. Bosio PM, McKenna PJ, Conroy R, O'Herlihy C. Maternal central hemodynamics in hypertensive disorders of pregnancy. Obstet Gynecol 1999; 94:978–984.
7. Dekker GA. Risk factors for preeclampsia. Clin Obstet Gynecol 1999; 42:422–435.
8. Eras JL, Saftlas AF, Triche E, Hsu CD, Risch HA, Bracken MB. Abortion and its effects on risks of preeclampsia and transient hypertension. Epidemiology 2000; 11: 36–43.
9. Robillard PY, Hulsey TC, Alexander GR, Keenan A, de Caunes F, Papiernik E. Paternity patterns and risk of preeclampsia in the last pregnancy in multiparae. J Reprod Immunol 1993; 24:1–12.
10. Robillard PY, Hulsey TC, Dekker GA. Revisiting the epidemiological standard of preeclampsia: primigravidity or primipaternity? Euro J Obstet Gynecol Reprod Biol 1999; 84:37–41.
11. Tubbergen P, Lachmeijer AM, Althuisius SM, Vlak ME, Geijn HP van, Dekker GA. Change in paternity: a risk factor for preeclampsia in multiparous women? J Reprod Immunol 1999; 45:81–88.
12. Trupin LS, Simon LP, Eskenazi B. Change in paternity: a risk factor for preeclampsia in multiparas. Epidemiology 1996; 7:240–244.
13. Li DK, Wi S. Changing paternity and the risk of preeclampsia/eclampsia in the subsequent pregnancy. Am J Epidemiol 2000; 151:57–62.
14. Marti JJ, Herrmann U. Immunogestosis: a new etiologic concept of "essential" EPH gestosis, with special consideration of the primigravid patient. Am J Obstet Gynecol 1977; 128:489–493.
15. Klonoff Cohen HAS, Savitz DA, Cefalo RC, McCann MF. An epidemiologic study of contraception and preeclampsia. JAMA 1989; 262:3143–3147.
16. Robillard PY, Hulsey TC, Perianin J, Janky E, Miri EH, Papiernik E. Association of pregnancy-induced hypertension with duration of sexual cohabitation before conception. Lancet 1994; 344:973–975.
17. Morcos RN, Bourguet CC, Prabcharan PSG, Khawli O, Krew MA, Eucker J, Skarote P. Pregnancy-induced hypertension and duration of sexual cohabitation. J Reprod Med 2000; 45:207–212.
18. Brandtzaeg P. History of oral tolerance and mucosal immunity. Ann NY Acad Sci 1996; 13:1–27.
19. Koelman CA, Coumans ABC, Nijman HW, Doxiadis IIN, Dekker GA, Claas FHJ. Correlation between oral sex and a low incidence of preeclampsia: a role for soluble HLA in seminal fluid? (Hypothesis). J Reprod Med 2000; 46:155–166.
20. Dekker GA, Robillard PY, Hulsey TC. Immune maladaptation in the etiology of

preeclampsia: a review of corroborative epidemiologic studies. Obstet Gynecol Survey 1998; 53:377–382.

21. Need JA, Bell B, Meffin E, Jones WR. Pre-eclampsia in pregnancies from donor inseminations. J Reprod Immunol 1983; 5:329–338.

22. Hoy J, Venn A, Halliday J, Kovacs G, Waalwyk K. Perinatal and obstetric outcomes of donor insemination using cryopreserved semen in Victoria, Australia. Hum Reprod 1999; 14:1760–1764.

23. Abdalla HL, Billet A, Kan AKS, et al. Obstetric outcome in 232 ovum donation pregnancies. Br J Obstet Gynaecol 1998; 105:332–337.

24. Salha O, Sharma V, Dada T, Nugent D, Rutherford AJ, Tomlinson AJ, Philips S, Allgar V, Walker JJ. The influence of donated gametes on the incidence of hypertensive disorders of pregnancy. Hum Reprod 1999; 14:2268–2273.

25. Lie RT, Rasmussen S, Brunborg H, Gjessing HK, Lie-Nielsen E, Irgens LM. Fetal and maternal contributions to risk of pre-eclampsia: a population based study. Br Med J 1998; 316:1343–1347.

26. Medawar PB. Some immunological and endocrinological problems raised by the evolution of viviparity in vertebrates. Symp Soc Exp Biol 1953; 11:320–338.

27. Mellor AL, Munn DH. Immunology at the maternal-fetal interface: lessons for T cell tolerance and suppression. Annu Rev Immunol 2000; 18:367–391.

28. Sprinks MT, Sellens MH, Dealtry GB, Fernandez N. Preimplantation mouse embryos express MHC class I genes before the first cleavage division. Immunogenetics 1993; 38:35–40.

29. Kovats S, Main EK, Librach C, Stubblemine M, Fisher SJ, DeMars R. A class I antigen, HLA-G, expressed in human trophoblasts. Science 1990; 248:220–222.

30. Clover LM, Sargent IL, Townsend A, Tampe R, Redman CW. Expression of TAP1 by human trophoblast. Eur J Immunol 1995; 25:543–553.

31. Goldman-Wohl DS, Ariel I, Greenfield C, Hochner-Celnikier D, Cross J, Fisher S, Yagel S. Lack of human leukocyte antigen-G expression in extravillous trophoblast is associated with pre-eclampsia. Mol Hum Reprod 2000; 6:88–95.

32. Aldrich C, Verp MS, Walker MA, Ober C. A null mutation in HLA-G is not associated with preeclampsia or intrauterine growth retardation. J Reprod Biol 2000; 47:41–48.

33. Wegman TG, Lin H, Guilbert L, Mosmann TR. Bidirectional cytokine interactions in the maternal-fetal relationship: is successful pregnancy a Th2 phenomenon? Immunol Today 1993; 15:353–356.

34. Mosmann TR, Cherwinski H, Bond MW. Two types of murine helper T cell clone. I. Definition according to profiles of lymphokine activities and secreted proteins. J Immunol 1986; 136:2348–2357.

35. Tafurie A, Alferink J, Moller P, Hammerling GJ, Arnold B. T cell awareness of paternal alloantigens during pregnancy. Science 1995; 270:630–633.

36. Clark DA. HLA-G finally does something! Am J Reprod Biol 1997; 38:75–78.

37. Hennessy A, Pilmore HL, Simmons LA, Painter DM. A deficiency of placental IL-10 in preeclampsia. J Immunol 1999; 163:3491–3495.

38. Marzi M, Vigano A, Trabattoni D, et al. Characterization of type 1 and type 2 cytokine production in physiologic and pathologic pregnancy. Clin Exp Immunol 1996; 106:127–133.

39. Taylor R. Immunobiology of preeclampsia. Am J Reprod Immunol 1997; 37:79–86.

40. Hamai Y, Fujii T, Yamashita T, et al. Pathogenetic implication of interleukin-2 expressed in preeclamptic decidual tissues. A possible mechanism of deranged vasculature of the placenta associated with preeclampsia. Am J Reprod Biol 1997; 38:83–88.

41. Hamai Y, Fujii T, Yamashita T, et al. Evidence for an elevation in serum interleukin-2 and tumor necrosis factor-α levels before the clinical manifestations of preeclampsia. Am J Reprod Biol 1997; 38:89–93.

42. Saito S, Sakai M, Sasaki Y, Tanebe K, Tsuda H, Michimata T. Quantitative analysis of peripheral Th0, Th1, Th2 and the Th1: Th2 cell ratio during normal pregnancy and preeclampsia. Clin Exp Immunol 1999; 117:550–555.

43. Sacks G, Sargent I, Redman C. An innate view of human pregnancy. Immunol Today 1999; 20:114–118.

44. Dadelszen van P, Watson RW, Noorwalli F, Marshall JC, Parodo J, Farine D, Lye SJ, Ritchie JW, Rotstein OD. Maternal neutrophil apoptosis in normal pregnancy, preeclampsia, and normotensive intra-uterine growth restriction. Am J Obstet Gynecol 1999; 181:408–414.

45. Sayegh MH, Turka LA. The role of T-cell costimulatory activation pathways in transplant rejection. N Engl J Med 1998; 338:1813–1821.

46. Ober C. HLA and pregnancy: the paradox of the fetal allograft. Am J Hum Genet 1998; 62:1–5.

47. Jiang SP, Vacchio MS. Multiple mechanisms of peripheral T cell tolerance to the fetal "allograft". J Immunol 1998; 160:3086–3090.

48. Bonney EA, Matzinger P. The maternal immune system's interaction with circulating fetal cells. J Immunol 1997; 158:40–47.

49. Schuiling GA, Koiter T, Faas MM. Pre-eclampsia. Why pre-eclampsia? Hum Reprod 1997; 12:2087–2092.

50. Tremellen KP, Seamark RF, Robertson SA. Seminal transforming growth factor β1 stimulates granulocyte-macrophage colony-stimulating factor production and inflammatory cell recruitment in the murine uterus. Biol Reprod 1998; 58:1217–1225.

51. Zavazava N, Kronke M. sHLA class I molecules induce apoptosis in alloreactive cytotoxic T cells. Nat Med 1996; 2:1005–1011.

52. Clark DA. Cytokines, decidua, and early pregnancy. Oxf Rev Reprod Biol 1993; 15: 83–111.

53. Yang L, DuTemple B, Gorczynski RM, Levy G, Zhang L. Evidence for epitope spreading and active suppression in skin graft tolerance after donor-specific transfusion. Transplantation 1999; 67:1404–1410.

54. Smith GN, Walker M, Tessier JL, Millar KG. Increased incidence of pre-eclampsia in women conceiving by intrauterine insemination with donor versus partner sperm for the treatment of primary infertility. Am J Obstet Gynecol 1997; 177:455–458.

55. Watson JG, Carroll J, Chaykin S. Reproduction in mice: the fate of spermatozoa not involved in fertilization. Gamete Res 1983; 7:75–84.

56. Hiby SE, King A, Sharkey A, Loke YW. Molecular studies of trophoblast HLA-G: polymorphisms, isoforms, imprinting and expression in preimplantation embryo. Tissue Antigens 1999; 53:1–13.

57. Dadelszen von P, Ornstein MP, Bull SB, Logan AG, Koren G, Magee LA. Fall in mean arterial pressure and fetal growth restriction in pregnancy hypertension: a meta-analysis. Lancet 2000; 355:87–92.

58. Kilpatrick DC, Gibson F, Livingston J, Liston WA. Pre-eclampsia is associated with HLA-DR4 sharing between mother and fetus. Tissue Antigens 1990; 35:178–181.
59. Wilton AN, Barendse WJ, Donald JA, Marshall P, Trudinger B, Gallery EDM, Brennecke SP, Cooper DW. HLA-DRB types in pre-eclampsia and eclampsia. Tissue Antigens 1991; 38:137–141.
60. Kilpatrick DC. Influence of human leukocyte antigen and tumour necrosis factor genes on the development of preeclampsia. Hum Reprod Update 1999; 5:94–102.
61. Haig D. Genomic imprinting and the theory of parent-offspring conflict. Semin Dev Biol 1992; 3:153–160.

4

The Differential Diagnosis of Preeclampsia and Eclampsia

Michael W. Varner
University of Utah, Salt Lake City, Utah, U.S.A.

Preeclampsia is among the most common complications of human pregnancy. It occurs in 6 to 8% of pregnancies in the United States and remains a significant cause of maternal mortality. Unfortunately, preeclampsia and eclampsia remain syndromes, in that their ultimate etiologies continue to be undefined. However, it is apparent that these syndromes clearly represent a final common pathway for multiple etiologies. It is well known that the preeclampsia that develops in a previously healthy young primigravida is a different entity than the preeclampsia that develops in a 40-year-old multigravida. Beyond this, there exist a surprising number of medical and surgical diseases that develop in women of reproductive age that can have their onset during pregnancy and thus be misdiagnosed as preeclampsia or eclampsia. Conversely, preeclampsia and eclampsia can be misdiagnosed as other medical or surgical disease. This chapter addresses the more common differential diagnoses that can mimic this pregnancy complication, with emphasis on those conditions more likely to be associated with clinically significant end-organ involvement.

As outlined elsewhere in this volume (Chapter 1), standard definitions for preeclampsia have been published and refined for many years. The American College of Obstetricians and Gynecologists has a generally endorsed list of clinical manifestations (Table 1) that identifies women with severe preeclampsia and eclampsia (1). These criteria have been developed because they identify a subset of women with preeclampsia shown to be at increased risk for maternal and/or fetal complications. In the absence of any of these signs or symptoms, the likelihood of maternal and/or fetal complications is remote. It is thus the purpose of this chapter to discuss the differential diagnoses in late pregnancy of the criteria list in Table 1.

Table 1 Clinical Manifestations of Severe Disease in Patients with Pregnancy-Induced Hypertension

I.	Blood pressure > 160–180 mmHg systolic or >110 mmHg diastolic
II.	Proteinuria > 5 g/24 h (normal < 300 mg/24 h)
III.	Elevated serum creatinine
IV.	Grand mal seizures (eclampsia)
V.	Pulmonary edema
VI.	Oliguria < 500 mL/24 h
VII.	Microangiopathic hemolysis
VIII.	Thrombocytopenia
IX.	Hepatocellular dysfunction (elevated alanine aminotransferase, aspartase aminotransferase)
X.	Intrauterine growth retardation or oligohydramnios
XI.	Symptoms suggesting significant end-organ involvement: headache, visual disturbances, or epigastric or right-upper quadrant pain

Source: Ref. 1.

I. BLOOD PRESSURE >160 to 180 mmHg SYSTOLIC OR >110 mmHg DIASTOLIC

A substantial body of evidence now exists to say that blood pressure ≥160 mmHg systolic and/or ≥110 mmHg diastolic represents a break point above which danger to mother and baby increases (2). While this level of blood pressure elevation may well be the sole result of preeclampsia, the possibility of other underlying causes of hypertension must always be considered. This is especially so in pregnant women whose hypertension is present prior to 20 weeks, who develop pre-eclampsia in other than their first viable pregnancy, or whose preeclampsia is early in onset and associated with other signs/symptoms that are severe in nature. Differential diagnostic considerations are outlined in Table 2.

A. Chronic Hypertension

Chronic hypertension, also called essential hypertension, is arterial hypertension of unknown cause. Chronic hypertension is generally diagnosed with persistent blood pressures above 140/90 mmHg with no identifiable cause. Chronic hypertension during pregnancy is diagnosed when a women is known to be hypertensive prior to pregnancy or else remains persistently hypertensive in the first 20 weeks of pregnancy. Sometimes the diagnosis is made only after the patient remains hypertensive for longer than 6 weeks after delivery, although whether this is an effect rather than the cause of the pregnancy-associated hypertension may still be unclear.

Table 2 Differential Diagnosis of Severe Hypertension (> 160/110 mmHg) in Late Pregnancy

Condition	Symptoms/signs
Chronic hypertension	Positive family history
Renal disease	
Renovascular hypertension	Sudden acceleration of benign hypertension
	Failed response to standard medical therapy
Primary aldosteronism	Weakness
	Muscle cramps
	Polyuria
	Refractory hypertension
Cushing's syndrome	Truncal obesity
	"Buffalo hump"
	Thin skin with striae
	Weakness
	Glucose intolerance
	Hypercalcuria
	Emotional or psychiatric problems
Pheochromocytoma	Intermittent or paroxysmal hypertension
	Visual disturbances
	Abdominal or chest pain
Coarctation of the aorta	

Many individuals with chronic hypertension will have a positive family history of hypertension and its complications, including congestive heart failure, coronary artery disease, stroke, and renal dysfunction.

B. Renal Disease

Preeclampsia and chronic renal disease share the characteristic of often remaining asymptomatic until their respective conditions are advanced. However, preeclampsia per se does not characteristically result in alteration of serum creatinine or blood urea nitrogen (BUN) until the condition is far advanced. Thus, underlying renal disease should be suspected when there is an elevated serum creatinine (≥ 1.0 mg/dL) or BUN (≥ 10 mg/dL). It should be remembered that because of the increased renal blood flow and glomerular filtration rate that occurs as a physiologic adaptation to pregnancy, the creatinine and BUN levels are significantly lower in pregnant than in nonpregnant women. Thus a creatinine of >1 mg/dL or a BUN >10 mg/dL, although frequently reported as within the normal range on most laboratory reports (since the nonpregnant range is stated), must be interpreted as high during pregnancy.

While proteinuria is common to both preeclampsia and chronic renal disease, preeclampsia per se does not result in diminished creatinine clearance until late in the disease. Thus, decreased creatinine clearance (<100 mL/min) should also raise the index of suspicion for underlying renal disease. A word of caution: This finding can often be the result of an incomplete urine sample collection. This can easily be detected by noting the amount of creatinine in the 24-hour urine collection. A pregnant woman of normal stature should have between 1.0 and 1.4 g of creatinine in a complete 24-hour urine collection.

On microscopic examination, the urinary sediment in acute or chronic renal disease frequently contains casts and/or cells. The urine of women with uncomplicated preeclampsia does not characteristically have these findings. Thus, the microscopic urinalysis findings may be of help in clarifying this differential consideration.

C. Renovascular Hypertension

Women most likely to have renovascular hypertension are those with hypertension of sudden onset, those with sudden acceleration of benign hypertension, and those who have failed to respond to standard medical therapy. Such patients characteristically have significant fixed diastolic hypertension. In the nonpregnant state an upper abdominal, high-pitched, continuous bruit is frequently heard. The physical changes of pregnancy make such a physical finding much less likely.

Definitive diagnosis of functionally significant renal artery stenosis requires selective renal angiography and differential renal vein renin measurements. The venous effluent from the involved kidney should have at least 1.5 times the renin activity of the uninvolved kidney. Outside of pregnancy, this difference can be enhanced with the administration of angiotensin converting enzyme (ACE) inhibitors. Because of their documented adverse fetal effects (3), ACE inhibitors should be avoided during pregnancy.

D. Primary Aldosteronism

A history of weakness, headaches, palpitations, muscle cramps, polydipsia, and polyuria associated with hypokalemia, glucose intolerance, and a metabolic alkalosis strongly suggests the possibility of hyperaldosteronism, particularly when associated with refractory hypertension. While the majority of individuals with primary aldosteronism (Conn's syndrome) will have either spontaneous or induced hypokalemia, as many of 20 to 25% of patients will require further testing to confirm the diagnosis. A high plasma aldosterone:renin ratio (greater than 20 in ng/dL) is very suggestive of the diagnosis. The definitive test for primary aldosteronism is the measurement of aldosterone excretion after 3 days of salt loading.

Patients with primary aldosteronism will have aldosterone excretion rates of at least 14 mg/24 h. Their glucocorticoid excretion will be normal. It is important to warn the laboratory if the patient has recently received any diuretics, ACE inhibitors, calcium antagonists or sympathetic system blocking drugs, since these agents may affect the renin-angiotensin-aldosterone axis.

The majority of patients with primary aldosteronism will have an adrenocortical adenoma, and most of the remainder will have bilateral adrenal hyperplasia. The patients with adenoma generally have more severe hypertension, more extreme aldosterone elevation, and more marked electrolyte imbalances. Adrenocortical adenomas can usually be visualized via adrenal computed tomography (CT) scanning, but sometimes selective adrenal venous sampling for aldosterone levels is required.

Treatment is usually surgical for unilateral aldosterone-producing cortical adenomas and medical for bilateral adrenal hyperplasia. The preferred medical treatments for bilateral adrenal hyperplasia (spironolactone and ACE inhibitors) are contraindicated in pregnancy. Alternative drugs that may be used include calcium channel antagonists and low-dose thiazide diuretics.

E. Cushing's Syndrome

Cushing's syndrome is defined as the presence of a chronic elevation of plasma cortisol. Most individuals with Cushing's syndrome exhibit truncal obesity, a prominent cervicodorsal fat pad ("buffalo hump"), thin skin with striae, progressive weakness as a result of muscular wasting, hypertension, glucose intolerance, and osteoporosis associated with hypercalcuria and nephrolithiasis. Many of these individuals also have emotional or psychiatric problems.

The physiological effects of increased corticosteroid-binding globulin (CBG) as well as the modest increase in free cortisol associated with normal pregnancy may obscure the laboratory diagnosis of Cushing's syndrome in pregnancy. However, a normal 24-hour urinary free cortisol level can easily exclude the disease, as can a normal plasma adrenocorticotropic hormone (ACTH). If the diagnosis of Cushing's syndrome is seriously considered during pregnancy, appropriate imaging studies of the pituitary and/or adrenal glands should be performed to exclude tumors.

Pregnancies complicated by Cushing's syndrome are known to be at increased risk for spontaneous premature labor and delivery. Cushing's syndrome is not associated with proteinuria or abnormalities of serum chemistries. This distinction can be of clinical value in assessing the possibility of superimposed preeclampsia.

Treatment is generally surgical when tumors are found. Medical therapy with agents such as ketoconazole, mitotane, and metyrapone may be required and should be administered only in consultation with an endocrinologist.

F. Pheochromocytoma

A history of intermittent and/or paroxysmal hypertension, headaches, palpitations, hyperhidrosis, or tremor associated with anxiety should suggest pheochromocytoma. Paradoxically, some patients with pheochromocytoma may exhibit orthostatic hypotension. These women may also suffer visual disturbances, intermittent fever, chest or abdominal pain, or unusual reactions to medications mediating catecholamines. With extreme hypertension, they may also experience convulsions or intracranial hemorrhage. Unexplained myocardial infarction in a pregnant woman should prompt a search for pheochromocytoma. Although most authorities suggest that pregnancy does not affect the disease, the increased cardiac output and blood volume as well as the mechanical effects of the third-trimester uterus may exacerbate the signs and symptoms of pheochromocytoma. The additional vascular stimulation and stress associated with labor and delivery may also induce a hypertensive crisis.

The laboratory criteria for the diagnosis of pheochromocytoma are not affected by the physiological changes of pregnancy. The hallmark laboratory findings are elevated vanillylmandelic acid, catecholamines, and metanephrines in a 24-hour urine collection. Importantly, these values may be affected by concurrent alpha-methyldopa, clonidine, labetalol, sotalol, tricyclic antidepressant, or levodopa administration; a full disclosure of all medications (and potential alcohol or illicit drug exposures) should be provided to the laboratory with the urine specimen. Other laboratory findings may include erythrocytosis, hyperglycemia, and hypercalcemia. As with Cushing's syndrome, pheochromocytoma is not characterized by progressive proteinuria. Because of the risk of associated conditions such as medullary thyroid carcinoma and hyperparathyroidism, an endocrinology workup is important.

Pheochromocytoma diagnosed in pregnancy may be treated either surgically or medically. Some 90% of these tumors are located in the adrenal medulla, but 10% are extra-adrenal and may be difficult to locate. Ten percent are malignant. Surgery is best reserved for the first half of pregnancy because visualization is better then, maternal vascular volume is less, and fetal well-being is less likely to be affected. Ten percent of pheochromocytomas will recur after surgical removal, and the patient should be made aware of this fact. The tumor can also be treated by alpha-adrenergic blockade using oral phenyoxybenzamine (starting at 10 mg/day and increasing every 2 days to a maximum of 1 mg/kg/day) for maintenance therapy and with IV phentolamine or nitroprusside for emergency blood pressure control. Combined alpha and beta blockade is recommended preoperatively. It is important that the alpha blockade be initiated prior to starting beta blockers for heart rate control (usually propranolol 10 mg every 6 hours). Beta blocker therapy is contraindicated in those patients with intrinsic beta sympathomimetic activity. Magnesium sulfate has been reported to be of use in the suppression of the intubation response and malignant hypertension during general anesthesia in women with pheochromocytoma. Cesarean section, with concurrent surgical removal of the tumor(s), is the recommended method of delivery.

G. Coarctation of the Aorta

Although previously undiagnosed coarctation of the aorta is a rare cause of hypertension in pregnancy, the identification of this condition in early pregnancy can be lifesaving. Women with sufficient aortic obstruction to cause significant hypertension do not tolerate the dramatic vascular changes of pregnancy. The condition can be diagnosed on physical examination by documentation of significant blood pressure differences between the upper and lower extremities. Depending on the location of the coarctation, there may also be significant blood pressure differences between the upper extremities. Patients with uncorrected coarctation will also have a significant lag between their radial and femoral pulses. Depending on the severity of the situation, cardiothoracic surgery may be indicated; this carries a significant risk for both mother and fetus, especially if bypass is required.

II. PROTEINURIA >5 g/24 h

Although normal pregnancy is associated with increased urine protein excretion (up to 300 mg/24 h versus < 100 mg/24 h nonpregnant), clinically significant proteinuria, particularly in the first half of pregnancy, should suggest the possibility of underlying renal disease. Otherwise healthy young adults may have postural proteinuria, present when upright but absent when recumbent, but this seldom exceeds 750 to 1000 mg/24 h. Likewise, extreme exertion, fever, seizures (eclamptic or noneclamptic), antibiotic injury, or congestive heart failure may produce proteinuria. However, proteinuria in excess of 1000 mg/24 h in pregnancy should always be considered an indicator of parenchymal renal disease.

While preeclampsia is associated with parenchymal renal disease, it is not associated with an active urinary sediment. Hematuria is frequently associated with concurrent systemic disorders such as coagulopathies, sepsis, or hemoglobinopathies. It can also be the result of urinary tract trauma, tumors, or urolithiasis. Hematuria is often seen in acute-onset renal diseases, both interstitial and glomerular, and in renal infarction. Red cell casts are often seen with glomerular diseases.

Likewise, proteinuria associated with pyuria should suggest an inflammatory process, usually infectious in origin, in the urinary tract. If the pyuria is also accompanied by leukocyte casts, renal parenchymal inflammation is usually present.

The presence of proteinuria in the first half of pregnancy should always suggest the possibility of underlying renal disease. An obstetric ultrasound should be performed to exclude either gestational trophoblastic disease or multiple pregnancy, both of which have been reported to cause preeclampsia prior to 20 weeks' gestation. On the other hand, the presence of proteinuria and hypertension late in pregnancy in a woman who has not received prenatal care to that point presents a difficult differential diagnosis. This is particularly so if associated with other multisystem organ dysfunction (thrombocytopenia, acute liver failure, etc.); in these cases, the diagnosis of preeclampsia should be seriously considered. However, this diagnosis can be confirmed only by either renal biopsy or puerperal resolution of signs and symptoms.

A. Glomerulonephritis

Although very uncommon, acute glomerulonephritis may closely mimic preeclampsia, particularly with onset in the latter part of pregnancy. Both are characterized by hypertension, proteinuria, and edema. However, preeclampsia is exceedingly rare prior to 20 weeks except, as noted above, in the presence of gestational trophoblastic disease or multiple pregnancy. The exclusion of these obstetric conditions in women with these signs in early pregnancy should strongly suggest an intrinsic renal process. Likewise, preeclampsia is not characterized by an active urinary sediment.

A positive streptococcal culture/rapid test, elevated antistreptolysin O titer, and low C3 or C4 complement levels may aid in the diagnosis of an infectious cause. Hematuria is common with distorted red cells from glomerular bleeding (as opposed to red cells with normal morphology when the bleeding is from the lower urinary tract).

Pregnancy may also occur in women known to have glomerulonephritis prior to conception. These pregnancies are generally well tolerated if maternal blood pressure is normal and the creatinine clearance is at least 70 mL/min (4).

B. Other Renal Disease

The most common explanation for apparent preeclampsia with persistent postpartum hypertension is previously unrecognized chronic hypertension. However, evolving primary renal disease should also be considered, particularly focal and/or segmental glomerulosclerosis, IgA nephropathy, and membranoproliferative glomerulonephritis (5).

III. ELEVATED SERUM CREATININE

The increase in renal blood flow normally seen in pregnancy results in a decrease in serum markers of renal function (creatinine, blood urea nitrogen, uric acid) and an increase in creatinine clearance. The normal serum creatinine and blood urea nitrogen (BUN) decrease to approximately 0.5 and 10 mg/dL, respectively. Serum uric acid generally decreases to 3 to 4 mg/dL.

Women characteristically have renal findings during the development of preeclampsia. Besides the proteinuria discussed above, most patients will develop laboratory evidence of renal impairment. This is most commonly seen as hyperuricemia (>5 mg/dL), but elevated creatinine and BUN levels can also be seen. Capillary glomerular endotheliosis is frequently seen on renal biopsy specimens from women with preeclampsia.

Most authorities define the upper limits of serum creatinine in the latter half of pregnancy as 0.8 to 0.9 mg/dL. Thus, nonpregnant normative laboratory values notwithstanding, any serum creatinine of 0.9 mg/dL or higher should suggest the possibility of underlying renal disease or renal compromise. In women whose serum creatinine is ≥1.5 mg/dL in the first trimester, the possibilities of fetal loss and accelerated deterioration of maternal function progressively increase (6).

Just as proteinuria may also signify underlying renal disease, elevated serum chemistries, especially if present in the first half of pregnancy, may also be a harbinger of underlying maternal renal disease. Indeed, the clinical triad of preeclampsia (hypertension, proteinuria, edema) is also seen in many nonpregnant women with intrinsic renal disease. If these findings are present before 20 weeks' gestation the likelihood of intrinsic renal disease is very high. The two potential obstetric confounders that can present at this early gestational age are multiple gestation and gestational trophoblastic disease.

The definitive initial diagnosis of renal disease usually requires renal biopsy. However, the aforementioned physiological changes during pregnancy make this procedure unacceptably dangerous; clinicians are therefore generally obliged to operate on a presumed clinical diagnosis. Previous renal biopsy studies have demonstrated that the majority of primigravidas with apparent preeclampsia have the characteristic biopsy findings. Although multigravidas may have preeclampsia alone (38%), a proportion also have underlying renal disease (26%) or chronic hypertension (24%) (7).

Intrinsic renal disease is not characteristically associated with abnormal liver function tests or thrombocytopenia. The association of these abnormalities with impaired renal function in the latter half of pregnancy further supports the suspicion of preeclampsia, although acute fatty metamorphosis of pregnancy (AFMP), hemolytic uremic syndrome (HUS), or thrombotic thrombocytopenic purpura (TTP) should be considered.

Although women with acute fatty metamorphosis of pregnancy (AFMP) may have significant renal impairment, they are also clinically jaundiced—a very uncommon sign in preeclampsia.

Although HUS is primarily seen in children, the condition can occur in women of reproductive age. Such women with HUS usually have prominent renal failure, impressive gastrointestinal features, and fewer neurological signs and symptoms. Women with TTP usually have mucous membrane bleeding and petechiae, fluctuating neurological symptoms, and jaundice. Laboratory evidence of microangiopathic hemolysis is present. Hematuria is often a prominent component—a complication not characteristically present in preeclampsia.

IV. GRAND MAL SEIZURES (ECLAMPSIA)

The grand mal seizures that distinguish eclampsia from preeclampsia are appropriately considered an indication to proceed with delivery. Eclamptic convulsions are not associated with an aura and, in the absence of associated hemorrhage, do not result in localizing neurological deficits. Eclamptic convulsions do not characteristically result in prolonged obtundation or coma or status epilepticus.

When these or other signs or symptoms are present, other causes of grand mal seizures must be considered in the late-pregnant woman. Likewise, grand mal seizures in the recently delivered woman, particularly those more than 24 hours postpartum, have an extended differential diagnosis. The following conditions must be considered, particularly if the woman has any localizing neurological deficit(s) or suffers prolonged obtundation or coma (see also Table 3).

A. Cerebral Venous Thrombosis

Cerebral venous thrombosis is a notorious imitator of eclampsia. Pregnancy, and particularly the immediate puerperium, is a hypercoagulable state. Pregnant women with underlying microvascular diseases, trauma, or infection are at particularly increased risk. Depending on the extent and location of the lesion(s), cerebral venous thrombosis can produce increased intracranial pressure, multifocal regions of brain ischemia, or cerebral infarction. Superior sagittal sinus thrombosis often presents with generalized or focal seizures that alternatively involve one and then the other side of the body. Motor deficits are common. These women often also have fever, headache, papilledema and various opthalmoplegias, visual field deficits, or expressive/receptive neurological deficits.

Cerebral venous thrombosis is best diagnosed via magnetic resonance venography. Cerebral CT scan is often the first imaging procedure performed in consideration of possible intracranial hemorrhage. Cerebral CT demonstrates hemorrhage, linear hyperdensities consistent with thrombosed veins on precontrast scans, and filling defects with contrast enhancement. Cerebral angiography is more invasive and is now uncommonly employed. When it is performed, specific attention should be directed to delayed filling of the venous sinuses and veins.

Table 3 Differential Diagnosis of Grand Mal Seizures in Pregnancy

Condition	Symptoms/signs
Eclampsia	Convulsions; no aura
	Occur in pregnant (or recently delivered) women with preeclampsia
Cerebral venous thrombosis	Quite variable, depending on location of thrombosis or thromboses
	May include headache, expressive or receptive deficits, opthamoplegias, visual field defects
Intracranial hemorrhage	Sudden onset of either "the worst headache of my life" or loss of consciousness
	Convulsions due to berry aneurysms more likely associated with antecedent dizziness or vomiting
Vasculitis	Quite variable
Epilepsy	Seizures may be evoked by known stimulatory factors
	Often accompanied by characteristic aura
Behavioral disturbances	

B. Intracranial Hemorrhage

The primary symptom associated with intracranial hemorrhage is the sudden onset of either "the worst headache of my life" or of loss of consciousness. Intracranial hemorrhage in women of reproductive age is usually due either to arteriovenous malformations (AVMs) or arterial aneurysms, with AVMs being relatively more common in younger pregnant women and aneurysms being more common in the mature spectrum of the reproductive years.

AVMs are relatively more likely to have produced antecedent central nervous system symptoms than other considerations in the eclampsia differential diagnosis. They often present as recurrent unilateral migraine headaches or progressive neurological disorders. The increase in blood volume and cardiac output as well as the progressive arteriolar collagen reorganization are widely thought to make AVMs more likely to become symptomatic in pregnancy.

Berry aneurysms should be particularly considered in women with atherosclerotic vascular disease who might become pregnant. They are also associated with polycystic kidney disease and certain connective tissue disorders such as Marfan's syndrome or Ehlers-Dahlos syndrome. These patients frequently report an awareness of dizziness or vertigo or of vomiting prior to the actual convulsion. This can be a valuable clinical distinction.

Unless accompanied by preexisting preeclampsia, the blood pressure in pregnant women with AVMs and berry aneurysms is often normal until the bleed and then rises suddenly and persistently. Likewise, these individuals will have localizing symptoms related to the location and volume of their intracranial bleeding. Nuchal rigidity is a very common physical finding that should also increase the suspicion of intracranial hemorrhage. As with cerebral venous thrombosis, a CT scan of the head should be performed promptly when intracranial hemorrhage is considered. It remains the diagnostic procedure of choice both because of its accuracy and widespread availability.

C. Vasculitis

Vasculitis can also mimic eclampsia, being potentially associated with hypertension, proteinuria and convulsions. Systemic lupus is the most common such vasculitis in women of reproductive age. Convulsions with lupus are usually associated with extreme hypertension (lupus cerebritis flare). Vasculitis can also be the result of long-term recreational drug abuse, particularly methamphetamine.

D. Epilepsy

Women with preexisting grand mal seizure disorders or epilepsy will usually be known or identified at the time of their seizure. In such women, the association of the seizure with known stimulatory factors such as flashing lights, music, video games, or sleep deprivation may also be of diagnostic value.

While it is possible to have the initial onset of epilepsy in pregnancy, this most commonly occurs in early pregnancy. Importantly, epileptic convulsions are not associated with hypertension, proteinuria, or other microvascular dysfunction.

The initial onset of seizures in a nonpreeclamptic woman should raise the questions of head trauma, central nervous system (CNS) infection, poisoning or metabolic disturbances, or vascular disease. CNS trauma sufficient to cause seizures should be self-evident. Brain abscess should be considered in the presence of other chronic infections, especially those near the brain (chronic middle ear disease, sinusitis) and those associated with a high risk of bacteremia such as endocarditis. Known histories of alcohol or other recreational substance abuse should raise the possibility of withdrawal symptoms. Acute meningitis and/or encephalitis are characteristically accompanied by high fever, malaise or myalgia, and other systemic complaints that frequently focus on the respiratory or gastrointestinal tracts.

The widespread use and mixing of nonprescription narcotics, cocaine, amphetamines, and alcohol should raise the suspicion of substance abuse. A toxicology screen is always a consideration, keeping in mind the regulations of the jurisdiction in which the patient is being evaluated.

E. Behavioral Disturbances

Somatization disorders can occasionally be confused with grand mal seizures. While these conditions may be accompanied by other appropriate complaints such as headache or epigastric pain, they are not associated with other physical findings. Hypertension, proteinuria, edema, or other laboratory abnormalities are not characteristically present.

These patients often also have childhood histories of neglect and/or abuse, and domestic violence is common. Personal and family histories of alcoholism and/or substance abuse, multiple divorces, or multiple surgeries are also common in such patients.

V. PULMONARY EDEMA

Pulmonary edema is among the least frequently diagnosed criteria for severe preeclampsia. While this may reflect the propensity to deliver preeclamptic women before they develop this complication, it may also reflect the infrequency with which obstetric care providers search for and recognize this problem. Pulmonary edema most commonly occurs postpartum, particularly when the patient begins her diuresis phase and when other signs and symptoms are abating.

Pulmonary edema usually presents with a nonproductive cough, wheezing, tachypnea, and dyspnea. As fluid further accumulates in the capillaries, rales and rhonchi can be heard, initially in the lower lobes, then extending upward as the severity of the disease increases. By this point, women are usually acutely dyspneic, pale, sweating, agitated, and producing pink or blood-tinged sputum.

The differential diagnosis of pulmonary edema includes iatrogenic fluid overload, heart failure, or transudation of fluid into the alveoli as a result of the progressive reduction of colloid osmotic pressure associated with progressive urinary protein loss.

Preeclamptic women must always have careful attention paid to fluid intake and output. They are perfect candidates for single-page bedside flow sheets on which all of the patient's providers can record and follow her fluid status. This will minimize the risk of iatrogenic fluid overload.

Preeclamptic patients with suspected pulmonary edema require intensive monitoring and represent one of the few generally agreed indications for pulmonary artery catheterization. Initial examination with an echocardiogram will quickly reveal those patients with a poor ejection fraction and systolic dysfunction (i.e., hypertensive cardiomyopathy) or those with diastolic dysfunction and high filling pressures. Undiagnosed valvular disease can also be elucidated with echocardiography. In those women with cardiogenic pulmonary edema, adult respiratory distress syndrome (ARDS), or sepsis, or who are hemodynamically unstable, a pulmonary artery catheter is essential. Those patients who are hemodynamically stable but have noncardiogenic pulmonary edema may be managed with appropriate noninvasive monitoring if available.

With normal colloid osmotic pressure, pulmonary catheter wedge pressure (PCWP) readings below 18 to 20 mmHg should not be associated with pulmonary edema. With PCWP readings between 18 and 25 mmHg, progressive pulmonary congestion will be seen. Clinically apparent pulmonary edema can be expected with PCWPs above 25 mmHg. As a result of decreased colloid osmotic pressures, clinical consequences in preeclamptic women will frequently occur at relatively lower PCWPs.

VI. OLIGURIA (<500 mL/24 h)

The differential diagnosis of oliguria in a preeclamptic woman may involve prerenal, intrinsic renal, or postrenal causes. These considerations are outlined in Table 4.

Prerenal oliguria will be seen more commonly in women who have other concurrent fluid losses (fever, hemorrhage, vomiting, diarrhea, etc.). The urine specific gravity is characteristically high (often >1.030) and urinary sodium concentrations are low, usually <10 mEq/L. Urinary creatinine is elevated (>40 mg/100 mL). The urinary sediment does not usually contain cellular elements.

Intrinsic renal disease, usually acute tubular necrosis (ATN), may develop following ischemic insults, classically following thrombin microemboli seen with abruptio placentae and disseminated intravascular coagulation. ATN may also develop following prolonged dehydration or massive blood loss. Intrinsic renal disease is characterized by high urinary sodium concentrations (usually >50 mEq/L) and low urinary creatinine concentrations (<15 mg/100 mL). Cellular elements, including casts, are commonly seen with intrinsic renal disease.

Postrenal causes of oliguria most commonly involve either a mechanical obstruction in a urinary catheter or else a postoperative unrecognized urinary tract injury (bladder and/or ureter) that is producing urinary ascites and/or a urinoma. Physical examination, perhaps augmented by an ultrasound imaging, can usually exclude these causes.

Table 4 Differential Diagnosis of Oliguria (< 500 mL/24 h)

Condition	Symptoms/signs
Prerenal	Usually associated with concurrent fluid loss (fever, hemorrhage, vomiting, diarrhea, etc.)
Intrinsic renal disease	Often associated with concurrent obstetric complications such as abruption and/or disseminated intravascular coagulation
Postrenal	

VII. MICROANGIOPATHIC HEMOLYSIS

Thrombotic thrombocytopenic purpura (TTP) and hemolytic uremic syndrome (HUS) are life-threatening causes of microangiopathic hemolysis that can masquerade as severe preeclampsia. These conditions have many features in common and may well be different manifestations of a single underlying pathophysiology, with those cases largely confined to the kidney being diagnosed as HUS and those with more generalized findings being diagnosed as TTP.

A. Thrombotic Thrombocytopenic Purpura

TTP is a condition that has recently been shown to be related to increased circulating von Willebrand multimers. Von Willebrand multimers are normally present in small amounts and their circulating level is regulated by an enzyme that breaks them down, von Willebrand factor metalloproteinase. Two of the functions of von Willebrand factor (vWf) multimers are to prolong the half-life of factor VIII and to promote platelet aggregation to subendothelial collagen. If vWf levels increase, systemic platelet aggregation occurs, with obstruction of the microcirculation and noninflammatory necrosis in organs such as the brain, heart, kidney, pancreas, and adrenal gland. Two types of TTP have been classified, (a) chronic relapsing TTP (a very rare autosomal recessive condition that relapses every 3 weeks indefinitely), caused by an absolute deficiency of vWf metalloproteinase, and (b) acute idiopathic TTP (a more severe and less predictable form) caused by IgG autoantibodies to vWf.

TTP is characterized by hemolytic anemia, thrombocytopenia, neurological symptoms, renal abnormalities, and fever. Women with this condition usually have mucous membrane bleeding and petechiae, fluctuating neurological symptoms, and jaundice. There is prominent laboratory evidence of microangiopathic hemolysis, including moderate to severe anemia with polychromatophilia, fragmented and nucleated red blood cells, moderate leukocytosis, and thrombocytopenia ($<50,000/\mu l$). This hemolysis leads to elevated indirect bilirubin and lactate dehydrogenase levels. Some degree of renal failure is usually present, with elevated serum BUN and creatinine as well as proteinuria developing early in the disease. Hematuria is often a prominent component, a complication not characteristically present in preeclampsia. Neurological findings are variable but can include paresis, aphasia, headache, obtundation, and seizures. Although patients early in the disease often do not have evidence of disseminated intravascular coagulation (DIC), progression of the disease to hepatic and renal failure is frequently associated with DIC.

The pathognomonic lesion of TTP is arteriolar and/or capillary hyaline thrombi. These thrombi are not associated with inflammatory reaction or vasculitis. The lesions are thought to consist of dense platelet aggregates surrounded by fibrin and can usually be found in biopsies of petechial sites.

Optimal treatment of TTP consists of plasma administration in the rare cases of relapsing chronic familial TTP and plasmapheresis in the more commonly encountered acute idiopathic TTP. High-dose steroid therapy is also important, as is the avoidance of platelet transfusions or the use of heparin or DDAVP (vasopressin). Consultation with a hematologist experienced in the management of this disease is important.

B. Hemolytic Uremic Syndrome

Although similar in many respects to TTP, HUS is characterized by more prominent hypertension and renal failure with fewer neurological signs and symptoms. HUS occurs primarily in children and is often preceded by gastroenteritis or viral upper respiratory tract infection within the preceding 7 to 10 days. The elevated liver function tests are primarily the result of microangiopathic hemolysis. Elevated fibrin split products are seen more commonly in HUS than in TTP.

Although most children with HUS recover completely in the course of a few weeks with supportive treatment alone, adults with HUS have a relatively worse prognosis because of their characteristically more severe renal involvement, often progressing to bilateral cortical necrosis.

It is not clear that any therapies are effective for HUS, although plasma exchange, steroids, antiplatelet agents, and aspirin may all be of benefit.

VIII. THROMBOCYTOPENIA

Thrombocytopenia (defined as a platelet count of less than the normal range of 150,000–400,000/μL) is very common in late pregnancy, the largest series reporting an incidence of 7.6% (8). The most common differential consideration of isolated thrombocytopenia in pregnancy is gestational thrombocytopenia. Although there are no specific diagnostic criteria for this condition, it characteristically has its onset earlier in gestation than does preeclampsia. It is commonly detected as part of routine prenatal screening. The thrombocytopenia is generally mild and only rarely falls below 70,000/μL.

Thrombocytopenia in preeclamptic women is most commonly the result of thrombus formation and/or membrane damage from contact with abnormal surfaces, resulting in premature removal of platelets from the circulation. The thrombocytopenia in severe preeclampsia does not commonly fall below 50,000/μL (9) and when the platelet count is below this level, other diagnoses should be considered.

The single most common differential consideration for thrombocytopenia in preeclampsia is disseminated intravascular coagulation (DIC). Because DIC is always a secondary phenomenon, the management should be directed to the identification and resolution of the instigating condition. Relatively common concurrent obstetric complications predisposing to DIC include hemorrhage and infection. These conditions must be appropriately and aggressively treated.

As outlined in the preceding section, conditions associated with microangiopathic hemolytic anemia (TTP, HUS) must also be considered.

Another relatively common [0.2% of pregnancies (10)] differential consideration of thrombocytopenia in young women is immune thrombocytopenic purpura (also called autoimmune thrombocytopenic purpura). This condition is the result of immune-mediated platelet destruction and is often but not always associated with maternal IgG antiplatelet antibodies. It is clinically characterized by persistent thrombocytopenia, normal or increased numbers of megakaryocytes on bone marrow examination, exclusion of other systemic disorders or drugs known to be associated with thrombocytopenia, and absence of splenomegaly (11). The majority of these women will have had this diagnosis established prior to pregnancy, usually as a result of easy bruising, petechiae, epistaxis, gingival bleeding or meno- or metrorrhagia. This condition is not usually exacerbated by pregnancy and is not associated with hypertension or proteinuria.

Systemic lupus erythematosus can masquerade as preeclampsia and may be associated with thrombocytopenia. In fact, thrombocytopenia may be the initial presenting feature and may antedate other manifestations by months or years. The antiphospholipid- and anticardiolipin-antibody syndromes must also be considered, particularly in women with an early onset of severe preeclampsia.

Certain medications can also cause thrombocytopenia. These include but are not limited to heparin, quinine, quinidine, zidovudine, and sulfonamides (11).

Sepsis must also be considered in the differential diagnosis of thrombocytopenia and preeclampsia. Besides bacterial sepsis, concurrent viral infections, including HIV, should also be considered.

Other less common differential diagnostic considerations of thrombocytopenia in preeclampsia include megaloblastic anemia and neoplasia. These conditions should have corresponding abnormalities in red cell numbers and indices.

IX. HEPATOCELLULAR DYSFUNCTION

Hepatocellular dysfunction in late pregnancy is characterized by elevations of the transaminase enzymes with or without hyperbilirubinemia. There are no changes in either of these serum chemistries in normal pregnancy. Severe preeclampsia may be associated with moderate (<10-fold) increases in transaminases as well as lactate dehydrogenase. Some cases are also accompanied by modest hyperbilirubinemia, almost always less than 5 mg/100 mL.

A. HELLP Syndrome

Over the preceding two decades a subset of women with severe preeclampsia presenting with *h*emolysis, *e*levated *l*iver function tests and thrombocytopenia (*low p*latelets) has come to be widely known as the HELLP syndrome (12). These women are frequently symptomatic, often presenting with upper abdominal pain, nausea, and vomiting. Although multiple specific thresholds of serum chemistry abnormality exist for the HELLP syndrome, the transaminase elevations are characteristically mild to moderate (less than 10 times normal), there is evidence of hemolysis (elevated lactate dehydrogenase and bilirubin), and platelet counts are generally below $100,000/mm^2$. On liver biopsy, the HELLP syndrome is characterized by deposition of fibrin in the periportal regions and sinusoids, focal parenchymal necrosis, but no inflammatory infiltration (13).

Despite the widespread appreciation of the HELLP syndrome, it is far from the only cause of hepatocellular dysfunction in late pregnancy. There are two other pregnancy-specific causes—as well as an extensive list of concurrent medical problems—that must be considered in the differential diagnosis of hepatocellular dysfunction associated with hypertension in late pregnancy (Table 5). Severe folic acid deficiency has been confused with HELLP syndrome and has resulted in preterm delivery with poor neonatal outcome. If megaloblastic anemia is a real possibility in someone who presents with early pregnancy anemia, thrombocytopenia, elevated liver enzymes, and abdominal pain, a bone marrow evaluation may be required to make the diagnosis. This is because in severe disease, red cell folate levels may lag behind the clinical course, and if there is concomitant iron deficiency megaloblastosis may be masked (14).

B. Acute Fatty Metamorphosis of Pregnancy (AFMP)

This condition, frequently called acute fatty liver of pregnancy, is actually a multiorgan abnormality that characteristically has its onset in the third trimester. It is frequently also associated with abdominal pain, malaise, confusion or encephalopathy, hypertension, and proteinuria. Liver production of clotting factors and glucose are severely affected by fulminant liver failure, and these patients may present with bleeding diatheses and hypoglycemia. Women with AFMP are clinically jaundiced, often to a marked degree. This is accompanied by hyperbilirubinuria, a finding not present in preeclampsia. Liver enzymes are generally moderately elevated (300–500 IU range) and ammonia levels are high. Diabetes insipidus is common and polyuria and polydipsia may be prominent. These women are at increased risk for death due to acute hepatic failure, the best single predictor of which is their ability to maintain their serum glucose values within the normal range. Up to 50% of these patients will also develop renal failure and pancreatitis. As with preeclampsia, the only known cure for AFMP is delivery.

Table 5 The Differential Diagnosis of Hepatocellular Dysfunction in Late Pregnancy

Condition	Symptoms/signs
HELLP (hemolysis, elevated liver enzymes, low platelets) syndrome	Upper abdominal pain Nausea and vomiting
Acute fatty metamorphosis of pregnancy	Abdominal pain Malaise Hypertension Proteinuria
Preeclampsia-associated hepatic rupture	Sudden right-upper-quadrant abdominal pain Nausea and vomiting Right shoulder pain from diaphragmatic irritation
Long-chain 3-hydroxyacyl-coenzyme A dehydrogenase (LCHAD) deficiency	
Viral hepatitis	Fatigue, anorexia, nausea and vomiting; pruritis, jaundice, and steatorrhea
Cholecystitis	Right-upper-quadrant pain that sometimes radiates to the back Postprandial nausea and vomiting
Systemic lupus erythematosus	
Sepsis	Usually associated with localized pain
Cocaine/abuse	Often associated with hypertension, convulsions, abruption, or preterm labor
Budd-Chiari syndrome	Most common in the first few weeks postpartum Painless ascites and rapid abdominal distention

C. Preeclampsia-Associated Hepatic Rupture

Spontaneous rupture of the liver is estimated to occur approximately one in every 45,000 pregnancies and is a true surgical emergency. Although the precise mechanisms remain unclear, it involves the right lobe of the liver in 90% of cases. Patients characteristically experience sudden right-upper-quadrant pain, nausea, and vomiting followed rapidly by obtundation and shock. They often also have referred pain to the right shoulder as a result of diaphragmatic irritation.

Spontaneous hepatic rupture and/or infarction occurs primarily in association with preeclampsia (15), although other uncommon associations have been reported including vascular malformations, autoimmune disorders, abscesses, and tumors. These women have grossly elevated transaminases but also a progressive coagulopathy and are often profoundly hypoglycemic.

Spontaneous rupture of the liver may be initially misdiagnosed as an abruption, ruptured uterus, or perforated maternal viscus.

Hepatic infarction will also be associated with very high serum levels of transaminases. These patients are characteristically more stable from a hemodynamic perspective.

This subject is covered in greater detail in Chapter 11.

D. Long-Chain 3-Hydroxyacyl-Coenzyme A Dehydrogenase Deficiency (LCHAD Deficiency)

Women carrying a fetus with a LCHAD deficiency frequently develop a syndrome resembling HELLP syndrome (16). This condition may also resemble acute fatty metamorphosis or persistent hyperemesis gravidarum.

E. Viral Hepatitis

At least in North America and western Europe, viral hepatitis is no more severe when it occurs during pregnancy than outside of pregnancy. The causes of viral hepatitis during pregnancy are the same as might be expected in nonpregnant women of reproductive age and include the hepatitis viruses (A through E), the herpesviruses (cytomegalovirus, Epstein-Barr virus, herpes virus and varicella virus) and HIV. Hepatitis A and B are the most common causes of viral hepatitis in North America and western Europe, with hepatitis B being the predominant cause of viral hepatitis elsewhere in the world. Although in North America and western Europe hepatitis A and B are no more severe when occurring in a pregnant woman than in other nonpregnant women of reproductive age, certain other causes of viral hepatitis have been reported to be more severe when occurring in pregnant women. These include hepatitis E, herpes simplex, and Epstein-Barr viral hepatitis.

Presenting symptoms usually include fatigue, anorexia, nausea, and vomiting. Pruritus, jaundice, hyperbilirubinuria, and steatorrhea usually follow shortly thereafter. Of note, viral hepatitis cannot be distinguished on clinical grounds from acute hepatitis caused by drugs, alcohol, or autoimmune diseases.

In contrast to preeclampsia, pregnant women with viral hepatitis are almost always obviously jaundiced with extremely high serum transaminases, with levels often in the thousands of international units (IU). Hypoglycemia is common and may be severe. Hypoglycemia portends an ominous prognosis and remains associated with a high incidence of fetal and maternal death. Specific diagnosis requires serological identification of the specific acute or chronic infection.

Hypertension and proteinuria are not present in otherwise uncomplicated viral hepatitis. However, hypertension may develop in response to the maternal cerebral edema that can occur in severe cases progressing to acute hepatic failure. Hepatorenal failure is also a severe complication.

F. Cholecystitis

Acute cholecystitis is a common cause for nonobstetric surgical intervention during pregnancy. The symptoms generally include right-upper-quadrant abdominal pain that sometimes radiates to the back, nausea, and vomiting. Clinically apparent jaundice occurs in about 20% of cholecystitis/cholelithiasis cases but is usually mild. Cholecystitis is frequently accompanied by pruritus, a symptom that may suggest intrahepatic cholestasis. Unlike intrahepatic cholestasis, however, the serum chemistries in cholecystitis reveal primarily conjugated hyperbilirubinemia, reflecting the obstetric nature of cholecystitis. Of clinical note, acute obstructive cholecystitis is often followed by secondary bacterial infection, particularly if symptoms persist for over 1 week.

G. Systemic Lupus Erythematosus (SLE)

Because the manifestations of SLE are related to the reaction between serum antigen-antibody complexes and fixed tissue antigens in vessel walls, this disease can produce signs and symptoms in almost any organ system. Hepatic involvement by SLE frequently results in hepatomegaly and can, in the absence of therapy, result in nonspecific liver enzyme elevations. Multiorgan SLE involvement frequently produces findings not associated with preeclampsia, such as arthropathy, skin rash, photosensitivity, alopecia, mucosal ulcers, Raynaud's phenomenon and myalgias.

H. Sepsis

Most perinatal infections are promptly resolved with antibiotic treatment and have no effects on hepatocellular function. However, there are several particularly serious but fortunately uncommon perinatal infections that may mimic the HELLP syndrome. Foremost among these is *Clostridium perfringens* sepsis. If associated with a surgical incision or laceration, the affected area initially develops a cellulitis with a watery discharge, followed by a bronze discoloration of the skin and crepitus near the incision. If it is associated only with endometritis, vaginal bleeding will be prominent, usually in association with nonviable retained tissue. A Gram's stain from either the margin of the infection or the endometrial contents should demonstrate Gram-positive rods. In either situation, clostridial sepsis is associated with inordinate pain and is not characteristically associated with hypertension or proteinuria.

Sepsis due to group A beta-hemolytic *Streptococcus* may also include evidence of hepatocellular dysfunction, although the primary symptomatology will be at the area of infection. Gram's stains from the margin of the infection will reveal Gram-positive cocci. In addition to aggressive antibiotic therapy, aggressive debridement and excision of nonviable tissue may be necessary.

I. Cocaine Abuse

Cocaine usage is associated with an increase in blood pressure and a risk of seizures. During pregnancy, cocaine abuse is also associated with an increased risk of preterm labor and placental abruption; the latter may also be associated with evidence of hepatocellular dysfunction, particularly if the abruption is sub-acute or chronic in nature.

J. Budd-Chiari Syndrome

This syndrome is the result of hepatic vein obstruction with resultant congestion and necrosis of the liver. As with most venous thromboembolic complications of pregnancy, Budd-Chiari syndrome is most likely to occur in the first few weeks postpartum. It presents with painless ascites and rapid abdominal distention. Serum chemistries are variably elevated. The diagnosis is best accomplished with Doppler ultrasound imaging of the hepatic veins, with percutaneous hepatic venous catheterization being employed for those situations where ultrasound is inconclusive. Any pregnant or puerperal woman with Budd-Chiari syndrome must be thoroughly evaluated for pregnancy-associated thrombophilias.

X. INTRAUTERINE GROWTH RETARDATION OR OLIGOHYDRAMNIOS

The small-for-gestational age newborn has long been associated with increased perinatal morbidity and mortality (17). These observations were originally based on birth weight alone and then evolved to correlate birth weight with gestational age. More recently, normative ultrasonographic estimates of fetal weight have allowed the diagnosis of intrauterine growth retardation (more commonly called intrauterine growth restriction in current parlance). These estimates generally refer to the lowest decile of fetal weights and should be corrected for fetal gender and for the population under study. Any diagnosis of intrauterine growth restriction presupposed an accurate knowledge of gestational age. Although there is a demonstrable increase in perinatal complications even at the tenth percentile, the likelihood of perinatal complications increases more rapidly below the fifth percentile and even more dramatically below the third percentile (18).

Significant growth restriction at term is an indication for delivery even in pregnancies with no evidence of preeclampsia. The decision to deliver a pre-eclamptic pregnancy remote from term solely on the basis of intrauterine growth restriction must consider both the possibility of other nonrelated causes for the growth restriction and the well-being of the fetus. In the absence of other markers of severe disease (Table 1), it is also possible for a pregnancy to be complicated by mild preeclampsia and an unrelated cause of growth restriction for which early delivery may not be beneficial. Among the more common causes of growth restriction for which delivery may not be necessary are maternal cigarette smoking, multiple gestation, and fetal genetic disorders/anomalies.

A. Smoking

Women who smoke have a three to four times greater likelihood of having a growth-restricted infant (19). Cigarette smoking remains among the most common identifiable causes of growth restriction and is one of the few that is amenable to prenatal treatment. Women who stop smoking as late as the early third trimester can still have significantly higher birth weights than those who continue to smoke throughout the pregnancy. In the setting of nonsevere preeclampsia that has developed remote from term in a woman who smokes and who has a growth-restricted baby, it would be appropriate to pursue smoking cessation efforts aggressively, while following the course of the evolving preeclampsia noninterventionally. Interestingly, women who smoke cigarettes during pregnancy are relatively less likely to develop preeclampsia.

B. Multiple Gestation

Twin pregnancy is known to be associated with an increased likelihood of growth restriction by 30 to 32 weeks of gestation. This is more frequent and more severe with monozygotic twins. Growth restriction is also more frequent and earlier in onset with higher-order multiple gestations. In the face of reassuring fetal surveillance, women pregnant with multiple gestations remote from term could be managed expectantly when one or more fetuses have estimated weights in the fifth to tenth percentiles and preeclampsia develops but there are no other severe criteria (Table 1).

C. Fetal Genetic Disorders/Anomalies

Many pregnancies complicated by significant fetal genetic disorders and/or congenital anomalies will result in growth restriction by the third trimester. This should be particularly suspected when fetal structural abnormalities and/or polyhydramnios is present. Many such pregnancies can realistically be expected to have suboptimal outcomes irrespective of the gestational age at which delivery occurs. However, if the fetal condition is nonlethal (gastroschisis, congenital heart disease, spina bifida, etc.), the family wishes to pursue an initial aggressive resuscitation course, and the pregnancy develops nonsevere preeclampsia remote from term, it is reasonable to allow the pregnancy to continue, albeit with careful maternal/fetal surveillance.

D. Oligohydramnios

The most clinically relevant definition of oligohydramnios (a criterion below which perinatal morbidity increases) is the absence of any vertical pocket of amniotic fluid exceeding 2 cm in depth (20). However, the most widely used definition of oligohydramnios is the amniotic fluid index, in which abnormal results are defined in standard deviations from the mean rather than with correlation to adverse clinical outcomes (21).

Mild oligohydramnios in the face of otherwise reassuring fetal surveillance and mild preeclampsia remote from term should raise the question of underlying pregnancy complications for which delivery is not necessarily advantageous or appropriate. The single most common scenario in which this issue might arise would be the pregnancy complicated by preterm premature ruptured membranes remote from term where otherwise nonsevere preeclampsia has developed.

XI. SYMPTOMS SUGGESTING SIGNIFICANT END-ORGAN INVOLVEMENT

One of the primary objectives of prenatal care has been the identification of those pregnant women destined to develop preeclampsia sufficiently early in the course of their disease to allow optimization of maternal and fetal outcomes. When combined with the increasing frequency of prenatal visits as gestational age advances, the routine assessment of blood pressure, weight gain, and urinalysis for presence of proteinuria has dramatically reduced preeclampsia-associated maternal and perinatal morbidity and mortality. This improvement in outcomes has not been associated with any decrease in disease frequency and reemphasizes the historic observation that pregnant women developing preeclampsia generally feel well until the disease is far advanced. Indeed, a pregnant woman who is symptomatic from her preeclampsia has, by definition, developed severe disease.

In evaluating a preeclamptic patient, these symptoms are as important indicators of the severity of the disease as any of the previously discussed signs and laboratory values. Any symptoms in preeclamptic women must be considered to indicate severe disease—and an indication for delivery for maternal well-being—until reasonably proven otherwise. It is the intention of this section to discuss the differential diagnosis of the symptoms characteristically associated with preeclampsia.

A. Headache

Headache has long been recognized as a harbinger of eclampsia. The precise mechanism of these headaches is not certain, although hypertensive encephalopathy, cerebral vasospasm, and abnormal cerebral perfusion pressure are intimately involved (22). However, preeclampsia can develop in women with preexisting headache disorders. All preeclamptic women should be questioned about underlying or preexisting medical problems, including headaches. A previous history of headaches similar in kind to the present headache should suggest a primary headache syndrome. Vascular or tension headaches often begin in childhood, and migraine headaches most commonly have their onset around puberty. The temporal course of the preexisting headache syndrome may also be helpful for establishing or confirming a diagnosis. Migraine headaches usually begin while the patient is awake, often have a prodrome or aura, and characteristically build over minutes to hours. Vascular or tension headaches typically occur daily, progress through the day, and are often associated with depression and/or pharmacological rebound. The combination of a positive headache history and the absence of other signs or symptoms of severe preeclampsia (Table 1) could justify continued careful observation, particularly if remote from term.

The new onset of headache during pregnancy should increase the suspicion of underlying pathology. Subarachnoid hemorrhage causes the abrupt onset of severe pain, sometimes also associated with loss of consciousness. Cerebral venous thrombosis is often associated with fluctuating symptoms and levels of consciousness. Although more common in the puerperium, cerebral venous thrombosis does occur during pregnancy. Intracranial tumors may first become symptomatic during pregnancy, although this most commonly occurs in the first trimester. Intracranial tumors are also often associated with fluctuating symptoms that are affected by changes in position.

On physical examination, the presence of any localizing neurological symptom or physical finding should increase the suspicion of primary or associated CNS disease. The presence on fundoscopic examination of obvious papilledema should also suggest an accompanying central nervous system disorder. Persistent obtundation also warrants further evaluation.

B. Visual Disturbances

Visual disturbances in preeclamptic women—most commonly blurred vision, scotomatas, and visual field defects—are the result of underlying vasospasm and cerebral edema. Cortical blindness can occur as a result of preeclampsia but should never be assumed. The sudden onset of complete loss of vision is a medical emergency requiring prompt ophthalmological consultation and evaluation. As with headaches, a history of preexisting ophthalmological problems, especially if similar in nature to the current episode, can be valuable in clinical decision making.

C. Epigastric or Right-Upper-Quadrant Pain

Progressive visceral ischemia secondary to preeclampsia results in epigastric or right-upper-quadrant abdominal pain and is generally associated with serological evidence of hepatocellular dysfunction. These symptoms may also represent a developing hepatic hematoma, particularly if the liver is palpable on physical examination. An expanding or ruptured hepatic hematoma will often be associated with maternal shock and fetal distress.

As with other symptoms in preeclamptic women, epigastric or right-upper-quadrant abdominal pain may equally be the result of other obstetric or concurrent causes (Table 5).

With the increased interest in trials of labor for women with previous lower-uterine-segment cesarean deliveries, uterine rupture has become more common. In contrast to the gradual onset of preeclampsia, uterine rupture is an acute, often catastrophic event generally occurring in labor and associated with maternal shock, fetal distress, and vaginal bleeding. The sudden onset during labor and associated vaginal bleeding generally make this distinction obvious.

Preeclampsia clearly predisposes pregnant women to placental abruptions. Abruptions may also present as abdominal pain. However, physical examination generally identifies the uterus rather than the upper abdomen as the source of pain. Likewise, vaginal bleeding, although not invariably present, generally directs diagnostic consideration away from maternal visceral ischemia.

Viral hepatitis may be associated with right-upper-quadrant abdominal pain but almost always includes clinically apparent jaundice and is not characterized by proteinuria or hypertension.

Cholelithiasis may produce right-upper-quadrant pain in pregnant women but is not associated with hypertension or proteinuria. The symptoms of cholelithiasis are often exacerbated by oral intake. The pain associated with cholecystitis is more constant, may radiate to the back (should suggest secondary pancreatitis), and is often accompanied by fever. The right-upper-quadrant pain associated with preeclampsia is not characteristically affected by oral intake, does not radiate to the back, and is not accompanied by temperature elevation.

Pregnancy does not increase the risk of appendicitis over that expected in nonpregnant women of reproductive age. However, appendicitis in pregnant women is more likely to be associated with complications.

REFERENCES

1. American College of Obstetricians and Gynecologists. Hypertension in Pregnancy. ACOG Technical Bulletin 219. Washington, DC: ACOG, 1996.
2. National High Blood Pressure Education Program Working Group on High Blood Pressure in Pregnancy. Report of the National High Blood Pressure Education Program Working Group on High Blood Pressure in Pregnancy. Am J Obstet Gynecol 2000; 183:S1–S22.
3. Hanssens M, Keirse MJNC, Vankelecom F, Van Assche FA. Fetal and neonatal effects

of treatment with angiotensin-converting enzyme inhibitors in pregnancy. Obstet Gynecol 1991; 78:128–135.

4. Jungers P, Houillier P, Forget D, Labrunie M, Skhiri H, Giatras I, et al. Influence of pregnancy on the course of primary chronic glomerulonephritis. Lancet 1995; 346: 1122–1124.

5. Imbasciati E, Ponticelli C. Pregnancy and renal disease: predictors for fetal and maternal outcome. Am J Nephrol 1991; 11:353–362.

6. Cunningham FG, Cox SM, Harstad TW, Mason RA, Pritchard JA. Chronic renal disease and pregnancy outcome. Am J Obstet Gynecol 1990; 163:453–459.

7. Fisher K, Luger A, Spargo BH, Lindheimer MD. Hypertension in pregnancy: Clinical-pathological correlations and remote prognosis. Medicine 1981; 60:267–276.

8. Burrows RF, Kelton JG. Thrombocytopenia at delivery: a prospective survey of 6,715 deliveries. Am J Obstet Gynecol 1990; 162:731–734.

9. Pritchard JA, Cunningham FG, Mason RA. Coagulation changes in eclampsia: Their frequency and pathogenesis. Am J Obstet Gynecol 1976; 124:855–864.

10. Rouse DJ, Owen J, Goldenberg RL. Routine maternal platelet count: an assessment of technologically driven practice. Am J Obstet Gynecol 1998; 179:573–576.

11. American College of Obstetricians and Gynecologists. Thrombocytopenia in pregnancy. ACOG Practice Bulletin #6. Washington, DC: ACOG, 1999.

12. Weinstein L. Syndrome of hemolysis, elevated liver enzymes and low platelet count; a consequence of hypertension in pregnancy. Am J Obstet Gynecol 1982; 142:159–167.

13. Rolfes DB, Ishak KG. Liver disease in pregnancy. Histopathology 1986; 10:555–570.

14. Walker SP, Wein P, Ihle BU. Severe folate deficiency masquerading as the syndrome of hemolysis, elevated liver enzymes and low platelets. Obstet Gynecol 1997; 90: 655–657.

15. Smith LG, Moise KJ, Dildy GA, Carpenter RJ. Spontaneous rupture of the liver during pregnancy: current therapy. Obstet Gynecol 1991; 77:171–175.

16. Wilcken B, Leung KC, Hammond J, Kamath R, Leonard JV. Pregnancy and fetal long-chain 3-hydroxyacyl-CoA dehydrogenase deficiency. Lancet 1993; 341:407–408.

17. Low JA, Boston RW, Pancham SR. Fetal asphyxia during the intrapartum period in intrauterine growth retarded infants. Am J Obstet Gynecol 1972; 113:351–357.

18. McIntire DD, Bloom SL, Casey BM, Leveno KJ. Birth weight in relation to morbidity and mortality among new-born infants. N Engl J Med 1999; 340:1234–1238.

19. Ounsted M, Moar VA, Scott A. Risk factors associated with small-for-dates and large-for-dates infants. Br J Obstet Gynaecol 1985; 92:226–232.

20. Chamberlain PF, Manning FA, Morrison I, Harman CR, Lange IR. Ultrasound evaluation of amniotic fluid volume. I. The relationship of marginal and decreased amniotic fluid volumes to perinatal outcome. Am J Obstet Gynecol 1984; 150:245–249.

21. Rutherford SE, Phelan JP, Smith CV, Jacobs N. The four-quadrant assessment of amniotic fluid volume: an adjunct to antepartum fetal heart rate testing. Obstet Gynecol 1987; 70:353–356.

22. Belfort MA, Saade GR, Grunewald C, Dildy GA, Abedejos P, Herd JA, Nisell H. Association of cerebral perfusion pressure with headache in women with pre-eclampsia. Br J Obstet Gynaecol 1999; 106:814–821.

5

Severe Preeclampsia Remote from Term

Michael D. Hnat and Baha M. Sibai
University of Cincinnati College of Medicine, Cincinnati, Ohio, U.S.A.

Severe preeclampsia is a clinical syndrome embracing a wide spectrum of signs and symptoms that can rapidly progress to an obstetrical emergency. In healthy nulliparous women, the rate of severe preeclampsia is 2 to 3% (1). Preeclampsia accounts for a large proportion of indicated preterm deliveries and contributes to maternal and neonatal morbidity and mortality (2–4).

In the past, women with severe preeclampsia were delivered without delay regardless of gestational age. When preeclampsia occurred remote from term, both obstetricians and patients were faced with delivering a nonviable fetus or an extremely low birth weight infant. It was not until the early eighties that expectant management was considered for severe preeclampsia. Since neonatal complications were due to prematurity and not to preeclampsia (5,6), prolonging a pregnancy in a patient with early-onset severe preeclampsia for 1 to 2 weeks or even 1 to 2 days for corticosteroid benefit may improve neonatal outcome without increasing maternal morbidity or mortality. This chapter reviews the diagnosis, management, and perinatal outcome in early-onset severe preeclampsia so that physicians may feel comfortable with their decision to manage expectantly a patient with severe preeclampsia remote from term.

I. SEVERE PREECLAMPSIA: DEFINING THE SCOPE OF THE DISEASE

When preeclampsia manifests itself with blood pressures exceeding 160 mmHg systolic or 110 mmHg diastolic, it is classified as severe. Preeclampsia is also severe when elevated blood pressure ($\geq$140 mmHg systolic or $\geq$90 mmHg diastolic) are associated with abnormal hemostasis or end-organ dysfunction, such as headache, visual disturbances, or right-upper-quadrant pain with nausea or vomiting. In addition, preeclampsia is considered severe when it is superimposed on chronic hypertension. Criteria used to diagnose severe preeclampsia are listed in Table 1 (7). Intrauterine growth restriction (IUGR) has been excluded from the criteria by the International Society for the Study of Hypertension in Pregnancy in 1987 because of the inconsistencies of the definition of IUGR (8).

Although expectant management has played a role in decreasing neonatal morbidity, preeclampsia remains one of the leading causes of maternal and neonatal morbidity and mortality (4). Maternal and neonatal complications are listed in Table 2.

Severe preeclampsia was once thought to have a beneficial effect on the preterm fetus as a result of intrauterine stress, which was held to accelerate neonatal lung maturity and neurological development. However, Schiff and colleagues (9) reported no significant difference in the incidence of an immature lung in maturity tests between women with preeclampsia and matched controls. Surprisingly, the rate of respiratory distress syndrome was greater in the preeclampsia group than in the control group, but was not significant. In addition, fetal neurological and physical development as defined by the Ballard score was not found to be accelerated at the time of delivery in infants born of women with preeclampsia (10). Lastly, Friedman and coworkers (5) have shown in a matched cohort study that there was no significant differences between premature neonates born to women with preeclampsia at 24 to 35 weeks and those born to normotensive women with preterm labor with regards to neonatal death, respiratory distress syndrome, intraventricular hemorrhage (grades III and IV), necrotizing enterocolitis, and sepsis. In this study, results were also similar for severe preeclampsia (Table 3). These studies indicate that neonatal complications in preterm infants are related to prematurity rather than preeclampsia.

Table 1 Criteria for Severe Preeclampsia

Blood pressure of $\geq$ 160 mmHg systolic or $\geq$ 100 mmHg diastolic, on two occasions at least 6 h apart with the patient at bed rest
1. Proteinuria of $\geq$ 5 g collected in a 24-h urine
2. Oliguria ($<$ 500 mL/24 h)
3. Persistent and severe cerebral or visual disturbances
4. Persistent and severe right-upper-quadrant or epigastric pain
5. Cyanosis or pulmonary edema
6. HELLP (hemolysis, elevated liver enzymes, and low platelets) syndrome
7. Eclampsia

Source: Adapted from Ref. 7.

Table 2 Maternal and Fetal Complications of Severe Preeclampsia

Maternal	Fetal
Central nervous system	Intrauterine fetal growth retardation
Intracranial hemorrhage	Abruptio placentae
Central venous thrombosis	Intrauterine fetal death
Hypertensive encephalopathy	Neonatal death
Cerebral edema	Complications related to prematurity
Retinal edema	Respiratory distress syndrome
Macular or retinal detachment	Intraventricular hemorrhage
Cortical blindness	Necrotizing enterocolitis
Transient blindness	Sepsis
Gastrointestinal/hepatic	Cerebral palsy
Subcapsular hematomas of the liver	
Rupture of liver capsule	
Renal	
Acute renal failure	
Acute tubular necrosis	
Hematologic	
Disseminated intravascular coagulation	
Thrombocytopenia	
Wound hematoma	
Hemorrhage requiring transfusion	
Cardiopulmonary	
Pulmonary edema, cardiogenic and	
noncardiogenic	
Respiratory depression or arrest	
Cardiac arrest	
Myocardial ischemia	
Miscellaneous	
Maternal death	
Ascites	
Laryngeal edema	
Uncontrolled hypertension	

II. REVIEW OF THE LITERATURE

Several nonrandomized studies have described maternal and perinatal outcome after expectant management of severe preeclampsia (Table 4) (11–12). With bed rest, magnesium sulfate, phenobarbital, antihypertensive medications, and various other agents, pregnancies with severe preeclampsia were extended an average of 10 to 19 days. In one of their first studies, Visser and coworkers (17) compared

Table 3 Neonatal Outcomes of Pregnancies with Severe Preeclampsia Delivered at ≤ 35 Weeks

Outcome	Preeclampsia ($n = 160$)	Control ($n = 160$)	RR and 95% CI
Neonatal death (%)	5.6	5.6	1.00 (0.41–2.45)
Respiratory distress syndrome (%)	27.5	27.5	1.00 (0.70–1.43)
Intraventricular hemorrhage[a] (%)	3.1	3.1	1.00 (0.30–3.99)
Necrotizing enterocolitis[b] (%)	7.5	5.0	1.50 (0.63–3.57)
Sepsis (%)	10.0	11.9	0.84 (0.61–1.53)

[a]Grades 3 and 4.
[b]Grades 2 and 3.
Source: Adapted from Ref. 5.

women with severe preeclampsia treated with volume expanders, vasodilators, and invasive cardiac monitoring (study group) to those without such therapy (control group). Maternal or neonatal outcomes were not significantly different between the two groups. In a larger study by Visser and others (18) using hemodynamic treatment with plasma volume expanders, the perinatal mortality rate and prolongation of pregnancy were similar to those in other studies without such treatment.

In a nonrandomized, prospective observational study, Sibai and colleagues (23) evaluated a protocol for expectant management that was instituted at the University of Tennessee, Memphis, in 1985. Pregnancy outcomes in 109 patients with severe preeclampsia developing ≤27 weeks' gestation were reported. Women who required immediate delivery for maternal or fetal indications such as HELLP (hemolysis, elevated liver enzymes, low platelet count) syndrome, pulmonary edema, fetal distress, and oligohydramnios were excluded. Patients who were ≤24 weeks' gestation ($n = 25$) were offered termination or expectant management, among whom 15 elected to continue with their pregnancy. Another group was delivered 24 hours after receiving the last doses of steroids because of the patient's desire or physician's advice; this group consisted of 30 women with >24 weeks' gestation. The remaining women ($n = 54$) elected expectant management. Patients who were managed expectantly were monitored in the labor and delivery unit for a minimum of 24 hours and given IV magnesium sulfate. Various antihypertensive agents were given to maintain a diastolic blood pressure between 90 and 100 mmHg. Laboratory studies, antenatal testing, and ultrasound for growth were used for intensive monitoring of maternal and fetal status. Indications for delivery included eclampsia, thrombocytopenia, HELLP syndrome, pulmonary edema, vaginal bleeding with suspected abruptio placentae, persistent epigastric pain, and fetal distress (23).

For the women who were ≤24 weeks pregnant and opted for expectant management ($n = 15$), the mean pregnancy prolongation was 19.4 ± 11.6 days and the mean gestational age at delivery was 24.8 weeks. The number of perinatal deaths was 14 (93%). Table 5 compares women who were >24 weeks pregnant and managed conservatively to those delivered 24 hours after steroids. The perinatal mortality rate was significantly lower in the expectantly managed group (24%) than in the aggressively managed group (64%) (23).

In a retrospective case-controlled study to assess the effect on neonatal outcome of prolonging pregnancy with hemodynamic treatment, Withagen and others (22) matched 222 neonates who were born to women with severe preeclampsia between 24 and 34 weeks' gestation to two matched controls. Neonates in control groups I and II were matched for gestational age (±1 week) at initiation of treatment and for gestational age at delivery, respectively. The control neonates were from nonpreeclamptic women with preterm labor with or without premature rupture of membranes. Only 1.8% of the study group received antepartum steroids whereas 36% and 29% of control groups I and II, respectively, received steroids. Morbidity and mortality were similar between the groups, with similar causes of death. The study's power was insufficient to demonstrate any real difference between the groups.

With improvements in neonatal survival over the years (especially in infants weighing <1500 g), randomized clinical trials were needed to evaluate whether expectant management or expeditious delivery 48 hours after steroids yielded better outcomes in women who present with severe preeclampsia at <34 weeks' gestation. In the early 1990s, two randomized prospective clinical trials demonstrated lower adverse perinatal outcomes in women managed expectantly (24,25). Advances in neonatal care, aggressive use of surfactant, more intensive maternal and fetal surveillance, and careful selection of patients for expectant management were reasons for the improved outcomes. Odendaal and colleagues (24) randomly assigned 38 patients at 28 to 34 weeks with severe preeclampsia to aggressive management [corticosteroid therapy followed by delivery in 48 hours ($n = 20$)] or expectant management [corticosteroid treatment followed by delivery only for specific maternal or fetal indications ($n = 18$)]. There was no increase in maternal complications in the group managed expectantly as compared with the group managed aggressively. In addition, there was a statistically significant prolongation of the pregnancy (mean 7.1 days), a reduction in the number of neonates requiring ventilation (11 vs. 35%), and a reduction in total neonatal complications (33 vs. 75%) in the group with expectant management.

In another prospective randomized study, expectant management was compared with aggressive treatment of severe preeclampsia at 28 to 32 weeks' gestation and demonstrated a reduction in neonatal complications and neonatal stay in the newborn intensive care unit without a significant increase in maternal morbidity (25). Eligible patients for this study were carefully selected for random-

Table 4 Nonrandomized Studies

Study	Year	Number of subjects	Gestational age (weeks)	Mean prolongation of pregnancy (days)	Perinatal and neonatal outcome
Martin et al.[11]	1979	55	35.2[a]	19.2	50/58
Sibai et al.[12]	1979	60	26.5 ± 1.9[a]	11.4 ± 7.8	8/60
Odendall et al.[13]	1987	129	29.4 ± 4.6 on admission[a]	11 ± 11	87/121 (excludes 8 abortions)
Pattinson et al.[14]	1988	45	<24	18 ± 14 for survivors	0/11
			24–25	11 ± 9 for non-survivors	4/12
			26–27		9/22
Moodley[15]	1993	50	<26	12.3	0/12
			26–27		3/9
			28–29		5/14
			20–32		11/15
Olah[16]	1993	Expectant managed group: 28	35.7 ± 4.8	9.5 (2–26)	Expectant managed group: 26/28
		Matched controls: 28 delivered <48 h	28.6 ± 4.6	1.4 (0–2)	<48 h: 23/28

Reference	Year	Number	Gestational age		
Visser et al.[17]	1994	Study group: 57 Control group: 57	Study: 32.9 (27.7–38.6)[b] Control: 31 (24.9–35.0)[b]	Study: 10 (0–57)[c] Control: 11 (0–64)[c]	Study: 52/57 Control: 49/57
Visser and Wallenberg[18]	1995	254	31.2[b] (22.3–37.7)	14[c] (0–62)	194/254
Hall et al.[19,20]	2000	340	29.9 ± 2 on admission	11 ± 7	306/337 (3 abortions)
Hall et al.[21]	2001	39	28.0 ± 0.9	14 ± 9	7/36 (3 abortions)
Withagen et al.[22]	2001	222 in each group study group control group 1 control group 2	31.3 29.3 31.3	14 (for study group)	175/222 165/222 161/222

[a]Gestational age in weeks at delivery unless otherwise specified.
[b]Median and range of gestational age at delivery.
[c]Median and range of days.

Table 5 Pregnancy Outcome in Women with Severe Preeclampsia at ≥24
Weeks' Gestational Age (GA): Conservative vs. Aggressive Management

Variable	Conservative group (n = 54)	Aggressive group (n = 30)	p-Value
Admission GA (weeks)	26.1 ± 0.9	26.0 ± 0.9	
Delivery GA (weeks)	28.0 ± 1.2	26.3 ± 0.8	<0.0001
Prolongation (days)	13.2 ± 8.1	2.0 ± 0.2	<0.0001
Birth weight (g)	880 ± 212	709 ± 159	<0.0001
Perinatal death (no.)	13	20	<0.0005
Days in NICU	20 ± 32	115 ± 94	<0.02

Source: Adapted from Ref. 23.

ization and had to remain stable during the 24-hour observational period. Exclusion criteria included maternal medical disease (renal disease, diabetes, collagen vascular disease), multifetal gestation, bleeding, eclampsia, HELLP syndrome, and severe intrauterine growth restriction (IUGR). For the expectant management group, the average prolongation of pregnancy was 15.4 + 6.6 days and was not affected by the amount of proteinuria at randomization. Maternal indications for delivery were thrombocytopenia, uncontrolled severe hypertension, headache or blurred vision, epigastric pain, severe ascites, and maternal demand. Other indications included fetal compromise, reaching 34 weeks' gestation, preterm labor or rupture of membranes, and vaginal bleeding. There were no cases of fetal or neonatal deaths, eclampsia, pulmonary edema, renal failure, or disseminated coagulapathy in either group (25).

The majority of the studies mentioned have shown only that expectant management is possible and beneficial in a select group of patients with severe preeclampsia, excluding patients with severe IUGR and HELLP syndrome. The presence of IUGR appears to be detrimental rather than protective for neonatal survival in severe preeclampsia and limits expectant management (26,27). In a retrospective study, Witlin and others (26) reported that the rate of IUGR increased with an increase in gestational age and latency period during expectant management in a series of 195 neonates born of women with severe preeclampsia. In both multivariate ($p = 0.038$; OR, 13.2; 95% CI, 1.16–151.8) and univariate analysis ($p = 0.001$; OR, 5.88; 95% CI 1.81–1926), IUGR decreased survival. Because prolongation of an adverse intrauterine environment may worsen rather than improve fetal outcome, patients with IUGR, oligohydramnios, and nonreassuring antenatal testing should be excluded from expectant management.

Chammas and colleagues (27) recommend delivery of neonates with IUGR 48 hours after the first dose of betamethasone. In this retrospective study, patients with severe preeclampsia <34 weeks' gestation were managed expectantly at the authors' institution. On admission, 19% and 11% of the fetuses were below the fifth percentile and between the fifth and tenth percentiles for estimated fetal weights by ultrasound (28), which was within 10% of the actual birth weight. The mean gestational age on admission was 31.1 ± 1.9 for women suspected of having IUGR and 29.3 ± 2.8 ($p = 0.034$) for those without growth restriction. The mean latency interval was 3.1 ± 2.1 days for IUGR neonates, which was significantly shorter than the latency for neonates with no IUGR, 6.6 ± 6.1 days. The rates of maternal and fetal indications for delivery were similar in both groups. There were no differences in Apgar scores, cord pH, and length of stay in the neonatal intensive care unit between the groups. There were two neonatal deaths due to prematurity but none occurred in the IUGR group. Because the mean latency period for IUGR neonates was only 3.1 + 2.1 days, Chammas concluded that IUGR neonates did not benefit by delaying delivery for 1 to 2 days after steroids (27).

III. EXPECTANT MANAGEMENT: WHO IS A CANDIDATE?

Not all women with severe preeclampsia are candidates for expectant management and not all circumstances are conducive to prolonging pregnancy. Each patient and situation must be individualized. Additionally, the physician must use his or her clinical expertise and experience to select a patient for such therapy. Expectant management should be carried out only at a tertiary perinatal care center where adequately trained personnel and appropriate equipment are available to handle the maternal and neonatal complications that can occur with severe preeclampsia (Table 2). Patients not at a tertiary institution must be stabilized and transferred. Tables 6 and 7 list the maternal and fetal criteria for expeditious delivery and expectant management (29). In a retrospective chart review of patients with severe preeclampsia at the University of Tennessee, 67% of the patients were eligible for expectant management based on the criteria previously described (29).

Management of severe preeclampsia is dependent on gestational age (Figure 1). Women at 34 weeks' gestation should be delivered upon initial presentation and at a facility that is capable of caring for the neonate, whereas women presenting between 32 and 34 weeks' gestation should be given corticosteroids and delivered 48 hours after the first dose if the situation permits. Another option in this group would be performing an amniocentesis for fetal lung maturity. If results of the amniocentesis suggest fetal lung maturity, then the fetus should be delivered. If the results suggest immaturity, steroids are administered and delivery is delayed until 48 hours after the first dose. In women at <32 weeks' gestation, it is important to delay delivery longer than 48 hours in hopes of decreasing the risks of prematurity. Women with severe preeclampsia with a nonviable fetus should be given the option to terminate the pregnancy. The lower limit of gestational age at

Table 6 Maternal Guidelines for Expeditious Delivery of Women with Severe Preeclampsia Remote from Term

Management	Clinical findings
Expeditious delivery (within 72 h)	One or more of the following: Uncontrolled severe hypertension[a] Eclampsia Platelet count < 100,000/μL AST or ALT > 2× upper limit of normal with epigastric pain or RUQ tenderness Pulmonary edema Compromised renal function[b] Abruptio placentae Persistent severe headache or visual changes
Consider expectant	One or more of the following: Controlled hypertension Urinary protein of any amount Oliguria (<0.5 mL/kg/h) that resolves with routine fluid intake AST or ALT > 2× upper limit of normal without epigastric pain or RUQ tenderness

AST = aspartate aminotransferase; ALT = alanine aminotransferase; RUQ = right upper quadrant
[a]Blood pressure persistently ≥ 160 mmHg systolic or ≥ 110 mmHg diastolic despite maximum recommended doses of two antihypertensive medications.
[b]Rise in serum creatinine of 1 mg dl over baseline levels.
Source: Ref. 29.

Table 7 Fetal Guidelines for Expedited Delivery and Expectant Management in Severe Preeclampsia Remote from Term

Management	Clinical findings
Expeditious delivery (within 72 h)	One or more of the following: Repetitive late or severe variable decelerations Biophysical profile ≤ 4 on two occasions 4 h apart Amniotic fluid index ≤ 2 cm Ultrasound estimated fetal weight ≤ 5th percentile Reverse umbilical artery diastolic flow
Consider expectant	All of the following: Biophysical profile ≥ 6 Amniotic fluid index > 2 cm Ultrasound estimated fetal weight > 5th percentile

Source: Ref. 29.

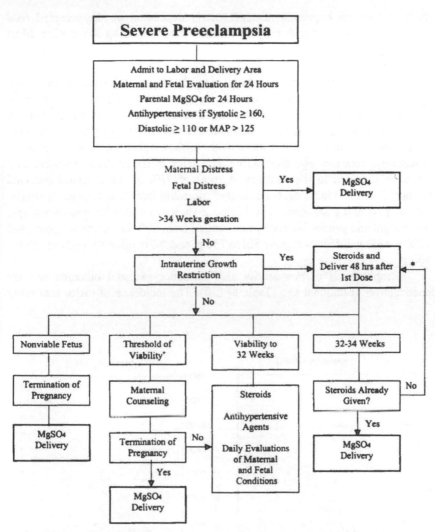

+Threshold of viability is dependent upon tertiary care center, and is usually around 23-24 weeks gestation.
*Alternate treatment may include amniocentesis for fetal lung maturity.

Figure 1   Recommended management of severe preeclampsia.

which to consider expectant management is dependent on the accepted fetal viability of the particular tertiary care center that is treating the mother. Most institutions in developed countries consider a fetus to be viable at approximately 23 weeks.

It is important to consider neonatal outcome in counseling the patients about expectant management. The gestational age, sex, and weight of the neonate influence neonatal outcome. The National Institute of Child Health and Human Development (NICHD) Neonatal Research Network (30) reported the mortality and morbidity rate for 4438 infants with birth weights from 501 to 1500 g. Importantly, neonates who died before admission to the neonatal intensive care unit were included in the analysis. A total of 71% of the neonates received antenatal steroids. Male infants had higher mortality rates than females of similar birth weights and gestational ages. Figure 2 shows mortality by gestational age, birth weight and gender. Mortality rate ranged from 89% in infants weighing 401 to 500 g, 48% in infants weighing 501 to 750 g, and 3% in infants weighing 1250 to 1500 g.

Complications of prematurity also influence neonatal outcome and are dependent on gestational age (Table 8) (30). The incidence of major morbidity

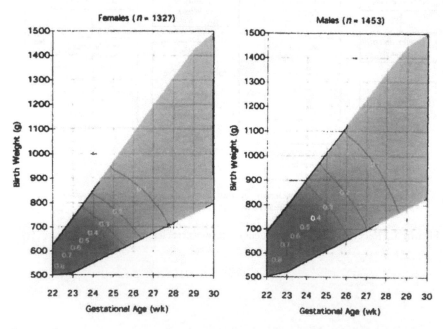

Figure 2   Mortality rates by gestational age, birthweight, and gender. (From Ref. 30.)

Table 8 Morbidity of Very Low Birth Weight Infants

Morbidity	501 to 750 g (n = 1002) (%)	751 to 1000 g (n = 1084) (%)	1001 to 1250 g (n = 1053) (%)	1251 to 1500 g (n = 1229) (%)
Respiratory distress syndrome	78	63	44	26
Chronic lung disease	52	34	15	7
IVH,[a] grade III	13	6	5	2
IVH,[a] grade IV	13	6	3	1
NEC[b] > stage II	14	9	5	3
Late-onset sepsis	48	33	18	7

[a]Intraventricular hemorrhage.
[b]Necrotizing enterocolitis.
Source: Adapted from Ref. 30.

(chronic lung disease, severe intraventricular hemorrhage and/or proven necrotizing enterocolitis) was 63% in the 501- to 750-g neonates; 42% in the 751- to 1000-g group; 23% in the 1001- to 1250-g group, and only 10% in the 1251- to 1500-g group (30).

In a separate report, neurodevelopmental and functional outcomes at 18 to 22 months' corrected age of 1151 infants weighing 401 to 1000 g at birth were described (31). Overall, 25% of the infants had an abnormal neurological examination, 17% had cerebral palsy, 3% were legally blind, and 11% had a hearing impairment, with 3% requiring hearing aids. Overall functional status demonstrated that 6% had not achieved normal head control, 7% were unable to walk without support, 86% had normal upper limb function, and 80% were able to feed themselves at 18 to 20 months. The deficits were the greatest in the 401- to 500-g group in that 29% had cerebral palsy, 21% had vision impairment, 14% had not achieved normal head control, and 21% were unable to walk without support. Normal upper limb function was present in 64%, and 67% could feed themselves.

In a cohort study, Woods and colleagues (32) reported outcomes of 4004 neonates born at 20 to 25 weeks. Of these, 1185 had signs of life at birth and 843 were admitted to the neonatal intensive care unit. Outcomes of the neonates born alive at 22 to 25 weeks' gestation are summarized in Table 9. At 30 months corrected age, neurological and developmental outcomes were available for 306 of the surviving neonates. Overall, 49% had no disabilities, 23% had severe disabilities classified as a need of physical assistance to perform daily activities, and 25% had other disabilities not classified as severe.

Neonatal survival and morbidity rates in 278 neonates between 22 to 25 weeks' gestation are listed in Table 10 (33). In this study, fetal deaths were also

Table 9 Outcomes of Neonates Born Alive at 22 to 25 Weeks' Gestation

Outcome	22 weeks ($n = 138$) (%)	23 weeks ($n = 241$) (%)	24 weeks ($n = 382$) (%)	25 weeks ($n = 424$) (%)
Died in delivery room	84	46	22	16
Admitted to NICU[a]	16	54	78	84
Died in NICU	14	44	52	40
Survived to discharge	1	11	26	44
Died after discharge	0	0.4	0.5	0.7
Had severe disability[b]	0.7	3	6	9
Had other disabilities[b]	0	6	7	10

[a]Neonatal intensive care unit.
[b]At 30 months' gestation.
Source: Adapted from Ref. 32.

included in the analysis. Physicians attempted to resuscitate all infants with a heart rate at birth with bag-and-mask ventilation and intubation, then reassessing the infants for further resuscitation measures. Of the 76 infants who were born alive, 46% survived to discharge. As expected, fetal morbidity and mortality decreased with increasing gestational age. Of interest, 35% of the neonates at 24 weeks died despite aggressive resuscitation in the delivery room. At 22 weeks' gestation, 40% of the neonates were born alive and only 1.8% survived; whereas at 23 weeks' gestation, 73% were born alive and 34% survived.

For expectant management, informed consent must be obtained. The risk

Table 10 Outcome of Pregnancies in 22 to 25 Weeks' Gestation

Outcome	Gestational age			
	22 weeks	23 weeks	24 weeks	25 weeks
Deliveries (n)	55	56	73	94
Live births (%)	40	73	84	92
Neonatal deaths (n)	21	22	25	16
Survival (%)	1.8	34	49	76
No resuscitation (%)	57	9	0	0
Died in delivery room[a] (%)	13	0	9	0
Died in NICU[a] (%)	4	36	25	7

[a]Resuscitated and died.
Source: Adapted from Ref. 33.

and benefits of expectant management versus aggressive treatment must be explained. It must be made clear that even though the infant may survive, it may not be neurologically intact, compromising its quality of life. This is especially important when a mother chooses to delay her pregnancy very early in gestation. A neonate born at a gestational age of 23 to 24 weeks has a high rate of intraventricular hemorrhage, cerebral palsy, and other complications of prematurity. Expectant management in a well-informed patient who refuses such management is contraindicated.

IV. ASSESSING MATERNAL AND FETAL STATUS

Hematological changes of preeclampsia vary as much as the signs and symptoms of the disease. These changes can be reflected in the battery of tests ordered for the assessment of the progression and severity of the disease. Clinical tests include (but are not limited to) complete blood count with platelets, uric acid, renal-hepatic profile, and coagulation studies along with a urinalysis and/or 24-hour urine for protein and creatinine clearance. Agreement does not always exist on when and how many tests should be ordered.

A baseline complete blood count (CBC) with platelets is useful in initially assessing preeclampsia and deciding which additional tests are necessary. Hemoconcentration or hemolysis of preeclampsia is reflected in the hemoglobin and hematocrit levels. In severe preeclampsia, hemoglobin levels are inversely related to the weight of the newborn and perinatal distress (34). Thrombocytopenia may also occur in preeclampsia and most likely results from platelet activation and consumption (35). Management is influenced by the severity of the thrombocytopenia. A rapid decline in platelet count or thrombocytopenia of $<100,000/mm^3$ is an indication for delivery. Additionally, Leduc and colleagues (36) reported that thrombocytopenia is related to perinatal morbidity and mortality. Because the disease can be manifest by a rapid decline in platelets, patients with severe preeclampsia should be monitored frequently.

Evaluation of other hematological parameters also depends on the presentation of the disease and the initial CBC results. Patients with low platelet counts should have a hepatic chemistry profile (37). In addition, liver function tests and platelet counts need to be performed on patients complaining of epigastric pain or nausea and vomiting. Liver function tests alone are not good predictors of severity or outcome of the disease except when associated with hemolysis or thrombocytopenia (38,39). In one study, lactate dehydrogenase (LDH) levels >600 IU/L were found in 89% of patients with epigastric pain, compared with 78% of patients who were symptom-free (38). In addition, LDH levels were significantly higher in patients with epigastric pain or nausea and vomiting as compared with symptom-free patients.

Barron and colleagues (41) assessed normal and abnormal coagulation profiles in patients with preeclampsia and recommended testing for prothrombin time (PT), activated partial thromboplastin time (aPPT), and fibrinogen in patients with an elevated LDH with thrombocytopenia as well as those with evidence of bleeding or abruptio placentae. A normal platelet count and a normal LDH had a negative predictive value of 100% and 99% for a prolonged PT or aPTT values and a low fibrinogen level.

Hyperuricemia is associated with renal dysfunction, especially decreased renal tubular secretion, and has multiple correlations with preeclampsia. Hyperuricemic levels have been consistently associated with glomerular endotheliosis (42) and have also been linked with increased oxidative stress in preeclampsia (43). Additional studies have associated serum uric acid levels with the severity of the diseases and with poor neonatal outcome, such as preterm delivery, poor fetal growth, perinatal distress, and even perinatal death (44–46). In one study, uric acid was found to be a better predictor than hypertension for neonates small for gestational age. In contrast, other investigators have not found an association between uric acid and poor perinatal outcome (47,48).

Lim and colleagues (49) studied uric acid findings in 344 women with hypertensive disorders of pregnancy and categorized them in groups according to criteria of the National Working Group on Hypertension in Pregnancy. Table 11 lists serum uric acid levels in the groups. There was considerable overlap of values among the groups. To diagnose preeclampsia, a cutoff of 5.5 mg/dL is only 69% sensitive and 51% specific. Although uric acid has been suggested to be the most sensitive indicator of preeclampsia (39), it should not be used as an indication for delivery (37).

Like uric acid, serum creatinine, blood urea nitrogen (BUN), and creatinine clearance reflect changes in glomerular filtration rate (GFR). BUN changes are influenced by protein intake and liver function. Thus, an abnormal BUN can be related to abnormal liver function while kidney function is normal. In additional serum creatinine levels may be elevated in severe preeclampsia. A serum creati-

Table 11 Uric Acid Levels in Pregnancy

	Number	Serum uric acid level (mean) (mg/dL)
Normal	93	4.3 ± 0.8
Transient hypertension	69	5.6 ± 1.7
Preeclampsia	130	6.2 ± 1.4
Chronic hypertension	23	4.9 ± 1.0
Superimposed preeclampsia	29	5.8 ± 1.4

Source: Ref. 49.

nine level of >0.8 mg/dL in pregnancy is considered abnormal. In the final weeks of pregnancy, creatinine clearance usually declines to near nonpregnant levels after demonstrating a rise during the second trimester.

Proteinuria is a hallmark of preeclampsia, usually found by dipstick and confirmed by a 24-hour urine. Conventional screening for proteinuria uses a dipstick that is sensitive to albumin. It is important to appreciate that false reactions may occur. False-positive results for protein can be due to concentrated urine, multiple white blood cells, or vaginal secretions with epithelial cells. Fever, stress, and exercise can also cause transient proteinuria.

Unfortunately, the degree of proteinuria diagnosed by dipstick does not always correlate with the same degree of proteinuria in a 24-hour urine and cannot be relied on to identify or eliminate the presence of proteinuria in women with gestational hypertension (50,51). Meyer and coworkers (50) demonstrated that urine dipstick values of ≥1+ had a positive predictive value of 92% for predicting >300 mg of protein in a 24-hour urine obtained in women hospitalized because of hypertension/preeclampsia. However, values of 3+ to 4+ had a positive predictive value of only 36% for proteinuria of ≥5 g/24 h, and a dipstick that is negative or trace has a poor negative predictive value of 34%. In addition, Kuo (51) demonstrated a high interobserver disparity in assessment of proteinuria by dipstick with both false-positive and false-negative results. The amount of protein was significantly underestimated in 20% of urine samples containing 500 mg/dL. Saudan and colleagues (52) showed that the false-positive rate could be reduced with the use of an automated urinalysis device for detection of proteinuria.

Proteinuria in pregnancy should be evaluated using a 24-hour urine and the result should not be considered pathological until it exceeds 300 to 500 mg/24 h (53). Higby and coworkers (52) showed that the upper limit of normal was 260 mg for urinary protein and 29 mg for albumin in a 24-hour period. Both total urinary protein and albumin increased after 20 weeks gestation.

The amount of proteinuria is not an indication for delivery. Schiff and colleagues (55) found no differences in maternal or fetal outcomes during expectant management of women with severe preeclampsia in the group who had increased proteinuria as compared with those with modest or no increase. In addition, the amount of proteinuria during expectant management did not correlate with the admission-to-delivery interval, the incidence of intervening maternal complications (eclampsia, HELLP syndrome, abruptio placentae), markers of fetal distress, or stillbirth rate (55). Therefore, obtaining a 24-hour urine to reassess proteinuria during the observation period of expectant management is not clinically helpful. In addition, increasing protein excretion with advancing gestation associated with known renal disease does not necessarily indicate significant progression of the disease and may be attributed to the increase in the GFR secondary to pregnancy.

An association of antiphospholipid antibodies and thrombophilias was found with early-onset severe preeclampsia (56–59). However, The National

Institute of Child Health and Human Development, Maternal-Fetal Medicine Units Network (60) obtained second-trimester serum samples from 317 women with a history of preeclampsia in a previous pregnancy for five antiphospholipid antibodies. They found no association of positive antiphospholipid with recurrent preeclampsia and concluded that testing for antibodies "is of little prognostic value in the assessment of the risk for recurrent preeclampsia among women with a history of preeclampsia" (60). Likewise, screening for acquired or inherited thrombophilias is not necessary and has not been proven to be significantly associated with severe preeclampsia remote from term (61–64).

V. FETAL EVALUATION

Uteroplacental blood flow may be reduced by about 50% in women with severe preeclampsia; therefore ultrasonography is performed on admission to assess fetal growth and amniotic fluid status. Reduced amniotic fluid volume is an indication of chronic placental insufficiency and must be measured. It is also necessary to confirm that fetal biometry is appropriate for gestational age, with no evidence of IUGR, and to rule out any congenital anomalies.

In a retrospective study, Schucker and others (65) assessed oligohydramnios in women with severe preeclampsia and conservative management as an indicator for fetal compromise and need for delivery. Of 136 patients, oligohydramnios was present in 20.4% to 47.4% of women, depending on which definition (≤5 or ≤7 cm) was used. Delivery was performed for fetal reasons in 45% and for maternal reasons in the remaining. There was no association between oligohydramnios and nonreassuring fetal testing requiring a cesarean section. Lastly, IUGR was present in 37% of the patients. The positive and negative predictive values for IUGR on admission were 78% and 66% respectively; at delivery, they were 57% and 68% respectively. However, the overall sensitivity of an amniotic fluid index ≤5 cm in detecting IUGR is ≤26%.

Measurements of Doppler flow velocity may be useful in pregnancy and in preeclampsia (66). In women with preeclampsia, umbilical artery and middle cerebral artery velocity waveform (FVW) is helpful in assessing fetal well-being when IUGR is present. The use of umbilical artery FVW in IUGR fetuses clearly reduces perinatal mortality (67,68). The correlation of abnormal FVW with fetal hypoxemia and acidemia in IUGR fetuses has also been well documented (68,69).

Doppler flow studies may assist in the management of IUGR fetuses in mothers with severe preeclampsia. A normal umbilical artery pulsatility index is reassuring for continuation of expectant management. Absent end-diastolic flow indicates closer monitoring, whereas the presence of reverse end-diastolic flow may necessitate urgent delivery. A greater than 50% mortality rate is associated with reverse end-diastolic flow. DuPlessis and associates (71) delayed delivery in

6 patients with reverse end-diastolic FVW by 24 to 48 hours to achieve corticosteroid benefits. There were no stillbirths and 5 minute Apgars ranged from 7 to 10.

Absent end-diastolic FVW with normal fetal heart rate variability in a preterm infant is not an indication for delivery (37). Results of the FVW Doppler must always be combined with the clinical presentation and findings of the fetal heart rate for management. Doppler FVW is followed weekly or more frequently if abnormal. A transition from a low vascular impedance to a high impedance with reverse end-diastolic flow in the middle cerebral artery may suggest an impending intrauterine fetal demise, signifying the end to expectant management.

Authorities differ on the frequency of fetal assessment (37,72). Frequent monitoring decreases the perinatal mortality rate. Odendaal (37) recommends fetal monitoring for fetal heart rate variability every 6 hours. Monitoring for variability only can be performed in approximately 25 to 50% less time than it takes to do a complete nonstress test (NST). In addition, a fetal heart rate (FHR) with good baseline variability is not associated with fetal asphyxia at birth. If variability is absent without any explanation, such as narcotics, Odendaal (37) recommends extended fetal monitoring and delivery if no FHR variability remains for 2 hours. Also, acoustic stimulation or a contraction stress test may aid in evaluating the fetus without variability.

Chari (72) and coworkers have shown that daily antenatal testing reduces the stillbirth or fetal compromise rate at delivery in severe preeclampsia. Friedman recommends NST every day along with fetal biophysical profiles (BPP). Once the patient is considered stable, BPP can be performed twice weekly. A nonreassuring fetal heart tracing indicating fetal distress or a biophysical profile score of ≤ 2 may require delivery without the neonate receiving the full benefit of corticosteroids.

VI. MEDICATIONS USED IN PREECLAMPSIA

Magnesium sulfate, antihypertensive medications and corticosteroids are the majority of medications used in the management of early-onset preeclampsia.

A. Corticosteroids

These have two roles in severe preeclampsia, improving fetal lung maturity (73) and possibly improving the hematological abnormalities associated with HELLP syndrome (74–78). It is well known that the incidence of respiratory distress syndrome can be improved by accelerating fetal lung maturity with the administration of steroids to mothers at <32 weeks' gestation (79,80). In a randomized, double-blind trial of 218 patients with severe preeclampsia between 26 and 34 weeks' gestation, Amorin (73) and coworkers demonstrated an incidence of respiratory distress syndrome in 23% of neonates who received antenatal steroids (adjusted RR 0.56, 95% CI 0.37–0.83) as compared with 43% in the placebo group. With a respiratory distress syndrome incidence of 40%, 182 patients were needed to obtain a power of 80% and an α error of 5% to detect a 50% reduction in the rate of respiratory distress syndrome. After randomization, betamethasone (12 mg) or placebo was administered on admission and repeated 24 hours later and weekly thereafter. No patient delivered <12 hours, and only six neonates were delivered between 12 and 24 hours after initiation of treatment. In addition, the rates of intraventricular hemorrhage, patent ductus arteriosus, and neonatal death were significantly reduced in the corticosteroid group as compared with the placebo. The rates of necrotizing enterocolitis and bronchopulmonary dysplasia were lower in the steroid group but not significant. There were no significant differences between the two groups with regard to the rates of the maternal complications (severe hypertension, pulmonary edema, acute renal failure, coagulopathy, HELLP syndrome, and imminent eclampsia). There were two maternal deaths. One death in the control group was attributed to a pulmonary embolism and the other, in the steroid group, was due to disseminated intravascular coagulation. The only maternal complication secondary to corticosteroids was gestational diabetes (RR 2.71, 95% CI 11.14–6.46).

Indicated preterm delivery may also be delayed for 48 hours after the first dose of steroids in patients with HELLP syndrome. With expectant management, maternal morbidity and perinatal mortality rates in women who had severe preeclampsia with HELLP syndrome were similar to those in women who did not have HELLP. High-dose corticosteroids used for accelerating fetal lung maturity will temporarily improve the hematological abnormalities associated with HELLP syndrome (74–78). Additional benefits of corticosteroids include maternal stabilization for transport to a tertiary care center, delaying of the delivery to achieve blood pressure control, and an increase in platelets to allow the use of regional anesthesia.

B. Magnesium Sulfate

Magnesium sulfate is administered to prevent eclampsia and has been proven to be more effective than phenytoin (81,82). It is given for the first 24 hours (when evaluating the patient) and then intrapartum and postpartum. Various protocols have been suggested, but a 6-g bolus followed by 2 g/h attains serum magnesium levels in the range of 4 to 8 mg/dL (83). For patients with renal compromise, the total bolus is given but the maintenance dose reduced. Magnesium levels are assessed when the patient's patellar reflexes are absent or she has renal insufficiency. A metanalysis of the literature regarding the use of magnesium sulfate therapy in preeclampsia and eclampsia demonstrated strong support for the routine use of magnesium for seizure prophylaxis in women with severe preeclampsia

(85). In a randomized double-blinded study, magnesium sulfate was shown to effectively decrease the rate of eclampsia when compared with placebo in women with severe preeclampsia (85). A total of 12 women (1.8%) experienced eclampsia. The rate of eclampsia was 0.3% in the magnesium sulfate group ($n = 345$) and 3.2% in the placebo ($n = 340$) group. Respiratory depression was experienced by one patient who was given an incorrect dosage of magnesium sulfate.

C. Antihypertensive Medications

Antihypertensive medications are administered for the rapid treatment of high blood pressure in pregnancy and for maintenance during expectant management. The primary aim of treatment is to prevent maternal cerebral hemorrhage (86). Blood pressures are reduced in a controlled manner to avoid harmful hypotensive effects in the mother and hypoxic effects in the fetus. Persistent systolic pressures of >160 mmHg and diastolic pressures of >110 mmHg may result in damage to the blood vessel wall (87). Marx and coworkers (88) suggest calculation of mean arterial pressure (MAP) to treat hypertension. A MAP exceeding 150 causes a loss of cerebral autoregulation. In order to allow for a margin of safety, Strandgaard and colleagues (86) suggest treating hypertension when the MAP is greater than 125 mmHg. Unfortunately, maternal side effects of many hypertensive medications, such as headache and nausea, are similar to those of pending eclampsia and may confuse the clinical presentation.

Duley and Henderson-Smart (89) performed a literature review involving only randomized trials to compare antihypertensive agents administered for rapid treatment of severe hypertension during pregnancy. The review included 14 studies with eight comparisons. Except for diazoxide and ketanserin, all agents were shown to reduce blood pressure in pregnancy and none proved to be better than another. Diazoxide was associated with hypotension and an increased risk of cesarean delivery when compared with labetalol. Ketanserin was associated with persistent hypertension when compared with hydralazine. It was concluded that the best choice of an antihypertensive agent depends on the physician's experience and familiarity with the medication. Medications used in the treatment of preeclampsia are listed in Table 12.

A common antihypertensive agent used to control severe hypertension in preeclampsia is hydralazine, a potent vasodilator that acts directly on vascular smooth muscle. Hydralazine may cause hypotension in preeclamptic patients who are hypovolemic. Therefore, patients should be given an intravenous bolus of fluids prior to hydralazine. A 5-mg bolus has been demonstrated to be effective and safe in treating severe hypertension in pregnancy (90). When given IV, the drug gradually takes effect over 15 to 30 minutes and peaks at 20 minutes. The half-life of hydralazine is 3 hours. Boluses of 5 or 10 mg can be given every 20 to

Table 12 Medications Used in Severe Preeclampsia

Magnesium sulfate	Calcium antagonist Seizure prophylaxis	6 g IV over 20 min, followed by 2 g/h Onset: immediate
Hydralazine	Arteriole vasodilator Blood pressure (BP) control	5–10 mg IV every 20 min (maximum dose: 30 mg) Onset: 10–20 min
Nifedipine	Calcium antagonist BP control	10 mg PO, can be repeated in 30 min, then 10–20 mg every 4–6 h (maximum dose 240 mg) Onset: 5–10 min
Labetalol	Mixed α_1/β blocker β_2 agonist BP control	20 mg IV, then 40–80 mg every 10 min (maximum dose of 300 mg/24 h IV or 240 mg/24 h PO) Onset: 5–10 min
Betamethasone	Corticosteroid Accelerate fetal lung maturity	12 mg IM every 24 h × 2 doses

30 minutes. Adverse reactions include fluid retention, tachycardia, palpitation, headache, a lupus-like syndrome, and neonatal thrombocytopenia.

Labetalol is a nonselective beta-blocker and postsynaptic $alpha_1$ blocker combining the effects of propranolol and prazosin (91). Oral labetalol has a beta/ alpha blockade ratio of 3:1 and intravenously has a ratio 7:1. In a randomized prospective study, Mabie and colleagues (91) compared the safety and efficacy of labetalol with that of hydralazine. Onset of action was more rapid for labetalol than for hydralazine. Although the fall in blood pressures was significantly greater with labetalol from 5 to 15 minutes, the decrease in pressure was greater for hydralazine from 45 to 120 minutes. There was no difference between adverse effects—especially hypoglycemia, hypotension, or bradycardia—in neonates born to women who received labetalol and those in neonates born to women who receive hydralazine. Labetalol should not be used in patients with hypertension secondary to cocaine. In addition, beta blockers may not lower blood pressure adequately in African Americans with hypertension.

In a randomized controlled trial, nifedipine was compared to prazosin in early-onset severe preeclampsia or hypertension in pregnancy (93). Nifedipine or prazosin was added to methyldopa (2 g/day) if blood pressure was not controlled. The number of days gained on either agent with methyldopa was similar. However, more cases of pulmonary edema and nonviable mid-trimester and third trimester intrauterine fetal death occurred with prazosin.

A promising drug for treating severe hypertension in preeclampsia is ketan-serin, a selective $serotonin_2$-receptor antagonist with minor $alpha_1$-receptor blocking properties. Ketanserin blocks vasoconstriction and platelet aggregation induced by serotonin, which has been shown to be elevated in preeclampsia (94). It also prohibits thrombus formation (94). Ketanserin has been shown to effectively reduce blood pressure in pregnancy (94,95). A randomized prospective multicenter trial compared the hemodynamic effects of ketanserin to hydralazine (94). Ketanserin was observed to act quickly and to gradually decrease MAP without reflex tachycardia or changes in cardiac output. In addition, ketanserin produced a gradual and minor decrease in systemic vascular resistance, unlike dihydralazine, which significantly lowered the systemic resistance. A less peripheral vasodilatory effect will maintain uteroplacental blood flow. Therefore ketanserin will not shift blood from the placental to the peripheral circulation and will maintain uteroplacental blood flow, and IUGR fetuses may benefit from the use of ketanserin rather than dihydralazine. In a retrospective study comparing women with preeclampsia who were treated with ketanserin ($n = 169$) with those who receive dihydralazine ($n = 146$), Bolte and associates (95) observed fewer maternal complications in women who received ketanserin. However, Steyn and Odendaal (96) found that ketanserin did not control blood pressure as effectively as dihydralazine and attributed the results to a suboptimal dose of ketanserin.

VII. MANAGEMENT

Once the diagnosis of severe preeclampsia has been made, the patient is admitted to the labor and delivery unit to determine whether she is a candidate for expectant management. Both maternal and fetal conditions are assessed and the diagnosis confirmed. Magnesium sulfate is administered for seizure prophylaxis and corticosteroids are administered to improve fetal outcome. If there are no indications for delivery and if the mother's safety is not jeopardized, expectant management is the treatment of choice when the fetus is below 34 weeks' gestational age. Termination may be offered to women at or below the threshold of viability. When the neonate is remote from term, perinatal outcome improves by delaying delivery for at least 48 hours after the first dose of steroids. Perinatal outcome can be improved if delivery can also be delayed for 1 to 2 weeks, especially at 24 to 26 weeks' gestation. The parents should be counseled on the intact perinatal survival rate appropriate for the gestational age on admission. Tables 4 and 5 list maternal and fetal conditions indicative of expedient delivery in 48 hours from the first dose of steroids and of expectant management, respectively.

During the observational period, the patient's oral intake is limited to ice chips and oral medications. Intravenous fluid of Ringer's lactate with 5% dextrose is administered at a rate of 100 to 125 mL/h. Accurate fluid input and output are recorded. Antihypertensive medications are given as needed to maintain a systolic blood pressure below 160 mmHg or a diastolic between 90 and 110 mmHg (MAP

< 125) to prevent cerebral complications such as encephalopathy or hemorrhage. Lowering the blood pressure below a diastolic of 90 mmHg may decrease utero-placental perfusion, precipitating fetal distress. Intravenous hydralazine and/or labetalol or oral nifedipine and/or labetalol are given to maximum dosages to control blood pressure (Table 12). Diuretics are used only to treat pulmonary edema.

Laboratory assessment includes a complete blood count with platelets, serum levels of creatinine, uric acid, aspartate aminotransferase (AST), lactate dehydrogenase (LDH), and a 24-hour urine collection for total protein. Once proteinuria is documented, another 24-hour urine does not need to be repeated since outcome in severely preeclamptic women with increasing proteinuria is the same as outcome in women with stable or decreasing proteinuria (55). A coagulation profile (partial thromboplastin time, prothrombin time, and fibrinogen) is not checked on a routine basis unless abruptio placentae is suspected or there is a fetal demise. The patient is observed in labor and delivery for 24 hours. Once the mother and fetus are proven to be eligible for expectant management, magnesium sulfate is discontinued and the patient is observed closely on the antepartum ward until delivery. Blood pressure is monitored every 4 to 6 hours. Certain women will have marked improvement in blood pressure after hospitalization but still warrant hospitalization. The platelet count may be done every day or every other day. AST and creatinine may be repeated every other day or weekly according to need.

Severe preeclampsia may progress rapidly and be accompanied by various systemic manifestations with different degrees of severity. Therefore the mother and the fetus must be evaluated frequently for signs and symptoms of worsening preeclampsia. The patient is asked to report any signs of worsening preeclampsia or imminent eclampsia. A headache should be treated with acetaminophen (paracetamol) and bed rest. If the patient has no history of migraine headaches but the headache persists for greater than 6 hours or remains severe in intensity when the blood pressure is meticulously controlled and magnesium sulfate is started, delivery should be considered.

The patient is delivered if any contraindications to expectant management arise during hospitalization or if she requests not to continue with expectant management. Other indications for delivery include reaching 34 weeks' gestation or if lung maturity is documented by amniocentesis between 32 and 34 weeks.

A trial of labor should be attempted and a cesarean section reserved for the usual obstetrical indications. Glazender (97) reviewed perinatal outcome for "small babies" who underwent an elective cesarean section versus those delivered vaginally. There were no significant differences between groups in neonatal outcome. However, maternal complications occurred more frequently in women who had a cesarean section. Severe preeclampsia is not an indication for a cesarean section. In patients with an unfavorable cervix and at a gestational age of less than 30 weeks, it is appropriate to consider an elective cesarean section or cervical ripening agents. When delivery is warranted in 24 to 48 hours, cervical ripening agents may be used while waiting the effect of the corticosteroids.

The rate of cesarean section is higher in patients with preeclampsia than those without. Women with very low birth weight infants who attempted labor were compared with those who had a cesarean section without a trial of labor (98). Seventy-five percent of the patients who had a successful vaginal delivery had an unfavorable Bishop score. The cesarean section rate was 68%, including 47% of cesarean sections due to fetal intolerance of labor. There was no significant difference between the groups for immediate and long-term outcome variables except for a lower rate of respiratory distress syndrome in the neonate who experienced labor. Magann and colleagues (99) had a 76% cesarean section rate in patients <34 weeks gestation complicated by the HELLP syndrome. For women ≥30 weeks' gestation, induction of labor was significantly more successful (48%) than for those <30 weeks' gestation (15%). In addition, 22% of women with a Bishop score ≤2 and 45% of patients with a score >2 delivered vaginally (odds ratio 0.5, 95% CI 0.2 to 1.3, $p = 0.16$).

In severe preeclampsia, platelet transfusion has a limited role. Transfusion is indicated if the platelet count is lower than $10,000/mm^3$ or if the patient experiences abnormal bleeding and is thrombocytopenic. At the time of cesarean section, a platelet count below $50,000/mm^3$ requires a transfusion of approximately 6 to 10 units of platelets. Repetitive transfusions are unnecessary because consumption of platelets is rapid and the effect transient.

Epidural anesthesia is the anesthetic of choice in women with preeclampsia. Adequate plasma volume expansion of 500 to 1000 mL of crystalloids is administered prior to the epidural. Conduction anesthesia is contraindicated for the usual reasons, such as an infection at the puncture site, a coagulopathy, or refusal of the mother.

Patients are at risk of eclampsia in the postpartum period and are monitored closely for at least 24 hours. Magnesium sulfate is continued until diuresis has occurred and blood pressure is controlled with nifedipine or labetalol. Resolution of the disease process usually occurs within 48 to 72 hours after delivery. Women who recover more slowly or who deteriorate are at risk for development of pulmonary edema from fluid mobilization, transfusion of blood products, and compromised renal function. Oxytocin is added to the IV fluids to prevent uterine atony, which can be aggravated by magnesium sulfate. Methylergonovine maleate (Methergine, ergometrine) is contraindicated in patients with hypertension.

VIII. SUMMARY

Although delivery is always appropriate therapy for women with severe preeclampsia, it may not be optimal for the fetus remote from term. Therefore there are two other management options that can be used to improve neonatal outcome. These are either expectant management or a 48-hour delay to allow for corticosteroid benefits. Assurance of both maternal and fetal well-being is essential before considering a delay in delivery, and intense monitoring of both the mother and fetus should continue throughout the pregnancy at a tertiary care center. Deterioration in the status of either necessitates delivery. The ultimate goals of therapy must always be safety of the mother first and then the delivery of a live, mature newborn that will not require intensive and prolonged neonatal care. This management scheme is only a guideline and should be combined with clinical judgment, which plays a considerable role in the management of these patients. After all, every patient is as unique as is the presentation of preeclampsia.

REFERENCES

1. Sibai BM, Caritis SN, Thom E, Klebanoff M, McNellis D, et al. Prevention of preeclampsia with low-dose aspirin in healthy, nulliparous pregnant women. N Engl J Med 1999; 329:1213–1218.
2. Kurkinen-Raty M, Koivisto M, Jouppila P. Preterm delivery for maternal or fetal indications: maternal morbidity, neonatal outcome and late sequelae in infants. Br J Obstet Gynaecol 2000; 137:616–622.
3. Mackay AP, Berg CJ, Atrash HK. Pregnancy-related mortality from preeclampsia and eclampsia. Obstet Gynecol 2001; 97:533–583.
4. Waterstone M, Bewley S, Wolfe C. Incidence and predictors of severe obstetric morbidity: case-control study. Br Med J 2001; 322:1089–1094.
5. Friedman SA, Schiff E, Koa L, Sibai BM. Neonatal outcome after preterm delivery for preeclampsia. Am J Obstet Gynecol 1995; 172:1785–1792.
6. Derham RJ, Hawkins DR, de Vries LS, Aber VR, Elder MG. Outcome of pregnancies complicated by severe hypertension and delivered before 34 weeks: stepwise logistic regression analysis of prognostic factors. Br J Obstet Gynaecol 1989; 96:1173–1181.
7. American College of Obstetricians and Gynecologists. Diagnosis and management of preeclampsia and eclampsia. Technical Bulletin No. 33. Washington, DC: ACOG, 2002.
8. World Health Organization Study Group. The hypertensive disorders of pregnancy. WHO Technical Report Series No. 758. Geneva: World Health Organization, 1987.
9. Schiff E, Friedman SA, Mercer BM, Sibai BM. Fetal lung maturity is not accelerated in preeclamptic pregnancies. Am J Obstet Gynecol 1993; 169:1096–1101.
10. Chari RS, Friedman SA, Schiff E, Frangieh AT, Sibai BM. Is fetal neurologic and physical development accelerated in preeclampsia? Am J Obstet Gynecol 1996; 174: 829–832.
11. Martin TR, Tupper WRC. The management of severe toxemia in patients at less than 36 weeks' gestation. Obstet Gynecol 1979; 54:602–605.
12. Sibai BM, Taslimi M, Abdella TN, Brooks TF, Spinnato JA, Anderson GD. Maternal and perinatal outcome of conservative management of severe preeclampsia in mid-trimester. Am J Obstet Gynecol 1985; 152:32–37.

13. Odendaal HJ, Pattinson RC, du Toit R. Fetal and neonatal outcome in patients with severe preeclampsia before 34 weeks. S Afr Med J 1987; 71:555–558.
14. Pattinson RC, Odendaal HJ, du Toit R. Conservative management of severe proteinuric hypertension before 28 weeks gestation. S Afr Med J 1988; 73:516–518.
15. Moodley J, Koranteeng SA, Rout C. Expectant management of early onset of severe preeclampsia in Durban. S. Afr Med J 1993; 83:584–587.
16. Olah KS, Redman CW, Gee H. Management of severe, early pre-eclampsia: is conservative management justified? Eur J Obstet Gynecol Reprod Biol 1993; 51: 175–180.
17. Visser W, van Pampus MG, Treffers PE, Wallenburg HC. Perinatal results of hemodynamic and conservative temporizing treatment in severe pre-eclampsia. Eur J Obstet Gynecol Reprod Biol 1994; 53:175–181.
18. Visser W, Wallenburg HCS. Maternal and perinatal outcome of temporizing management in 254 consecutive patients with severe preeclampsia remote from term. Eur J Obstet Gynecol Reprod Biol 1995; 63:147–154.
19. Hall DR, Odendaal HJ, Dirster GF, Smith J, Grove D. Expectant management of early onset, severe pre-eclampsia: maternal outcome. Br J Obstet Gynaecol 2000; 10:1252–1257.
20. Hall DR, Odendaal HJ, Kirsten GF, Smith J, Grove D. Expectant management of early onset, severe pre-eclampsia: perinatal outcome. Br J Obstet Gynaecol 2000; 107:1258–1264.
21. Hall DR, Odendaal HJ, Steyn W. Expectant management of severe pre-eclampsia in the mid-trimester. Eur J Obstet Gynecol Reprod Biol 2001; 96:168–172.
22. Withagen MI, Visser W, Wallenburg HCS. Neonatal outcome of temporizing treatment in early-onset preeclampsia. Eur Obstet Gynecol Reprod Biol 2001; 94:211–215.
23. Sibai BM, Akl S, Fairlie F, Moreti M. A protocol for managing severe preeclampsia in the second trimester. Am J Obstet Gynecol 1990; 163:733–738.
24. Odendaal HJ, Pattinson RC, Bam R, Grove D, Kotze TJvW. Aggressive or expectant management for patients with severe preeclampsia at 28–34 weeks' gestation: a randomized controlled trial. Obstet Gynecol 1990; 76:1070–1075.
25. Sibai BM, Mercer BM, Schiff E, Friedman SA. Aggressive versus expectant management of severe preeclampsia at 28 to 32 weeks' gestation: a randomized controlled trial. Am J Obstet Gynecol 1994; 171:818–822.
26. Witlin AG, Saade GR, Mattar F, Sibai BM. Predictors of neonatal outcome in women with severe preeclampsia or eclampsia between 24 and 33 weeks' gestation. Am J Obstet Gynecol 2000; 182:607–611.
27. Chammas MF, Nguyen TM, Li MA, Nuwayhid BS, Castro LC. Expectant management of severe preterm preeclampsia: is intrauterine growth restriction an indication for immediate delivery? Am J Obstet Gynecol 2000; 183:853–858.
28. Alexander GB, Himes JM, Kaufman RB, Mor J, Kogan M. A United States national reference of fetal growth. Obstet Gynecol 1996; 87:163–168.
29. Friedman SA, Schiff E, Lubarsky SI, Sibai BM. Expectant management of severe preeclampsia remote from term. In: Pitkin RM, ed. Clinical Obstetrics and Gynecology. Philadelphia: Lippincott Williams & Wilkins, 1999:470–478.
30. Lemons JA, Bauer CR, Oh W, Korones SB, Papile, Stil BJ, et al. Very low birth weight outcomes of the National Institute of Child Health and Human Development Neonatal Research Network, January 1995 through December 1996. Pediatrics 2001; 107:e1–8.

31. Vohr BR, Wright LL, Dusick AM, Mele L, Verter J, Steichen JJ, et al. Neurodevelopmental and functional outcomes of extremely low birth weight infants in the National Institute of Child Health and Human Development Neonatal Research Network, 1993–94. Pediatrics 2000; 105:1216–1226.

32. Wood NS, Marlow DM, Costeloe K, Chir B, Gibson AL, Wilkinson AR. Neurologic and developmental disability after extremely preterm birth. N Engl J Med 2000; 343: 378–384.

33. El-Metwally D, Vohr B, Tucker R. Survival and neonatal morbidity at the limits of viability in the mid 1990s: 22 to 25 weeks. J Pediatr 2000; 137:616–622.

34. Sagen N, Koller O, Haram K. Haemoconcentration in severe pre-eclampsia. Br J Obstet Gynaecol 1982; 89:802–805.

35. Redman CW, Bonnar J, Beilin L. Early platelet consumption in pre-eclampsia. Br Med J 1978; 1:467–469.

36. Leduc L, Wheeler JM, Kirshon B, Mitchell P, Cotton DB. Coagulation profile in severe preeclampsia. Obstet Gynecol 1992; 79:14–18.

37. Odendaal HJ. Severe preeclampsia and eclampsia. In: Sibai BM, ed. Hypertensive Disorders in Women. Philadelphia: Saunders, 2001:41–59.

38. Martin JN, Blake PG, Perry KG, McCaul JF, Hess LW, Martin RW. The natural history of HELLP syndrome: patterns of disease progression and regression. Am J Obstet Gynecol 1991; 164:1500–1509.

39. Roberts JM. Pregnancy-related hypertension. In: Creasy RK, Resnik R, eds. Maternal-Fetal Medicine. Philadelphia: Saunders, 1999:833–872.

40. Martin JN, May WL, Magann EF, Terrone DA, Rinehart BK, Blake PG. Early risk assessment of severe preeclampsia: admission battery of symptoms and laboratory tests to predict likelihood of subsequent significant maternal morbidity. Am J Obstet Gynecol 1999; 180:147.

41. Barron WM, Heckerling P, Hibbard JU, Fisher S. Reducing unnecessary coagulation testing in hypertensive disorders of pregnancy. Obstet Gynecol 1999; 94:364–370.

42. Nochy D, Birembaut P, Hinglais H, Freund M, Idatte JM, Jacquot C, Chartier M, Bariety J. Renal lesions in the hypertensive syndromes of pregnancy: immunomorphological and ultrastructural studies in 114 cases. Clin Nephrol 1980; 13:155–162.

43. Many A, Hubel CA, Roberts JM. Hyperuricemia and xanthine oxidase in preeclampsia, revisited. Am J Obstet Gynecol 1996; 174:288–291.

44. Sagen H, Haram K, Nilsen ST. Serum urate as a predictor of fetal outcome in severe pre-eclampsia. Acta Obstet Gynaecol Scand 1984; 63:71–75.

45. Schuster E, Weppelmann B. Plasma urate measurement and fetal outcome in preeclampsia. Gynecol Obstet Invest 1981; 12:162–167.

46. Redman CW, Beilin LJ, Bonnar J, Wilkinson RH. Plasma-urate measurements in predicting fetal death in hypertensive pregnancy. Lancet 1976; 7949:1370–1373.

47. Odendaal HJ, Pienaar ME. Are high uric acid levels in patients with early preeclampsia an indication for delivery? (Abstract.) S Afr Med J 1997; 87:213–218.

48. Sibai BM, Anderson GD, McCubbin JH. Eclampsia II. Clinical significance of laboratory findings. Obstet Gynecol 1982; 58:153–157.

49. Lim KH, Friedman SA, Ecker JK, Kao L, Kilpatrick SJ. The clinical utility of serum uric acid measurements in hypertensive diseases of pregnancy. Am J Obstet Gynecol 1998; 178:1067–1071.

50. Meyer NL, Mercer BM, Friedman SA, Sibai BM. Urinary dipstick protein: a poor predictor of absent or severe proteinuria. Am J Obstet Gynecol 1994; 170:137–141.
51. Kou VS, Koumantakis G, Gallery ED. Proteinuria and its assessment in normal and hypertensive pregnancy. Am J Obstet Gynecol 1992; 167:723–728.
52. Saudan PJ, Brown MA, Farrell T, Shaw L. Improved methods of assessing proteinuria in hypertensive pregnancy. Br J Obstet Gynaecol 1997; 104:1159–1164.
53. Lindheimer MD, Katz AI. Renal physiology and disease in pregnancy. In: Seldin DW, Giebisch G, eds. The Kidney: Physiology and Pathophysiology. Philadelphia: Lippincott Williams & Wilkins, 2000:2597–2644.
54. Higby K, Suiter CR, Siler-Khodr T. A comparison between two screening methods for detection of microproteinuria. Am J Obstet Gynecol 1995; 173:1111–1114.
55. Schiff E, Friedman SA, Kao L, Sibai BM. The importance of urinary protein excretion during conservative management of severe preeclampsia. Am J Obstet Gynecol 1996; 175:1313–1316.
56. Dekker GA, de Vries JI, Doelitzsch PM, Huijgens PC, von Blomberg BM, Jakobs C, van Geijn HP. Underlying disorders associated with severe early-onset preeclampsia. Am J Obstet Gynecol 1995; 173:1042–1048.
57. Branch DW, Andres R, Digre KB, Rote NS, Scott JR. The association of antiphospholipid antibodies with severe preeclampsia. Obstet Gynecol 1989; 73:541–545.
58. Kupferminc MJ, Fait G, Many A, Gordon D, Eldor A, Lessing JB. Severe preeclampsia and high frequency of genetic thrombophilic mutations. Obstet Gynecol 2000; 96:45–49.
59. Cotter A, Molloy A, Scott JM, Daly SF. Elevated plasma homoscysteine in early pregnancy: a risk factor for the development of severe preeclampsia. Am J Obstet Gynecol 2001; 184:S11.
60. Branch DW, Porter TF, Rittenhouse L, Caritis S, Sibai B, Hogg B. Antiphospholipid antibodies in women at risk for preeclampsia. Am J Obstet Gynecol 2001; 184:832–834.
61. Livingston JC, Barton JR, Park V, Haddad B, Chahine R, Phillips O, Sibai BM. Maternal and fetal genetic thrombophilias are not associated with severe preeclampsia. Am J Obstet Gynecol 2000; 182:S25.
62. Alfirevic Z, Mousa HA, Martlew V, Briscoe L, Perez-Casa M, Toh CH. Postnatal screening for thrombophilia in women with severe pregnancy complications. Obstet Gynecol 2001; 97:753–759.
63. Kim YJ, Williamson RA, Murray JC, Andrews, J, Pietscher JJ, Peraud PJ, Merrill DC. Genetic susceptibility to preeclampsia: roles of cytosine-to-thymine substitution at nucleotide 677 of the gene for methylenetetrahydrofolate reductase, 68–base pair insertion at nucleotide 844 of the gene for crystathionine beta-synthase and factor V Leiden mutation. Am J Obstet Gynecol 2001; 184(6):1211–1217.
64. Ozcan T, Rinder HM, Murphy J, Kohn C, Copel JA, Magriples U. Genetic thrombophilia and hypertensive complications of pregnancy. Obstet Gynecol 2001; 97:S40.
65. Schucker JL, Mercer BM, Audibert F, Lewis RL, Friedman SA, Sibai BM. Serial amniotic fluid index in severe preeclampsia: a poor predictor of adverse outcome. Am J Obstet Gynecol 1996; 175:1018–1023.
66. Divon MY. Umbilical artery Doppler velocimetry: Clinical utility in high-risk pregnancies. Am J Obstet Gynecol 1996; 174:10–14.

67. Neilson JP, Alfirevic Z. Doppler ultrasound for fetal assessment in high risk pregnancies (Cochrane Review). In: The Cochrane Library, 2, 2001. Oxford: Update Software.
68. Bilardo CM, Nicolaides KH, Campbell S. Doppler measurements of fetal and uteroplacental circulations: relationship with umbilical venous blood gases measured at cordocentesis. Am J Obstet Gynecol 1990; 162:115–120.
69. Tekay A, Campbell S. Doppler ultrasonography in obstetrics. In: Callen PW, ed. Ultrasonography in Obstetric and Gynecology. Philadelphia: Saunders, 2000:677–723.
70. Wang KG, Chen CP, Yang JM, Su TH. Impact of reverse end diastolic flow velocity in the umbilical artery on pregnancy outcome after 28 gestational weeks. Acta Obstet Gynaecol Scand 1998; 77:527–531.
71. DuPlessis JM, Hall DR, Norman K, Odendaal HJ. Reversed end diastolic flow velocity in viable fetuses: is there time to wait for the effect of corticosteroids before delivery? Int J Gynecol Obstet 2001; 72:187–188.
72. Chari RS, Friedman SA, O'Brien JM, Sibai BM. Daily antenatal testing in women with severe preeclampsia. Am J Obstet Gynecol 1995; 173:1207–1210.
73. Amorim MM, Santos LC, Faundes A. Corticosteroid therapy for prevention of respiratory distress syndrome in severe preeclampsia. Am J Obstet Gynecol 1999; 180:1283–1288.
74. Magann EF, Martin JN Jr. Critical care of HELLP syndrome with corticosteroids. Am J Prenatol 2000; 17(8):417–422.
75. Magann EF, Bass D, Chauhan SP, Sullivan DL, Martin RW, Martin JN Jr. Antepartum corticosteroids: disease stabilization in patients with the syndrome of hemolysis, elevated liver enzymes, and low platelets (HELLP). Am J Obstet Gynecol 1994; 171(4):1148–1153.
76. Martin JN Jr, Perry KG Jr, Blake PG, May WA, Moore A, Robinette L. Better maternal outcomes are achieved with dexamethasone therapy for postpartum HELLP (hemolysis, elevated liver enzymes, and thrombocytopenia) syndrome. Am J Obstet Gynecol 1997; 177(5):1011–1017.
77. O'Brien JM, Milligan DA, Barton JR. Impact of high-dose corticosteroid therapy for patients with HELLP (hemolysis, elevated liver enzymes, and low platelet count) syndrome. Am J Obstet Gynecol 2000; 183(4):921–924.
78. Tompkins MJ, Thiagarajah S. HELLP (hemolysis, elevated liver enzymes, and low platelet count) syndrome: the benefit of corticosteroids. Am J Obstet Gynecol 1999; 181:304–309.
79. Liggins GC, Howie RN. A controlled trial of antepartum glucocorticoid treatment for prevention of the respiratory distress syndrome in preterm infants. Pediatrics 1972; 50:515–525.
80. Anonymous. Effect of corticosteroids for fetal maturation on perinatal outcome. NIH Consensus Development Panel on the effect of corticosteroids for fetal maturation on perinatal outcome. JAMA 1995; 273:413–418.
81. Lucas MJ, Leveno KJ, Cunningham FG. A comparison of magnesium sulfate with phenytoin for the prevention of eclampsia. N Engl J Med 1995; 333:201–221.
82. Duley L, Gulmezoglu AM, Henderson-Smart DJ. Anticonvulsants for women with pre-eclampsia (Cochrane Review). In: The Cochrane Library, Issue 2, 2001. Oxford: Update Software.

83. Sibai BM. Magnesium sulfate is the ideal anticonvulsant in preeclampsia-eclampsia. Am J Obstet Gynecol 1990; 162:1141–1145.

84. Witlin AG, Sibai BM. Magnesium sulfate therapy in preeclampsia and eclampsia. Obstet Gynecol 1998; 92:883–889.

85. Coetzee EJ, Commisse J, Anthony J. A randomized controlled trial of intravenous magnesium sulphate versus placebo in the management of women with severe preeclampsia. Br J Obstet Gynaecol 1998; 105:300–303.

86. Strandgaard S, Olesen J, Skinhoj E, Lassen NA. Autoregulation of brain circulation in severe arterial hypertension. Br Med J 1973; 1:507–510.

87. Redman CW, Roberts JM. Management of preeclampsia. Lancet 1993; 341:1451–1454.

88. Marx GF, Schwalbe SS, Cho E, Whitty JE. Automated blood pressure measurements in laboring women: are they reliable? Am J Obstet Gynecol 1993; 168:796–798.

89. Duley L, Henderson-Smart DJ. Drugs for rapid treatment of very high blood pressure during pregnancy (Cochrane Review). In: The Cochrane Library, Issue 2, 2000. Oxford: Update Software.

90. Paterson-Brown S, Robson SC, Redfern N, Walkinshaw SA, de Swiet M. Hydralazine boluses for the treatment of severe hypertension in pre-eclampsia. Br J Obstet Gynaecol 1994; 101:409–413.

91. Mabie WC, Gonzalez AR, Sibai BM, Amon E. A comparative trial of labetalol and hydralazine in the acute management of severe hypertension complicating pregnancy. Obstet Gynecol 1987; 70:328–333.

92. MacCarthy EP, Bloomfield SS. Labetalol: A review of its pharmacology, pharmacokinetics, clinical uses and adverse effects. Pharmacotherapy 1983; 3:193–219.

93. Hall DR, Odendaal HJ, Steyn DW, Smith M. Nifedipine or prazosin as a second agent to control early severe hypertension in pregnancy: a randomized controlled trial. Br J Obstet Gynaecol 2000; 107:759–765.

94. Bolte AC, van Eyck J, Strackvan Schijndel RJ, van Geijn HP, Dekker GA. The haemodynamic effects of ketanserin versus dihydralazine in severe early-onset hypertension in pregnancy. Br J Obstet Gynaecol 1998; 105:723–731.

95. Bolte AC, van Eyck J, Gaffar SF, van Geijn HP, Dekker GA. Ketanserin for the treatment of preeclampsia. J Perinat Med 2001; 29(1):14–22.

96. Steyn DW, Odendaal HJ. Dihydralazine or ketanserin for severe hypertension in pregnancy? Preliminary results. Eur J Obstet Gynecol Reprod Biol 1997; 75:155–159.

97. Grant A, Glazener CMA. Elective caesarean section versus expectant management for delivery of the small baby (Cochrane Review). In: The Cochrane Library, Issue 2, 2001. Oxford: Update Software.

98. Regenstein AC, Laros RK, Wakeley A, Kitterman JA, Tooley WH. Mode of delivery in pregnancies complicated by preeclampsia with very low birth weight infant. J Perinatol 1995; 15:2–6.

99. Magann EF, Roberts WE, Perry KG, Chauhan SP, Blake PG, Martin JN. Factors relevant to mode of preterm delivery with syndrome of HELLP (hemolysis, elevated liver enzymes, and low platelets). Am J Obstet Gynecol 1994; 170:1828–1832.

6
Preeclampsia in Pregnant Women with Chronic Hypertension and Renal Disease

Justine C. Norman and John M. Davison
University of Newcastle Upon Tyne, Newcastle Upon Tyne, England

Preeclampsia is an important cause of maternal and fetal morbidity and mortality, complicating 5–10% of all pregnancies. It has been described as a maternal syndrome at the extreme end of the spectrum of the gestational inflammatory disturbance that affects all vascular compartment cells and causes widespread maternal endothelial dysfunction (1). The considerable overlap between normal pregnancy and preeclampsia accounts for the lack of an ideal screening test and/or prophylactic strategy. Whatever the etiology of preeclampsia, the ultimate target is the maternal endothelium, which leads to a multiorgan disorder with widespread enhanced vascular reactivity, activation of the coagulation cascade, and disrupted volume homeostasis (1–4).

The exact pattern of end-organ damage dictates the subsequent signs and symptoms. The superimposition of vasoconstriction, disordered coagulation, and a contracted intravascular volume on a previously normal cardiovascular system is bad enough, but when superimposed on a systemic circulation and/or renal vasculature already compromised, the sequelae are much more serious. From the obstetric viewpoint, there are major diagnostic difficulties in distinguishing preeclampsia, chronic hypertension, renal disease, and combinations of these separate entities. This chapter focuses on defining hypertension in pregnancy in relation to preexisting pathology, identifying the pitfalls in the detection and diagnosis of preeclampsia in women with chronic hypertension and/or renal disease, and highlighting the controversies surrounding the antenatal care and obstetric problems in these women.

I.   WHAT CONSTITUTES HYPERTENSION IN PREGNANCY AND HOW IS IT CLASSIFIED?

Hypertension relies on an arbitrary line dividing normal from abnormal blood pressure. Classification systems aim to compare like with like while distinguishing normal pregnancy changes from those that put the mother and fetus at increased risk. For pregnancy, this is defined as a systolic blood pressure (SBP) >140 mmHg and/or diastolic blood pressure (DBP) >90 mmHg (two or more recordings 6 hours apart) and as such complicates approximately 10% of pregnancies (5). It must be remembered, however, that all hypertensive states confer additional risks.

The classification of hypertension in pregnancy is currently under review in many countries, with the International Society for the Study of Hypertension (ISSHP) coordinating these efforts (see Chapters 1 and 7). Basically, three broad categories exist: *chronic hypertension, gestational hypertension* and *preeclampsia* (5). In the United States, a clinically orientated framework uses four categories: *chronic hypertension, preeclampsia/eclampsia, preeclampsia superimposed upon chronic hypertension*, and *transient (late-gestational) hypertension* (4). A review by the National Institutes of Health and the National High Blood Pressure Education Programme is under way, drawing on the rapidly growing databases from recently completed and ongoing multicenter trials that include longitudinal determination of blood pressure. The prime concerns of this chapter are the problems of chronic hypertension of whatever cause and the superimposition of preeclampsia upon that chronic hypertension.

II.   HOW IS BLOOD PRESSURE (BP) MEASURED?

With the woman seated and her arm at rest, the BP is taken at the level of the heart. The first beat heard (Korotkoff phase 1) gives the systolic pressure. Phase V, the disappearance of all sounds, has now been generally accepted as most accurately reflecting the diastolic BP. In only a very small number of patients, phase V is never reached. In the majority of women, phases IV and V are within 5 mmHg (6). Automated machines measure phases I and V, and an extensive literature is available on the role and pitfalls of ambulatory BP monitoring. Hypertension will be overdiagnosed in obese women unless a large cuff is used (bladder size 15 × 33 cm). The initial prenatal visit provides a convenient baseline, but it must be remembered that even at this time diastolic BP is typically 7 to 10 mmHg below prepregnancy values. It then reaches a nadir in the second trimester, thereafter steadily increasing to prepregnancy levels. Thus a single reading of 140/90 mmHg defines approximately 2% of the population before 20 weeks but more than 10% after that time (7). Such changes can often be exaggerated in women with chronic hypertension, creating diagnostic confusion with preeclampsia in the third trimester. The "white coat effect" is worthy of mention. This effect becomes apparent when a recording by an obstetric caregiver is higher than that seen when blood pressure is evaluated in the woman's usual environment (8). It is uncommon in women presenting for the management of hypertension in the second half of pregnancy, and it is doubtful that pregnancy as such is more likely to induce this effect (6,8).

III. WHAT IS CHRONIC HYPERTENSION?

Hypertension presenting before 20 weeks' gestation warrants further investigation for an underlying cause (9). Most cases (90%) will be essential hypertension, but secondary causes, especially renal disease, are important. By the end of the first trimester, many women with chronic hypertension will be relatively normotensive as a result of the expected decrease in BP at this time. The gradual rise to prepregnancy levels in the third trimester may reveal previously undocumented chronic hypertension. Superimposed preeclampsia may also present at this time, although a clear diagnosis of this condition may only be clarified in retrospect, when hypertension is noted to persist beyond 3 months postpartum.

IV. WHAT IS PREECLAMPSIA?

Preeclampsia can be defined as hypertension presenting after 20 weeks and resolving by 3 months postpartum with evidence of end-organ damage (10). All gravidas must be considered at risk despite the tendency just to dwell on the well-recognized predisposing factors, including chronic hypertension, previous preeclampsia, first pregnancy or a new partner, age extremes, and multiple pregnancy (11). The classic triad of hypertension, proteinuria, and edema is of little value in identifying those affected (7). Proteinuria (+1) on dipstick testing (which is frequently unreliable) (12) will not represent significant proteinuria in 50% of cases, and urinary tract infection always requires exclusion. Proteinuria is a relatively late sign (>300 mg in a 24-hour collection), and edema is common at some time in the majority of healthy pregnant women. Table 1 documents how the pattern of end-organ involvement dictates the resulting symptoms, signs, and biochemical disturbances (3,7). Importantly too, some women may remain asymptomatic; the condition may therefore go unrecognized unless further investigations are undertaken.

V. WHEN IS PREECLAMPSIA NOT PREECLAMPSIA?

As part of end-organ pathology, preeclamptic glomeruli undergo structural changes with pronounced endothelial vacuolization and hypertrophy of the cyto-

Table 1 The Symptoms, Signs, and Investigation of Preeclampsia

End-organ involvement	Symptoms	Signs	Investigation
CNS	Severe headache, visual disturbances	Hyperreflexia, clonus, eclampsia	Blood pressure Funduscopy; papilledema
Kidney		Proteinuria	Increasing urate (early indicator of renal involvement) Increased creatinine/urea (late feature of compromised renal perfusion) Proteinuria > 300 mg/24 h Oliguria
Vascular endothelium	Facial/finger edema	Hypertension	Thrombocytopenia (peripheral consumption) Prolonged clotting times (usually normal unless disseminated intravascular coagulation develops) Hypoalbuminemia (increasing risk of pulmonary edema) Increased hematocrit (hypovolemia)
Liver	Epigastric pain, nausea	Epigastric tenderness	Raised transaminases (indicate cellular damage) NB Alkaline phosphatase is produced by the placenta normally increased in pregnancy
Placenta—fetal compromise		None or clinically reduced fundal height, amniotic fluid volume	Ultrasound: fetal growth restriction with or without signs of placental insufficiency; reduced amniotic fluid volume, abnormal uterine artery Doppler and/or reduced umbilical artery Doppler blood flow
Placenta—abruptio placentae	Acute abdominal pain with or without vaginal bleeding	Tense, tender uterus ± pv bleeding ± fetal demise	Ultrasound: retroplacental hypoechoeic area; a normal ultrasound does not exclude a small abruption

Table 2 Renal Pathology in 176 Hypertensive Pregnant Women Diagnosed Clinically as Having Preeclampsia

Biopsy diagnosis	Number of patients	Primigravidas	Multiparas
Preeclampsia	96	79	17
With nephrosclerosis	13	6	7
With renal disease	3	1	2
With both	2	1	1
Nephrosclerosis	19	3	16
With renal disease	4	2	2
Renal disease	31	12	19
Normal histology	8	0	8

Source: Modified from Ref. 15.

plasmic organelles, first defined as glomerular capillary endotheliosis over 40 years ago by Spargo et al. (13). Such changes were thought to be pathognomonic of preeclampsia, but it is now accepted that no one feature is specific to preeclamptic nephropathy. It is also accepted that although these morphological features start to resolve within 48 hours after delivery, complete resolution may take 4 to 5 weeks or even as long as 6 months (14). Consequently, postpartum renal biopsy has been used to prove whether a patient has preeclampsia as opposed to chronic hypertension, renal disease, and/or various combinations. In the classic study of Fisher et al. (15), renal biopsies were undertaken within a few days of delivery after pregnancies complicated by hypertension, proteinuria, and edema. Table 2 documents the pathological diagnosis in 176 primagravid and multigravid women. The clinical diagnosis was "wrong" in 25% of primagravidas and, more often than not, in multigravidas. Comprehensive reviews of preeclamptic renal changes have been published elsewhere (16,17). Given the subtle interrelationships between "pure preeclampsia" and "renal deterioration in the presence of renal disease," the clinical label of preeclampsia may be confusing (7). This is discussed further below in relation to specific renal diseases.

VI. WHAT HAPPENS TO RENAL FUNCTION IN PREECLAMPSIA?

Glomerular capillary endotheliosis is accompanied by decreased renal hemodynamics, hypofiltration, disordered renal vascular sensitivity, and compromised glomerular barrier function with the appearance of nondiscriminatory "shunts" to explain nonselective proteinuria. Altered tubular function contributes to hyperuricemia and sodium retention. Occasionally functional impairment is very severe, with tubular and/or cortical necrosis; but if the renal failure is uncomplicated by preexisting renal disease, 80% will regain normal function, whereas it is 20% in those with underlying renal pathology.

More recent postdelivery renal biopsy studies (18,19) have linked the morphometric alterations with loss of glomerular charge selectivity and an attenuation in ultrafiltration coefficient as also being important in relation to proteinuria and hypofiltration, respectively. While the consensus is that there does not appear to be an early warning phase of microalbuminuria, there is now evidence of microalbuminuria (>14 mg/24 h) 3 to 5 years after preeclampsia, which may reflect residual glomerular damage from gestational protein trafficking and/or covert renal disease (20).

VII. WHAT IS THE RELATIONSHIP BETWEEN CHRONIC HYPERTENSION AND PREECLAMPSIA?

A. Background

The incidence of superimposed preeclampsia in chronic hypertension ranges from 4.7 to 18.4% for mild hypertension (DBP >90 mmHg) (21–24) up to 54 to 100% for severe hypertension (DBP >100 mmHg) (25). These figures are unaffected by the use of antihypertensives (24–28). Of interest, black women with chronic hypertension in pregnancy have a higher incidence of superimposed preeclampsia and prematurity than white women with chronic hypertension (29). Other predictors for the development of superimposed preeclampsia include preeclampsia during a previous pregnancy, hypertension for more than 4 years preconception, and the presence of a diastolic BP of at least 100 mmHg during the first trimester (11).

Severe hypertension in early pregnancy is certainly associated with diverse fetal and maternal outcomes irrespective of the development of superimposed preeclampsia. In a group of 338 pregnant women with chronic hypertension, there was a 10.9% incidence of small for gestational age (SGA) infants, compared with 4.1% for the normal population. The incidence was increased to 19.2% in women with superimposed preeclampsia (9). In another study of 298 chronic hypertensive women (SGA rate 15.5% in the absence and 35.4% in the presence of superimposed preeclampsia), there was no relationship with the first-trimester DBP (25).

In early studies of untreated gravidas with chronic hypertension, the perinatal survival rates varied between 19 and 50% and there was a correlation with the development of superimposed preeclampsia (27,28,30). Later studies have reported perinatal survival rates of approximately 75% despite similar rates of superimposed preeclampsia (24,26), indicative of better management strategies.

B. Management

Some consider the use of antihypertensive drugs as beneficial in preventing sudden increases in blood pressure, cerebral hemorrhage, or hypertensive encephalopathy (31,32). A clear benefit of antihypertensives, however, in mild to moderate chronic hypertension remains unproven, as treatment does not prevent placental abruption or superimposed preeclampsia or influence perinatal outcome. There is no consensus regarding thresholds for treatment. Some recommend medications if DBP exceeds 95 mmHg at any time during pregnancy, whereas others are less stringent. Multicenter controlled trials are urgently needed (33).

Alpha-methyldopa is the most commonly used agent for the control of blood pressure during pregnancy (34). Its safety is well established both in pregnancy and in the long-term follow up of infants (35). Other agents used to control blood pressure in pregnancy include labetalol (36) (a combined alpha- and beta-adrenoceptor blocker), calcium-channel blockers, and hydralazine. Angiotensin converting enzyme (ACE) inhibitors, angiotensin receptor blockers, and diuretics should be avoided in pregnancy. Diuretics may reduce uteroplacental perfusion, and ACE inhibitors have been associated with renal failure, neonatal anuria, intrauterine growth retardation (IUGR), and oliguria (37) (see Table 3). Angiotensin receptor blockers are newer agents, and although they have not been formally studied in pregnancy, they are best avoided, given their common pathway with ACE inhibitors.

A study in 156 pregnant women with chronic hypertension who were aggressively treated with antihypertensives if their diastolic blood pressure ex-

Table 3 Drugs Commonly Used for the Treatment of Hypertension in Pregnancy

Drug	Dose	Comment
Chronic treatment		
Methyldopa	750–3000 mg in 2–4 divided doses	Established safety record after the first trimester. Restricted use postpartum due to sedative and depressive side effects.
Labetalol	100–500 mg tid	Alpha and beta blocker. Vasodilates without impairing cardiac output. Avoid in asthma.
Nifedipine	10–40 mg slow release bid	Slow-release form best. Caution if combined with magnesium sulfate; risk of profound hypotension.
Acute treatment		
Hydralazine	5–10 mg IV or IM repeat if necessary	Agent of choice. Dose may be limited by maternal tachycardia.
Labetalol	20 mg IV repeat at 20-min intervals if necessary	Side effects include flushing and nausea.
Nifedipine	10 mg sublingually; repeat in 20 min if necessary	Risk of hypotension if combined with magnesium sulfate; headache, nausea.

ceeded 90 mmHg demonstrated a perinatal outcome similar to that in studies where antihypertensive medication was not administered (26). Neither did the use of medication in these studies alter the rate of superimposed preeclampsia (26). In general, therefore, antihypertensive therapy may be beneficial in cases of severe hypertension, but it is only one aspect of the management of chronic hypertension in pregnancy.

C. Prophylaxis

Low-dose aspirin (75–150 mg/day) has been used intermittently over the years to reduce the incidence of superimposed preeclampsia, IUGR, prematurity, and fetal death in pregnant women with chronic hypertension. A 1985 study examined 102 women at risk for preeclampsia, IUGR or fetal death, one-third of whom had chronic hypertension. Half were treated with aspirin and half received placebo. The aspirin group demonstrated a much lower incidence of IUGR than the control group and no cases of preeclampsia or fetal death were noted (38). This conclusion is endorsed by a recent literature review (39), but for most the data regarding the use of prophylactic low-dose aspirin in pregnancies complicated by chronic hypertension remain controversial (4,32,40). Oxidative stress may also play a role in the pathogenesis of preeclampsia (41); hence the study of prophylactic vitamins C and E, with encouraging initial results (42). Other proposed prophylactic measures include calcium supplementation and/or fish oil products, although these substances have not been shown to prevent preeclampsia in low-risk normal pregnant women (4,40).

VIII. WHAT IS THE RELATIONSHIP BETWEEN RENAL DISEASE AND PREECLAMPSIA?

A. Background

Pregnancy in women with chronic renal disease was previously discouraged or, if the patient was already pregnant, termination (and often sterilization) were advised due to the risk of maternal and fetal complications. Nowadays, it is easier to predict the effect of pregnancy on renal disease as well as the effect of renal disease on the pregnancy. Although counseling is more optimistic, there are still risks, which depend on the degree of renal impairment at conception (32,43), the presence of hypertension at conception or early in pregnancy (44,45), the type of underlying renal disease (46), and the degree of proteinuria (45,47).

B. Pregnancy When Renal Function Is Preserved/Mildly Impaired

The definition of preserved or mildly impaired renal function is a serum creatinine of less than or equal to 1.4 mg/dL (125 μmol/L). In the classic study of Katz et al.

(44), there were 121 pregnancies in 89 women in whom a diagnosis of renal disease was confirmed by renal biopsy. All had normal or mildly impaired renal function; two-thirds had chronic interstitial nephritis and focal and diffuse glomerulonephritis. Renal function declined mildly in 16% during pregnancy but reversed spontaneously postpartum. Proteinuria increased in 50% and tended to be severe but seemed to have little influence on the natural course of the renal disease. This study demonstrated that although renal function may worsen during pregnancy, its natural course is probably not affected by gestation in the absence of hypertension (44). At a mean follow-up of 62 months, only 5 of these women had progressed to end-stage renal disease; in most cases the severity of hypertension and renal impairment was lower than it had been during gestation. The live birthrate was 94%, but there was an increased incidence of preterm delivery and small-for-gestational-age infants as compared with the normal population. The incidence of superimposed preeclampsia within this group was also increased at 11% (44). These findings have been supported by other studies, which also indicate that women with mild renal disease should not be discouraged from becoming pregnant, because the complication rate is generally low and there is a successful outcome in over 95%. Moreover, pregnancy does not adversely influence the natural course of the disease process (46,48). Certain nephropathies, however, may be unpredictably adversely affected by pregnancy, as discussed further on (see Table 4).

C. Moderate-Severe Renal Insufficiency

Moderate renal insufficiency is defined as a serum creatinine 1.4 to 3.0 mg/dL (125–265 μmol/L) and severe insufficiency as a serum creatinine greater than 3.0 mg/dL (265 μmol/L). Early studies demonstrated that pregnancy resulted in high rates of deterioration in renal function (approximately 50%) and avoidance of pregnancy was advised (49,50). More recent data suggest that the risks may be less and, although there is the possibility of renal decline (25–50%), this does not occur in most women (51–54). In one study, serum creatinine did not increase during pregnancy in half of the women with moderate renal impairment and in no women with severe renal impairment (53). Other studies have shown that there may be a gestational deterioration in renal function that can persist or deteriorate postpartum if the levels of serum creatinine are greater than 180 μmol/L (2.0 mg/dL) (52,54,55). An important message is that maternal hypertension usually worsens and control of BP is required to achieve a good pregnancy outcome (54). Data are slow to accrue and are all retrospective (see Table 5).

With respect to the effect of renal disease on pregnancy, complications were higher than in pregnancies complicated only by mild hypertension. The perinatal mortality rate was approximately 16%; hypertension worsened in 30 to 50%, proteinuria increased in 30%, and superimposed preeclampsia occurred in 42% (51,53,54). At serum creatinine levels of greater than 220 μmol/L (2.5 mg/dL), the rates of prematurity and intrauterine growth retardation have been quoted as 73

Table 4 Specific Renal Diseases and Pregnancy

Renal disease	Effects and outcome	Risk of preeclampsia
Chronic glomerulonephritis	Usually no adverse effect in absence of hypertension UTI more frequent The renal lesion may be affected by the coagulation changes of pregnancy	Mild
IgA nephropathy	Risk of hypertension and worsening of renal function	Moderate-severe
Pyelonephritis	Bacteriuria in pregnancy may lead to exacerbation Multiple organ dysfunction can occur	Mild
Reflux nephropathy	Risks of hypertension/worsening or renal function	Mild-moderate
Urolithiasis	UTI more frequent Avoid lithotripsy Natural history not affected	Mild
Diabetic nephropathy	Increased UTI, edema Natural history not affected	Moderate-severe
Polyarteritis nodosa	Poor fetal prognosis Risk of maternal death	Severe
Polycystic disease	Minimal risk of functional impairment and hypertension	Mild at most
Systemic lupus erythematosus	More favorable prognosis if in remission > 6 months prior to conception Controversies regarding steroid dosing	Severe
Scleroderma	If onset during pregnancy; rapid deterioration may occur Reactivation of quiescent scleroderma may occur postpartum	Severe
Previous urinary tract surgery	Possible associations with other urinary tract malformations Renal function may worsen	Mild
After nephrectomy, solitary kidney and pelvic kidney	Possible associations with other malformations of urogenital tract Pregnancy well tolerated	Mild
Wegener's granulomatosis	Proteinuria (± hypertension) is common from early pregnancy Avoid cytotoxics but immunosupressives safe	Moderate-severe
Renal artery stenosis	May present as chronic hypertension or recurrent isolated preeclampsia Transluminal angioplasty in pregnancy if appropriate	Mild-moderate

Table 5 Moderate-Severe Renal
Disease and Pregnancy

Problems in pregnancy	90%
Successful obstetric outcome	84%
Problems long term	50%
End-stage renal failure	15%

Source: Refs. 54 and 56.

and 57%, respectively, compared with 55 and 31% with serum creatinine levels less than 220 μmol/L (2.5 mg/dL). The incidence of superimposed preeclampsia at serum creatinine levels above 220 μmol/L (2.5 mg/dL) can be as high as 80% (52–54,56). Furthermore, with moderate to severe renal impairment, hypertension in prepregnancy or in the first trimester is associated with a 10 times higher risk of fetal loss than in normotensive women with the same degree of renal impairment (56).

Although patients whose renal function is severely impaired often have amenorrhea or anovulatory menstrual cycles and are infertile, conception may occur and successful pregnancies have been documented (52). Although the combination of severe renal failure and hypertension presents a large risk for both mother and fetus, there is much controversy as to whether termination of pregnancy should be considered. One view is that women who demonstrate a significant decline in renal function can be offered dialysis and continue with the pregnancy, since dialysis commenced during pregnancy is associated with an 80% rate of live births. Women with advanced renal failure are at especially high risk of serious sequelae during gestation; therefore it is advisable to preserve what renal function there is and await transplantation before pregnancy is considered (43).

It is not known why pregnancy exacerbates renal disease. There may be increases in intraglomerular pressure, superimposition of platelets and fibrin onto already damaged glomerular vessels, or perhaps microvascular coagulopathy and/or endothelial dysfunction as part of the preeclamptic process (Figure 1).

IX. SPECIFIC RENAL DISORDERS WITH POTENTIAL ADVERSE OUTCOMES

A. Pregnancy in Women Undergoing Dialysis

For most patients undergoing dialysis, conception may be difficult because of amenorrhea or anovulatory cycles. Pregnancy is, however, still a possibility and tends to be recognized late (50,57). Fertility is reduced in women with end-stage renal disease, but correction of the associated anemia and improvements in dialysis can restore fertility (58). The incidence of conception has been quoted as 1 per

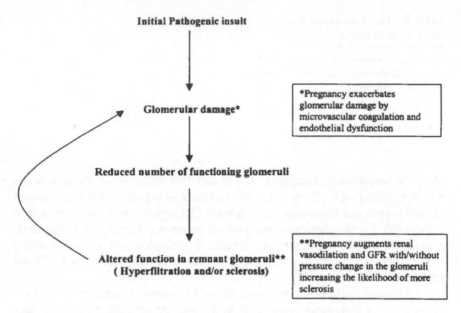

Figure 1 Glomerular injury: why pregnancy exacerbates renal disease.

200 patients, but this is difficult to assess, since spontaneous and therapeutic abortions are common among these women.

In pregnancy, dialysis should be employed earlier, as blood urea nitrogen (BUN) levels greater than 80 mg/dL are associated with an increased risk of fetal complications. Therefore, the aim of dialysis is to maintain BUN <80 mg/dL. It is also important to rigidly control blood pressure, limit intravascular volume changes, and control calcium levels (59). If dialysis is to be commenced in pregnancy, peritoneal dialysis is safe but most would use hemodialysis. There is currently an ongoing argument about whether to switch from hemo- to peritoneal dialysis in pregnancy (60), but actually there is no good evidence to suggest that peritoneal dialysis is better than hemodialysis or vice versa (61).

The frequency and duration of dialysis should be increased by approximately 50% during pregnancy (57). Anemia is often aggravated in women with chronic renal disease, and transfusion or recombinant erythropoietin therapy may be required. Peritonitis is a potential complication of peritoneal dialysis.

With respect to pregnancy complications, in 1980 the rate of live births in 115 pregnancies in women undergoing dialysis was only 23% (62). A further study in 1992 demonstrated a rate of live births of 30% in 22 women studied over the previous 5 years (63). By 1994 there was a rate of 83% live births in women undergoing peritoneal dialysis and 42% in those undergoing hemodialysis (59).

Prematurity is a major problem in dialysis patients, with the mean gestational age at delivery being approximately 32 weeks. The prematurity rate is possibly related to the increased incidence of polyhydramnios (59,61). In general, therefore, the likelihood of a successful live birth in patients undergoing dialysis is at best 40 to 50%, and patients should be counseled accordingly.

Hypertension and superimposed preeclampsia are significant risks in these women. These complications have an adverse effect on maternal and perinatal mortality and morbidity. Blood pressure should ideally be controlled with anti-hypertensive medication to maintain diastolic blood pressure <100 mmHg.

B. Pregnancy in Women Following Renal Transplantation

Renal function returns to normal rapidly after transplantation. About 1 in 20 women with a functioning transplant become pregnant, but early loss of pregnancy is common (spontaneous or therapeutic abortion) with about 75% progressing beyond the first trimester. However, of these pregnancies, 95% end successfully (32,50,64). A transplanted kidney will undergo the same pregnancy-associated increase in GFR as a normal kidney, and pregnancy does not affect the rate of rejection. A preconception serum creatinine of greater than 180 μmol/L (2.0 mg/dL), however, may be associated with a decline in renal function. It is advisable to avoid pregnancy for approximately 2 years after transplantation, until the patient's condition is stable (64).

The potential maternal complications of pregnancy following transplantation are hypertension, superimposed preeclampsia, a decline in renal function, and graft rejection. The risk of developing hypertension, preeclampsia, or both is 30%. As with all chronic renal disorders in pregnancy, hypertension must be aggressively treated and the possibility of superimposed preeclampsia considered (57). If complications occur before 28 weeks, the likelihood of a successful outcome is reduced to 70%. Serial assessments of renal function must be done to monitor for rejection; if rejection is suspected, renal biopsy may be necessary (65).

As shown in Table 6, gestational outcome and long-term prognosis relate to the prepregnancy transplant status. The upper level of serum creatinine associated with a successful outcome is 160 to 180 μmol/L (1.8–2.0 mg/dL) (66). Prepregnancy hypertension is associated with adverse perinatal outcomes (67). Repeated pregnancies in women with renal allografts have also demonstrated a good outcome with respect to graft function (68).

Long-term follow up of women who did and did not have pregnancies following transplantation reveals that the mean serum creatinine level did not differ significantly between the two groups. This suggests that pregnancy does not have an adverse effect on long-term graft function (50,67,69).

Fetal complications are relatively common. Preterm delivery occurs in 45 to 60% of transplant pregnancies and intrauterine growth restriction in at least 20%. Neonatal complications can also occur. Nevertheless, women with stable graft

Table 6 Renal Allograft Recipients: Pregnancy Implications, Problems and Success in Relation to Renal Status[a]

	Problems in pregnancy (%)	Successful obstetric outcome (%)	Long-term problems (%)
All cases	49	95	12
With nonpregnant renal status (Scr)			
< 125 μmol/L (< 1.4 mg/dL)	30	97	7
> 125 μmol/L (> 1.4 mg/dL)	82	75	27

[a]Unpublished literature review. Estimates based on 4220 women in 5370 pregnancies that attained at least 28 weeks' gestation (1961–1998).

function without hypertension have an approximately 90% chance of delivering a healthy child, and pregnancy does not adversely affect long-term renal function (70) (Table 6).

C. Reflux Nephropathy

This term describes renal changes relating to past vesicoureteral reflux and often complicated by recurrent infection. Reflux nephropathy is a frequent cause of tubulo-interstitial disease in women of childbearing age. Urinary tract infections should be routinely screened for during pregnancy in these women, and those with persistent reflux may benefit from prophylactic ureterovesical reimplantation (48,71,72). Pregnancy may be successful and does not seem to adversely affect renal function if the plasma creatinine is less than 180 μmol/L (2.0 mg/dL). The association of renal impairment together with hypertension and proteinuria, however, may cause the loss of renal function and has a fetal mortality rate of 73% (72–74).

D. Systemic Lupus Erythematosus (SLE)

SLE is a multisystem disease that frequently affects the kidneys and is often seen in women of childbearing age. SLE in pregnancy causes various problems, in part mediated by an effect on the immune system (75).

Pregnancy has been reported to have no effect, cause relapse, or be associated with a transient improvement in SLE (76). The 6 months prior to conception appear to be crucial, since women in disease remission have fewer and milder flare-ups than those with recently active disease (75,77). The course of pregnancy is also more problematic in women if SLE first appears during pregnancy or in those with active disease. Data are variable and in one study there was no deterioration in renal function in four out of five pregnancies complicated by SLE (78). A further study, however, demonstrated that SLE runs a variable and unpredictable course irrespective of disease activity preconception. In this, 7 out of 19 patients with SLE demonstrated significant worsening of renal function during gestation, and 2 women died of renal failure (79).

The effect of SLE on pregnancy is variable. Preterm delivery and spontaneous abortion are more common and fetal survival depends on preconception disease status. Survival rates range from 88 to 100% if the disease is in remission prior to pregnancy but only 50 to 80% when recent disease activity has been documented (80,81). Patients with renal disease or active SLE are at a higher risk of superimposed preeclampsia (80). Neonatal complications such as congenital heart block, connective tissue disease and neonatal lupus syndrome have also been documented.

Intrauterine fetal death is common in women with circulating lupus anticoagulant; it is therefore important to screen for this in all pregnant women with SLE (44). Lupus nephropathy may sometimes present during pregnancy and may be mistaken for preeclampsia, especially if accompanied by hypertension and renal impairment. These women are at a very high risk of fetal and maternal complications. Another serious complication of SLE in pregnancy is cerebritis; this should be suspected in cases where any type of cerebral symptom or sign appears. Further discussion of lupus cerebritis is beyond the scope of this chapter, but the reader is reminded to look for this deadly problem in all patients with complicated SLE. Most authorities recommend antenatal prophylactic aspirin therapy in pregnant patients with SLE, but data are few and inconsistent.

E. Diabetic Nephropathy

Diabetic nephropathy is a progressive glomerular disease characterized by glomerular scarring, increased protein permeability, and renal failure. It eventually affects approximately 30% of all patients with insulin-dependent diabetes mellitus but its incidence in pregnancy is approximately 3.8% (61,82).

Women with diabetic nephropathy typically have chronic hypertension and proteinuria, which may be difficult to differentiate from preeclampsia (50,82). In women with a preconception creatinine clearance <70 mL/min, there is an increased risk of acceleration of renal impairment and pregnancy should be discouraged (83,84). Nephrotic syndrome, hypertension, and first-trimester proteinuria >300 mg/24 h are adverse features. At the time of delivery, hypertension complicates 75% of pregnancies with diabetic nephropathy (85). The complications usually disappear postpartum (86) and in general there is little evidence to suggest that pregnancy hastens the progression of diabetic nephropathy (82). The development of insulin has significantly improved fetal and maternal survival. Maternal survival was 66% before and 100% after insulin was introduced. The respective fetal survival rates were 40 and 90% (87).

Although perinatal outcome is successful in approximately 90% of pregnancies complicated by maternal nephropathy, poor prognostic indicators include proteinuria >3 g/24 h, a mean arterial blood pressure >107 mmHg, or a serum creatinine >125 μmol/L (1.4 mg/dL) (85,88). Obstetric complications are not dissimilar in women with diabetic nephropathy than in those with other forms of chronic renal disease (88). Associated chronic hypertension is a poor prognostic indicator associated with a high incidence of fetal growth restriction, fetal distress, prematurity, and perinatal morbidity (82). Preeclampsia complicates 13.6% of type I diabetic pregnancies compared with 5% of nondiabetic pregnancies, and it affects more than 30% of women with diabetic nephropathy and associated hypertension. The perinatal mortality associated with the combination of preeclampsia and diabetes is 60 per 1000 live births, compared with 3.3 per 1000 live births in a normotensive diabetic pregnant population (85,89).

F. Primary Glomerular Diseases

These can be acute or chronic and include membranoproliferative glomerulonephritis, focal glomerulosclerosis, membranous nephropathy, focal glomerulonephritis, Alport's syndrome and IgA nephropathy. Acute glomerulonephritis is a rare complication in pregnancy but can present in a similar way to preeclampsia; hence its diagnosis can be missed or delayed, with potentially serious consequences (43,90).

The consensus of opinion in chronic glomerular disease is that in most cases pregnancy does not adversely affect the natural course of the disease (32,50,91–93). In a minority, accelerated renal impairment occurs, and this may be associated with certain types of glomerular disease, such as membranoproliferative glomerulonephritis (94).

Primary glomerular disease is associated with an increased incidence of spontaneous abortion, prematurity, low birth weight, and perinatal mortality. In general, however, the outcome is favorable, with a fetal viability of approximately 75% if renal function is preserved (91,95,96). Certain conditions are associated with a poorer outcome. Membranous nephropathy has a low incidence of complications (fetal loss rate of <10%) (95,97,98), but conditions such as membranoproliferative glomerulonephritis (MPGN) and focal glomerulosclerosis have higher rates of obstetric complications (94). Despite this, even in MPGN type II, which normally has a poor prognosis due to the development of end-stage renal disease, uneventful pregnancy has been reported in the absence of renal insufficiency or hypertension (99).

The coexistence of hypertension or impaired renal function with glomerular disease is associated with a poor obstetric outcome. Hypertension as a new complication occurs in 20% of pregnant women with glomerulonephritis and a worsening of preexisting hypertension is seen in approximately 15% (91,98,100).

Abe et al. confirmed that normal women and those with a GFR >70 mL/min had a normal delivery rate of 79% compared with 36 to 50% if the pregnancy was complicated by renal impairment of hypertension (95). They concluded that certain criteria were associated with a more favorable outcome such as blood pressure <140/90, GFR >70 mL/min, serum creatinine <1.1 mg/dL (100 μmol/L) and certain histological types of disease. The histological type of primary glomerulonephritis is not, however, thought to be as important a prognostic indicator as the presence of proteinuria, hypertension, and renal impairment (92).

Pregnancy does not appear to have a negative impact on the natural progression of IgA nephropathy (57,73,101) although worsening of renal function has been reported (102). In general, pregnancy complications or a decline in renal function are rare unless preconceptual GFR is <70 mL/min or hypertension is present. It should be noted that individual patients with IgA nephropathy may demonstrate an unpredictable or irreversible deterioration in renal function (103).

X. PREPREGNANCY COUNSELING AND ANTENATAL CARE OF WOMEN WITH CHRONIC RENAL DISEASE OR CHRONIC HYPERTENSION

Women with chronic renal disease and/or chronic hypertension should be encouraged not to delay pregnancy. Renal function declines with age, and the evidence suggests that fetal prognosis is good if renal function is not impaired. Pregnancy may not be advisable in women whose prepregnancy serum creatinine is >2.0 mg/dL (180 μmol/L) or those who have poorly controlled hypertension (DBP >100 mmHg). Termination of pregnancy may be advisable in cases of rapidly deteriorating renal function or with severe lupus nephropathy in the first trimester of pregnancy (43,57). Specific prepregnancy guidelines for renal allograft recipients are well documented (64) (see Table 7).

Table 7 Prepregnancy Counseling Guidelines for Renal Transplant Recipients

Good posttransplantation health for 2 years
No or minimal proteinuria
No (or well-controlled) hypertension
No evidence of graft rejection
No pelvicalyceal distention apparent on IVU/ultrasound
Stable renal function (serum creatinine < 180 μmol/L (2.0 mg/dL) and preferably < 125 μmol/L (1.4 mg/dL))
Maintenance prednisolone < 15 mg/day, azathioprine < 2 mg/kg/day and cyclosporine < 5 mg/kg/day
Stature compatible with good obstetric outcome

Ideally, a full physical examination should be performed before pregnancy or in early gestation along with routine baseline biochemistry and urinalysis. This should include urine culture, blood urea and electrolytes, urate, glucose, creatinine clearance and 24-hour urine protein excretion. Pheochromocytoma and Conn's syndrome (primary aldosteronism) should be excluded if the woman is hypertensive. In patients with significant proteinuria or hypertension, an electrocardiogram, chest x-ray, and/or echocardiogram may be required. A good prognostic indicator for hypertension in the later stages of pregnancy is the BP in the second trimester (10).

Women with chronic renal disease or chronic hypertension should ideally be seen every 2 weeks until 28 to 32 weeks and then weekly until term. Fetal growth and well-being should be assessed regularly by serial ultrasonography and biophysical monitoring. Hypertension must be controlled; alpha methyldopa or labetalol are suggested as the initial drug options, although other drugs may ultimately be required. Attempts must be made to identify the onset of superimposed preeclampsia and to differentiate it from worsening renal disease or chronic hypertension. Nephrotic syndrome is a known complication of renal disease and preeclampsia; in these cases a low-sodium diet may be appropriate.

If renal function deteriorates at any stage of pregnancy, reversible causes should be considered. Toward term, a 15 to 20% reduction in renal function is acceptable if there is only a minimal effect on serum creatinine (43,104). If a reversible cause is not evident, expediting delivery (often following steroid administration for fetal lung maturity) should be considered.

Vaginal delivery should be the aim, but cesarean section may be required for obstetric reasons. Given the reduced clearance of nonvolatile acid, fetuses of women with renal disease do not tolerate labor as well as those of women with normal kidneys. Fetal status should thus be continuously monitored during labor. Preterm delivery is common (45–60%); therefore good pediatric facilities should be available. Even after delivery, women with chronic renal disease, superimposed preeclampsia, and/or underlying cardiovascular disease are at especially high risk of complications such as renal failure, pulmonary edema, and encephalopathy.

REFERENCES

1. Redman CWG, Sacks GP, Sargent IL. Preeclampsia: An excessive maternal inflammatory response to pregnancy. Am J Obstet Gynecol 1999; 180:499–506.
2. Roberts JM, Taylor RN, Musci TJ, Rodgers GM, Hubel CA, McLaughlin MK. Preeclampsia: An endothelial cell disorder. Am J Obstet Gynecol 1989; 161:1200–1204.
3. Dekker GA, Sibai BM. Etiology and pathogenesis of preeclampsia: Current concepts. Am J Obstet Gynecol 1998; 179:1359–1375.

4. Norwitz ER, Repke JT. Preeclampsia prevention and management. J Soc Gynecol Invest 2000; 7:21–36.
5. Davey DA, MacGillivray I. The classification and definition of the hypertensive disorders of pregnancy. Clin Exp Hypertens 1986; B5:97–113.
6. Brown MA, Whitworth JA. Recording diastolic blood pressure in pregnancy. Br Med J 1991; 303:120–121.
7. Roberts JM, Redman CWG. Preeclampsia: More than pregnancy-induced hypertension. Lancet 1993; 341:1447–1454.
8. Rayburn WF, Schnoor TA, Brown DL, Smith CV. "White coat" hypertension during pregnancy. Hypertens Pregnancy 1993; 12(2):191–197.
9. McGowan LME, Buist RG, North RA, Gamble G. Perinatal morbidity in chronic hypertension. Br J Obstet Gynaecol 1996; 103:123–129.
10. Sibai BM. Diagnosis and management of chronic hypertension in pregnancy. Obstet Gynecol 1991; 78:451–461.
11. Sibai BM, Lindheimer M, Hauth J, Caritis S, VanDorsten P, Klebanoff M, et al. Risk factors for preeclampsia, abruptio placentae, and adverse neonatal outcomes among women with chronic hypertension. N Engl J Med 1998; 339(10):667–671.
12. Halligan AWF, Bell SC, Taylor DJ. Dipstick Proteinuria: Caveat emptor. Br J Obstet Gynaecol 1999; 106:1113–1115.
13. Spargo BH, McCartney C, Winemiller R. Glomerular capillary endotheliosis in toxaemia of pregnancy. Arch Pathol 1959; 13:593–599.
14. Furukawa T, Shigematsu H, Aizawa T, Oguchi H, Furuta S. Residual glomerular lesions in postpartum women with toxaemia of pregnancy. Acta Pathol Jpn 1983; 33: 1159–1169.
15. Fisher KA, Luger A, Spargo BH, Lindheimer MD. Hypertension in pregnancy: Clinico-pathological correlation and late prognosis. Medicine 1981; 60:267–276.
16. Gaber LW, Spargo BH, Lindheimer MD. Renal pathology in preeclampsia. In: Lindheimer MD, Davison JM, eds. Renal Disease in Pregnancy. Baillières Clinical Obstetrics and Gynecology. London: Baillière Tindall 1994; 443–468.
17. Conrad KP, Lindheimer MD. Renal and cardiovascular alterations. In: Lindheimer MD, Roberts JM, Cunningham FG, eds. Chesley's Hypertensive Disorders in Pregnancy, 2nd ed. Stamford, CT: Appleton & Lange, 1999: 263–326.
18. Naicker T, Randeree IGH, Moodley J, et al. Correlation between histological changes and loss of amnionic charge of the glomerular basement membrane in early onset preeclampsia. Nephron 1997; 75:201–207.
19. Lafayette RA, Malik T, Druzin M, Derby G, Myers BD. The dynamics of glomerular filtration after cesarean section. J Am Soc Nephrol 1999; 10:1561–1565.
20. Bar J, Kaplan B, Wittenberg C, et al. Microalbuminuria after pregnancy complicated by pre-eclampsia. Nephrol Dial Transplant 1999; 14:1129–1132.
21. Chesley LC. Remote prognosis. In: Hypertensive Disorders in Pregnancy. New York: Appleton-Century-Crofts, 1978: 421–443.
22. Sibai BM, Abdella TN, Anderson GD. Pregnancy outcome in 211 patients with mild chronic hypertension. Obstet Gynecol 1983; 61:571–576.
23. Redman CW, Beilin LJ, Bonnard J, Ounsted MK. Fetal outcome in trial of antihypertensive treatment in pregnancy. Lancet 1976; 2:753–756.

24. Sibai BM, Anderson GD. Pregnancy outcome of intensive therapy in severe hypertension in first trimester. Obstet Gynecol 1986; 67:517–522.
25. Rey E, Couturier A. The prognosis of pregnancy in women with chronic hypertension. Am J Obstet Gynecol 1994; 171:410–416.
26. Mabie WC, Pernoll ML, Biswas MK. Chronic hypertension in pregnancy. Obstet Gynecol 1986; 67:197–205.
27. Chesley LC, Annitto JE. Pregnancy in the patient with hypertensive disease. Am J Obstet Gynecol 1947; 53:372–381.
28. Landesman R, Holze W, Scherr L. Fetal mortality in essential hypertension. Obstet Gynecol 1955; 6:354–365.
29. Rey E. Preeclampsia and neonatal outcomes in chronic hypertension: Comparison between white and black women. Ethnicity Dis 1997; 7:5–11.
30. Taylor HC Jr, Tillman AJB, Blanchard J. Fetal losses in hypertension and preeclampsia. Part 1. Analysis of 4432 cases. Obstet Gynecol 1954; 3:225–239.
31. Redman CWG. Hypertension in pregnancy. In: De Swiet M, ed. Medical Disorders in Obstetric Practice, 3rd ed. Oxford: Blackwell Scientific, 1995: 182–225.
32. Lindheimer MD, Davison JM, Katz AI. The kidney and hypertension in pregnancy: Twenty exciting years. Semin Nephrol 2001; 21:173–189.
33. Von Dadelzen P, Ornstein MP, Bull SB, Logan AG, Koren G, Magee LA. Fall in mean arterial pressure and fetal growth restriction in pregnancy hypertension: a meta-analysis. Lancet 2000; 355:87–92.
34. Redman CWG, Roberts JM. Management of preeclampsia. Lancet 1993; 3:1451–1454.
35. Cockburn J, Moar VA, Ounsted M, Redman CWG. Final report of study on hypertension during pregnancy: the effects of specific treatment on the growth and development of the children. Lancet 1982; 1:647–649.
36. Hutton JD, James DK, Stirrat GM, et al. Management of severe preeclampsia and eclampsia by UK consultants. Br J Obstet Gynaecol 1992; 99:554–556.
37. Rossa FW, Bosco LA, Graham CF, et al. Neonatal anuria with maternal angiotensin converting enzyme inhibition. Obstet Gynecol 1989; 74:371–374.
38. Beaufils M, Uzan S, Donsimoni R, Colau JC. Prevention of preeclampsia by early platelet therapy. Lancet 1985; 2:840–842.
39. Duley L, Henderson-Smart D, Knight M, et al. Antiplatelet drugs for prevention of preeclampsia and its consequences: Systematic review. Br Med J 2001; 322: 329–333.
40. Lindheimer MD. Pre-eclampsia-eclampsia 1996: Preventable? Have disputes on its treatment been resolved? Curr Opin Nephrol Hypertens 1996; 5:452–458.
41. Roberts JM, Hubel CA. Is oxidative stress the link in the two-stage model of preeclampsia. Lancet 1999; 354:817.
42. Chappell LC, Seed PT, Briley AL, Kelly FJ, Lee R, Hunt BJ, et al. Effect of antioxidants on the occurrence of preeclampsia in women at increased risk: A randomised trial. Lancet 1999; 354:810–816.
43. Davison JM, Katz AI, Lindheimer MD. Kidney disease and pregnancy: Obstetric outcome and long-term renal prognosis. Clin Perinatol 1985; 12(3):497–519.
44. Katz AI, Davison JM, Hayslett JP, Singson E, Lindheimer MD. Pregnancy in women with kidney disease. Kidney Int 1980; 18:192–206.
45. Jungers P, Houillier P, Forget D, Henry-Amar M. Specific controversies concerning

the natural history of renal disease in pregnancy. Am J Kidney Dis 1991; 17(2): 116–122.

46. Abe S. Pregnancy in IgA nephropathy. Kidney Int 1991; 40:1098–1102.
47. Studd JWW, Blainey JD. Pregnancy and the nephrotic syndrome. Br Med J 1969; 1: 276–280.
48. Williams DJ. Renal disease in pregnancy. Curr Obstet Gynaecol 1997; 7:156–162.
49. Bear RA. Pregnancy in patients with renal disease: a study of 44 cases. Obstet Gynecol 1976; 48(1):13–18.
50. Davison JM. Renal disorders in pregnancy. Curr Opin Obstet Gynecol 2001; 13: 109–114.
51. Hou SH, Grossman SD, Madias NE. Pregnancy in women with renal disease and moderate renal insufficiency. Am J Med 1985; 78(2):185–194.
52. Imbasciati E, Pardi G, Capetta P, Ambroso G, Bozzetti P, Pagliari B, et al. Pregnancy in women with chronic renal failure. Am J Nephrol 1986; 6:193–198.
53. Cunningham G, Cox SM, Harstad TW, Mason RA, Pritchard JA. Chronic renal disease and pregnancy outcome. Am J Obstet Gynecol 1990; 163:453–459.
54. Jones DC, Hayslett JP. Outcome of pregnancy in women with moderate or severe renal insufficiency. N Engl J Med 1996; 335:226–232.
55. Epstein FH. Pregnancy and renal disease. N Engl J Med 1996; 335:277–278.
56. Jungers P, Chauveau D. Pregnancy in renal disease. Kidney Int 1997; 52:871–885.
57. Jones DC. Pregnancy complicated by chronic renal disease. Clin Perinatol 1997; 24(2):483–496.
58. Schaefer RM, Kokot F, Wernze H, Geiger H, Heidland A. Improved sexual function in hemodialysis patients on recombinant erythropoietin: A possible role for prolactin. Clin Nephrol 1989; 31:1–5.
59. Hou SH. Frequency and outcome of pregnancy in women on dialysis. Am J Kidney Dis 1994; 23:60.
60. Redrow M, Cherem L, Elliott J, et al. Dialysis in the management of pregnant patients with renal insufficiency. Medicine 1988; 67:199.
61. Williams DJ. The implications of pre-existing renal disease in pregnancy. Curr Obstet Gynaecol 1999; 9:75–81.
62. Registration Committee of the European Dialysis and transplant association: Successful pregnancies in women treated by dialysis and kidney transplantation. Br J Obstet Gynaecol 1980; 87:839–845.
63. Souqiyyeh MZ, Huraib SO, Saleh AG, Aswad S. Pregnancy in chronic hemodialysis patients in the kingdom of Saudi Arabia. Am J Kidney Dis 1992; 19:235–238.
64. Davison JM. Towards long-term graft survival in renal transplantation and pregnancy. Nephrol Dial Transplant 1995; 10:85–89.
65. Davison JM. Dialysis, transplantation and pregnancy. Am J Kidney Dis 1991; 17:127.
66. Davison JM. Pregnancy in renal allograft recipients: Problems, prognosis and practicalities. Baillières Clin Obstet Gynaecol 1994; 8:501–525.
67. Armenti VT, Moritz MJ, Davison JM, et al. Pregnancy and transplantation. Graft 2000; 3:49–63.
68. Ehrich JHH, Loirat C, Davison JM, Rizzoni G, Wittkop B, Selwood NH, et al. Repeated successful pregnancies after kidney transplantation in 102 women (Report by the EDTA registry). Nephrol Dial Transplant 1996; 11:1314–1317.

69. Sturgiss SN, Davison JM. Effect of pregnancy on long function of renal allografts: An update. Am J Kidney Dis 1995; 26:54–56.

70. Sturgiss SN, Davison JM. Perinatal outcome in renal allograft recipients: Prognostic significance of hypertension and renal function before and during pregnancy. Obstet Gynecol 1991; 78:573–577.

71. El-Khatib MT, Becker GJ, Kincaid-Smith PS. Reflux nephropathy and primary vesicoureteric reflux in adults. Q J Med 1990; 77:1241–1253.

72. Jungers P, Houillier P, Chaveau D, et al. Pregnancy in women with reflux nephropathy. Kidney Int 1996; 50:593–599.

73. Jungers P, Forget D, Houillier P, Henry-Amar M, Grunfeld JP. Pregnancy in IgA Nephropathy, reflux nephropathy, and focal glomerular sclerosis. Am J Kidney Dis 1987; 9(4):334–338.

74. Kincaid-Smith P, Fairley KF. Renal disease in pregnancy: Three controversial areas: mesangial IgA nephropathy, focal glomerular sclerosis (focal and segmental hyalinosis and sclerosis), and reflux nephropathy. Am J Kidney Dis 1987; 9:328.

75. Jungers P, Dougados M, Pelisseries C, et al. Lupus nephropathy and pregnancy. Arch Intern Med 1982; 142:771–776.

76. Out HJ, Derksen RHWM, Christiaens GCML. Systemic lupus erythematosus and pregnancy. Obstet Gynaecol Surv 1989; 44:585–591.

77. Hayslett JP, Lynn RI. Effect of pregnancy in patients with lupus nephropathy. Kidney Int 1980; 18:207.

78. Fine LG, Barnett EV, Danovitch GM, et al. Systemic lupus erythematosus in pregnancy. Ann Intern Med 1981; 94:667–677.

79. Imbasciati E, Surian M, Battino S, et al. Lupus nephropathy and pregnancy. A study of 26 pregnancies in patients with SLE and nephritis. Nephron 1984; 36:46–51.

80. Lê Thi Huong D, Wechsler B, Vauthier-Brouzes D, et al. Pregnancy in past or present lupus nephritis: A study of 32 pregnancies from a single center. Ann Rheum Dis 2001; 60:599–604.

81. Hayslett JP. The effect of SLE on pregnancy and pregnancy outcome. Am J Reprod Immunol 1992; 28:199.

82. Combs CA, Kitzmiller JL. Diabetic nephropathy and pregnancy. Obstet Gynecol 1991; 34(3):505–515.

83. Biesenbach G, Stoger H, Zazgornik J. Influence of pregnancy on progression of diabetic nephropathy and subsequent requirement of renal replacement therapy in female type 1 diabetic patients with impaired renal function. Nephrol Dial Transplant 1992; 7:105–109.

84. Biesenbach G, Grafinger P, Stoger H, Zazgornik J. How pregnancy influences renal function in nephropathic type 1 diabetic women depends on their pre-conceptual creatinine clearance. J Nephrol 1999; 12(1):41–46.

85. Garner P. Type 1 diabetes mellitus and pregnancy. Lancet 1995; 346:157–161.

86. Kitzmiller JL, Brown ER, Phillippe M, et al. Diabetic nephropathy and perinatal outcome. Am J Obstet Gynecol 1981; 141:741–751.

87. Hare JW, White P. Pregnancy in diabetes complicated by vascular disease. Diabetes 1977; 26:953–955.

88. Leguizaman G, Reece EA. Effect of medical therapy on progressive nephropathy: Influence of pregnancy, diabetes and hypertension. J Matern Fetal Med 2000; 9: 70–78.

89. Garner PR, D'Alton ME, Dudley DK, Huard P, Hardie M. Preeclampsia in diabetic
     pregnancies. Am J Obstet Gynecol 1990; 163:505–508.
90. Shepherd J, Shepherd C. Poststreptococcal glomerulonephritis: A rare complication
     of pregnancy. J Fam Pract 1992; 34:625–632.
91. Barcelo P, Lopez-Lillo J, Cabero L, Del Rio G. Successful pregnancy in primary
     glomerular disease. Kidney Int 1986; 30:914–919.
92. Abe S. An overview of pregnancy in women with underlying renal disease. Am J
     Kidney Dis 1991; 17(2):112–115.
93. Jungers P, Houillier P, Forget D, et al. Influence of pregnancy on the course of
     primary chronic glomerulonephritis. Lancet 1995; 346:1122.
94. Surian M, Imbasciati E, Cosci P, Banfi G, Barbiano di Belgiojoso G, Brancaccio D,
     et al. Glomerular disease and pregnancy: A study of 123 pregnancies in patients with
     primary and secondary glomerular diseases. Nephron 1984; 36:101–105.
95. Abe S, Amagasaki Y, Konishi K, Kato E, Sakaguchi H, Iyori S. The influence of
     antecedent renal disease on pregnancy. Am J Obstet Gynecol 1985; 153:508–514.
96. Alexopoulos E, Bili H, Tampakoudis P, Economidou D, Sakellariou G, Mantalenakis
     S, et al. Outcome of pregnancy in women with glomerular diseases. Renal Failure
     1996; 18(1):121–129.
97. Cameron JS, Hicks J. Pregnancy in patients with preexisting glomerular disease.
     Contr Nephrol 1984; 37:149–156.
98. Jungers P, Forget D, Henry-Amar M, Albouze G, Fournier P, Vischer U, et al.
     Chronic kidney disease and pregnancy. Adv Nephrol 1986; 15:103–141.
99. Inaba S, Tanizawa T, Igarashi T, Higuchi A, Satou H, Mase D, et al. Long-term
     follow-up of membranoproliferative glomerulonephritis type II and pregnancy: A
     case report. Clin Nephrol 1989; 32:10–13.
100. Packham DK, North R, Fairley KF, Kloss M, Whitworth JA, Kincaid-Smith P.
     Primary glomerulonephritis and pregnancy. Q J Med 1989; 71(266):537–553.
101. Abe S. The influence of pregnancy on the long-term renal prognosis of IgA nephrop-
     athy. Clin Nephrol 1994; 41(2):61–64.
102. Packham DK, North RA, Fairley KF, Whitworth JA, Kincaid-Smith P. IgA glomer-
     ulonephritis and pregnancy. Clin Nephrol 1988; 30(1):15–21.
103. Becker GJ, Fairley KF, Whitworth JA. Pregnancy exacerbates glomerular disease.
     Am J Kidney Dis 1985; 6:266–272.
104. Davison JM, Dunlop W. Changes in renal haemodynamics and tubular function
     induced by normal human pregnancy. Semin Nephrol 1984; 4:198–207.

7

HELLP Syndrome: The Scope of Disease and Treatment

James N. Martin, Jr.
University of Mississippi Medical Center, Jackson, Mississippi, U.S.A.

Everett F. Magann
University of Western Australia, Perth, Australia

Christy M. Isler
Brody School of Medicine, East Carolina University, Greenville, North Carolina, U.S.A.

I. INTRODUCTION

Considered to be part of the broad continuum of maternal disease inclusive within preeclampsia/eclampsia, HELLP syndrome is a serious pregnancy disorder characterized by laboratory evidence of abnormal interaction between the microvasculature and circulating constituents of blood. This produces thrombocytopenia, microangiopathic hemolytic anemia, and the release of cellular breakdown products, particularly from the liver, including transaminases and lactate dehydrogenase. It is a hallmark of critical illness in a pregnant patient with potentially serious sequelae. HELLP syndrome has been termed "atypical" preeclampsia, since the magnitude of maternal hypertension and proteinuria usually do not directly reflect the extent of the underlying pathophysiology.

II. BACKGROUND AND HISTORICAL

Weinstein is credited with naming this unique variant of severe preeclampsia in 1982 with the acronym HELLP syndrome (H, hemolysis; EL, elevated liver enzymes; LP, low platelets)(1). In reality, the entity of preeclampsia-eclampsia complicated by microthrombi and coagulopathy had been described as early as the nineteenth century as a condition affecting multiple organ systems, often with lethal outcome (2–13). In the three decades prior to Weinstein's report, a number of investigative groups reported patient experiences that would probably be recognized today as some form of atypical preeclampsia or HELLP syndrome. Dilemmas about diagnosis persist because the laboratory components of HELLP syndrome can be encountered not only as a primary expression of preeclampsia but also as a secondary phenomenon in patients with complicated sepsis, acute respiratory distress syndrome (ARDS)/acute lung injury, renal failure, and multiple organ disease with disseminated intravascular coagulopathy (DIC). Also potentially confounding the diagnosis are catastrophic obstetric misadventures including extensive placental abruption and amniotic fluid embolism in patients with underlying preeclampsia which, due to their inherent pathophysiology, can present confusing clinical pictures reminiscent of HELLP syndrome.

III. TERMINOLOGY AND LABORATORY DIAGNOSIS

The years since Weinstein's publication have seen a burgeoning literature and a growing knowledge base reflective of the great interest in this pregnancy complication. Terminology and diagnostic criteria used to describe and diagnose the syndrome have been inconsistent and confusing. This is in part due to differences in laboratory testing methods, disagreements regarding laboratory thresholds for disease diagnosis, heterogeneity among patient presentations, and variations in sampling times during the course of disease.

Fundamentally there are three general diagnostic criteria required to make the laboratory diagnosis of HELLP syndrome (Table 1) (14–16). First, most patients exhibit microangiopathic changes, which are evident on peripheral blood smear but do not necessarily correlate with clinical signs of disease severity such as degree of hypertension and/or proteinuria. The fragmented red cells observed are termed schistocytes, burr cells, and fragmentocytes. Their appearance is indistinguishable from that observed with other thrombotic microangiopathies such as thrombotic thrombocytopenic purpura (TTP) and hemolytic uremic syndrome (HUS). The degree of microangiopathic hemolytic anemia appears to correlate with the extent of small vessel involvement and subsequent endothelial dysfunction. Intravascular hemolysis is considered to result from mechanical damage to red blood cells, in part by intimal abnormalities of the microcirculation compounded by segmental vasospasm. Fibrin deposition along the swollen endothelial cells probably injures or destroys red blood cells that are passing through the affected vasculature at high velocity. A change in the membrane fluidity of erythrocytes by a decrease in deformability could play a role in the process (17).

As a consequence of hemolysis, serum indirect bilirubin and total lactate

Table 1 Diagnosis of HELLP Syndrome

Nonspecific signs/symptoms
  Nausea/vomiting/mild headache/malaise/exhaustion
Signs/symptoms of preeclampsia
  Epigastric pain/proteinuria/hypertension
  Hyperuricemia/edema
Evidence of intravascular hemolysis
  Increased LDH, AST, indirect bilirubin
  Decreased haptoglobin
  Peripheral smear demonstrates fragmented erythrocytes (burr/schistocytes)
  Urinary urobilinogen
Evidence of hepatocyte injury/dysfunction
  Increased ALT, AST, LDH
Thrombocytopenia
  Platelets ≤ 150,000/μL

---

dehydrogenase increase and serum haptoglobin decreases (18–23). Haptoglobin has been reported to decrease earlier than any other available lab parameter (24). Patients with elevated lactate dehydrogenase tend to have abnormal peripheral smears. A rise in the reticulocyte count is also expected. Other markers of hemolysis include elevated urine urobilinogen. In severe cases, evidence of fibrin consumption and developing disseminated intravascular coagulopathy (DIC) will coexist with the microangiopathic hemolytic anemia as a late, advanced phase of HELLP syndrome.

The second criterion for HELLP syndrome is elevated liver enzymes indicative of hepatic cell injury and dysfunction. The majority of investigators rely on elevated transaminases for this criterion, primarily aspartate aminotransferase (AST) (25). Both AST and alanine aminotransferase (ALT) are present in high concentration in hepatocytes, leaking into the circulation when hepatocytes or their cell membranes are damaged (25). ALT is the more specific marker of hepatocellular injury, since it is confined to the cytoplasm of hepatocytes. In contrast, AST is found in mitochondria and the cytoplasm of hepatocytes as well as heart, skeletal muscle, kidney, brain, pancreas and erythrocytes. Serum concentrations of AST and ALT are raised to different degrees in almost all forms of liver disease. Serum levels are highly variable and are determined by the intracellular concentration and source of the enzymes, the amount leaked from the cell, and the rate of clearance from the circulation. Serum concentrations are thus not necessarily a reliable index of the severity of hepatic injury, and neither of the aminotransferases alone is an ideal marker of hepatocyte injury. During active HELLP syndrome the ratio of AST to ALT is often 2:1 or higher, whereas with disease recovery the ratio returns to 1:1 or even reverses (23).

Differences among reference and hospital laboratories compound comparisons between published papers and individual practice environments (26). Most healthy pregnant patients do not develop transaminases in excess of 39 IU/L; therefore ⩾40 IU/L in our hospital system is considered borderline abnormal. Values of AST of ⩾70 IU/L are clearly abnormal and strong evidence of hepatic dysfunction in patients with suspected HELLP syndrome. The possibility that increased transaminases could result from extrahepatic sources may explain the mixed pattern seen in some patients (27–31). Although there is evidence to suggest that abnormalities in liver function tests do not reliably reflect the degree of liver injury, extreme elevations have been associated with increased risk for the development of significant maternal morbidity (32). The plasma concentration of human hepatocyte growth factor has been cited by one investigator as useful in the early detection of HELLP syndrome and as a laboratory marker of the clinical severity of the disorder (33).

The third criterion for HELLP syndrome is thrombocytopenia. It is the earliest laboratory change of the disease that can be detected by commonly available laboratory testing (23). The traditionally accepted definition of thrombocytopenia is a platelet count ⩽150,000/mL, subdivided into three subgroups of 100,000 to 150,000/mL for mild thrombocytopenia, 50,000 to 100,000/mL for moderate, and <50,000/mL for severe thrombocytopenia. Nevertheless, Sibai prefers that a threshold of ⩽100,000/mL be achieved to comfortably consider the diagnosis of HELLP syndrome. This is in part to differentiate HELLP syndrome from the more benign gestational thrombocytopenia, and in part because the threshold for significant peril to the mother and fetus with HELLP syndrome probably exists at a platelet count ≪100,000/mL (14).

IV. PATHOGENESIS

As with preeclampsia, the origins and essential pathogenesis of HELLP syndrome remain poorly understood (Table 2). Both are later pregnancy complications probably reflective of a gestational disruption of normal early events that begins with abnormal implantation and ends only after the placenta and its supporting

Table 2 Pathogenesis of HELLP Syndrome

Unknown specific triggering event
Perturbation of endothelial homeostasis
Altered platelet and erythrocyte activaton/endothelial interactions
Inflammatory response
Increased oxidative stress/decreased free radical scavenging capacity
Enhanced pressor sensitivity

decidua are removed from the mother. The uteroplacental unit is believed to become dysfunctional, presumably secondary to abnormalities in development of an adequate vascular base via decidualization of the spiral arteries. As a consequence, at some time in the second half of pregnancy, increasing ischemia of the placenta may produce oxidative stress, which triggers the release of factor(s) that systemically injure the endothelium with activation of platelets, vasoconstrictors, and loss of normal pregnancy vascular relaxation (34–40). Finger microcirculation studies with laser-Doppler fluxometry in patients with HELLP syndrome reveal lower basal skin blood flow and a high oscillation of skin blood flow postulated to be due to enhanced sensitivity to pressors (41).

Rates of progression of disease and the profile of clinical and laboratory expression of disease are highly variable among patients, but they are usually rapid and progressive after a slow initial phase. The extent of the decrease in total glutathione levels in maternal whole blood might correlate with the risk of developing the disease and its progression. Whole blood total glutathione levels are variably lower in pregnant women with HELLP syndrome, possibly indicating decreased detoxification or free radical scavenging capacity (42,43). In addition, intracellular retention of cadherin-5 appears to be increased in response to HELLP syndrome, thus decreasing the number of adhesion complexes in the cell membrane, and possibly increasing vascular permeability (44).

The pathogenesis of HELLP syndrome may involve complement-induced release of bioactive substances from activated leukocytes such as that observed in patients with sepsis, trauma, or acute lung injury (45–47). These vasoactive substances, including endothelin, probably cause the microvascular injury as well as the endothelial damage and dysfunction that underlie the myriad signs and symptoms of preeclampsia with or without HELLP syndrome (36–40,48,49). HELLP syndrome has been suggested to be an inflammatory process, in part because of the observed correlation between the degree of leukocytosis and the severity of the syndrome at initial clinical presentation (50). Abnormal cytokine expression in patients with HELLP syndrome has also been reported. It is hypothesized that cytokine- and neutrophil-mediated liver injury could be operative in patients with this disease process (51,52). The finding of increased bioactive tumor necrosis factor α in patients with HELLP syndrome raises the possibility of its involvement in the endothelial injury associated with this condition (53). In addition, decreased antioxidant activity may be one of the mediators of endothelial cell damage (54–56). Ibdah suggested that a recessively inherited disorder of mitochondrial fatty acid oxidation could manifest itself initially as HELLP syndrome or as acute fatty liver of pregnancy (57). Polymorphisms in the genes of biotransformation enzymes (detoxification/lipid peroxidation) do not seem to influence the risk of developing HELLP syndrome (58).

It is likely that HELLP syndrome represents a disordered immunologic process either as a primary or a secondary event (59–62). Increased plasma concentrations of anaphylatoxins C3a and C5a have been demonstrated in patients with preeclampsia/HELLP syndrome compared to controls (63). Depression of both T- and B-cell potential and impaired monocyte handling of intracellular pathogens have been reported in patients with HELLP syndrome preceding the diagnosis by 7 to 14 days (64). Moreover, platelet antibodies have been reported in a small number of patients and newborns. Passive transfer of the disease to the fetus has been claimed in some instances where fetal thrombocytopenia and microangiopathic hemolytic anemia have been diagnosed in the fetuses of mothers with HELLP syndrome (65). It is possible that immune thrombocytopenic purpura and HELLP syndrome may coexist to produce a confounding clinical picture for both mother and child.

In addition to the decreased platelet count, there appear to be qualitative as well as quantitative considerations to platelet assessment in HELLP syndrome. An increase in platelet aggregation and size predates the development of preeclampsia by 2 to 5 weeks (66–67). The normal life span of a platelet is 8 to 10 days; but in pregnancies complicated by preeclampsia, the life span can be reduced to 3 to 5 days (68,69). A further reduction in platelet life span, structural integrity, and altered platelet membrane function is observed in patients with HELLP syndrome, probably due to enhanced platelet adherence to damaged vascular endothelium (70,71). The cycle is likely to be self-perpetuating. Release of arachidonic acid and vasoactive amines during this pathological platelet-endothelium interaction leads to peripheral vasoconstriction and hypertension (71,72).

Although the serum concentration of platelet activating factor (PAF), a potent activator of platelet aggregation, is not altered by preeclampsia, the serum inhibition of its activity is reduced, with variable effects on systemic platelet aggregation (73).

Compensation by the bone marrow occurs with increased production and release of large young platelets into the vascular system. Ultimately, there is a decline in the platelet count because release cannot keep pace with consumption (74). During normal pregnancy the platelet count gradually decreases toward term, a phenomenon that may be dilutional without a compensatory thrombopoietic response (75). β-thromboglobulin, a platelet-specific protein increases with platelet aggregation. Increased serum β-thromboglobulin in patients with preeclampsia reflects both the extent of platelet consumption in the microvasculature and altered clearance by the kidney (76). Since antigenic levels of tissue-type plasminogen activator and type 1 plasminogen activator inhibitors are reportedly much higher in patients with HELLP syndrome compared to controls, it appears that platelet activation and alterations in plasminogen activation are involved (77). Following delivery, there is a slow rise in the platelet count as the exhausted and consumed platelets are replaced by new ones.

There is a growing body of evidence to suggest that marked perturbations in lipid and lipoprotein metabolism could be operative in the pathogenesis of HELLP syndrome as well as preeclampsia and acute fatty liver of pregnancy (78). A specific accumulation of large triglyceride-rich very low density lipoprotein (VLDL) in the circulation of women with preeclampsia has been reported. It is likely that triglycerides accumulate in hepatocytes when the liver's ability to produce VLDL is saturated, and these appear as microvesicular fat droplets more densely in HELLP syndrome patients than in those with preeclampsia. The density of hepatocellular fat is negatively correlated with the platelet count, and positively correlated with plasma urate. Other evidence to support the role of impaired hepatic function in the pathogenesis of HELLP syndrome includes (1) the possible association between Gilbert's syndrome and HELLP syndrome; (2) the increased incidence of preeclampsia in two Norwegian families with hereditary abnormal mitochondrial function; and (3) the observation that about 20% of patients with HELLP syndrome have persistent postpartum impairment of bilirubin-conjugation while other functions normalize (78).

The role of the red blood cell, if any, in HELLP syndrome has not been fully elucidated. There is a possibility that HELLP syndrome may result from abnormal erythrocyte and endothelial interaction. This hypothesis is supported by findings in the spontaneously hypertensive rat (79) and the work by Kaibara's group (80) in Japan who showed that the hypercoagulability of blood in preeclampsia is strongly related to red blood cell alterations.

The hematological and vascular changes that have been associated with HELLP syndrome may be the result of a genetically based disorder in vascular homeostasis that becomes unmasked or expressed during pregnancy (81). Activated protein C resistance resulting from a mutation in coagulation factor V has emerged as a leading cause of thrombosis in pregnancy, and one group has reported a link between HELLP syndrome and the factor V R506Q mutation (82–85). Others have not found evidence of hemostatic abnormalities in a large number of patients with HELLP syndrome (86). There may be other unrecognized genetic factors since approximately 20 to 40% of women with HELLP syndrome exhibit evidence of preeclampsia/HELLP syndrome in subsequent pregnancies (87–89). Ethnic variation related to HELLP syndrome may exist but due to small study samples this issue remains unresolved (90). There does not appear to be any significant degree of seasonal variation in disease occurrence (91). A thickened gallbladder wall has been claimed to be a progenitor of HELLP syndrome (92). Another group has evidence suggesting an association of HELLP syndrome with glucose intolerance and autoimmunity (93).

V. INCIDENCE

HELLP syndrome complicates up to 30% of pregnancies with severe pre-eclampsia or eclampsia encountered in a tertiary referral center. Due to referral bias, with most published studies from tertiary care centers, and because of difficulties with the diagnosis, the true incidence of HELLP syndrome is difficult to determine. We estimate from the available data that approximately 1 per 1000 pregnancies in the United States is affected.

VI. PATIENT SERIES AND DISEASE CLASSIFICATION

Investigators at the Universities of Mississippi (Jackson) and Tennessee (Memphis) in the United States have contributed the two largest published patient series and profiles of pregnancies complicated by HELLP syndrome (14,15,23,32,94–98). Much of what is known about this condition is based on this large patient experience, which constitutes a pair of retrospective case series descriptive of the maternal and perinatal outcomes of more than 1000 patients and their progeny (Tables 3 and 4). In both institutions, patients with preeclampsia/eclampsia are considered to have HELLP syndrome if the maternal platelet count is ≤100,000/μL, total serum lactic dehydrogenase is ≥600 IU/L (normal pregnancy range <<400 IU/L), and serum transaminase, either as aspartate (AST, SGOT) or alanine (ALT, SGPT), is ≥70 IU/L (normal pregnancy range <40 IU/L).

In the Mississippi classification system for HELLP syndrome, patients are further subdivided according to the lowest observed perinatal platelet count into class 1 HELLP syndrome if there is severe thrombocytopenia (nadir platelet count ≤50,000/μL) or class 2 HELLP syndrome if there is moderate thrombocytopenia (nadir platelet count between >50,000/μL and ≤100,000/μL). This classification scheme was formulated because the two commonly available laboratory tests of HELLP syndrome, maternal platelet count and, to a lesser extent, total serum

Table 3 Mississippi and Tennessee HELLP Series

	Series	
	Mississippi	Tennessee
Numbers of patients	Class 1, 201	Class 1 and 2, 509
	Class 2, 300	Partial, 71
	Class 3, 276	
	Severe PET, 193	Severe PET, 178
Years of study	1980–1997	1977–1995
Gestation	20–42 weeks	10% < 27 weeks,
		33% postpartum
Maternal deaths	3 (0.4%)	6 (1%)
References	AJOG 168: 386, 1993	AJOG 169: 1000, 1993
	AJOG 180: 1373, 1999	AJOG 175: 460, 1996

Table 4   HELLP Syndrome: Triple
Class System

Class 1
  Platelets ≤ 50,000/μL
  Total serum LDH ≥ 600 IU/L
  AST and/or ALT ≥ 70 IU/L
Class 2
  Platelets > 50,000 but ≤ 100,000/μL
  Total serum LDH ≥ 600 IU/L
  AST and/or ALT ≥ 70 IU/L
Class 3
  Platelets > 100,000 but ≤ 150,000/μL
  Total serum LDH ≥ 600 IU/L
  AST and/or ALT ≥ 40 IU/L

LDH, appear to be very reflective of HELLP syndrome disease severity and the rapidity of recovery (96). The threshold for abnormality of LDH at >600 IU/L is based upon the laboratory utilizing the pyruvate-to-lactate assay as opposed to the lactate-to-pyruvate system (threshold 200 IU/l), which we used until mid-1993 (26).

The Memphis and Mississippi groups both recognize the existence of a transitional group of patients: those at Mississippi with mild thrombocytopenia >100,000/μL but ≤150,000/μL, total serum LDH ≥600 IU/L, and transaminase(s) ≥40 IU/L are classified as having class 3 HELLP syndrome (98), whereas at Tennessee patients are considered to have incomplete or "partial" HELLP syndrome if any portion of the full laboratory criteria is incompletely met (99). HELLP syndrome patients identified as class 3 (or incomplete) generally exhibit disease that is mild and intermediate between patients with complete disease (class 1 and 2) and patients with severe preeclampsia without components of HELLP syndrome. Recently, Abbade and colleagues demonstrated that their 43 patients with partial HELLP syndrome treated between 1991 and 1995 developed more eclampsia, prematurity, small for gestational age, and low-birth-weight (LBW) babies than control patients with preeclampsia (100).

VII. SIGNS AND SYMPTOMS OF DISEASE

Faridi and Rath are correct in their assertion that "all pregnant women with upper abdominal pain irrespective of symptoms (and signs) of preeclampsia should be considered to have HELLP syndrome" so that laboratory evaluation can be initiated (101). The onset of HELLP syndrome can be insidious, while some patients with the disease present as very ill. The major symptoms are nausea, vomiting, headache, and malaise. Patients with advanced disease may present with eclamptic seizures. In the absence of seizures, disease symptomatology can be confused with many other conditions, including viral syndromes, regional musculoskeletal problems, gastroenteritis, peptic ulcer disease, gallbladder disorders, hepatitis, pancreatitis, pyelonephritis, kidney stones, connective tissue disorders, and thrombotic microangiopathies. The primary problem with the diagnosis of HELLP syndrome is that patients frequently do not exhibit hypertension, proteinuria, and/or edema until the disorder is advanced. A small percentage of patients may never experience the classical triad of features. Thus a high index of suspicion is sometimes required to make the diagnosis. HELLP syndrome should be considered in women in the third trimester or early puerperium with new-onset thrombocytopenia. Preeclampsia is a disorder of young, nulliparous patients, while HELLP syndrome most frequently is encountered in older, multiparous patients (98). Although HELLP syndrome disease severity appears not to be influenced by parity, multiparous patients with eclampsia have a more complicated course when HELLP syndrome supervenes (102). While obesity appears to be a risk factor for preeclampsia, this is not the case with HELLP syndrome (103).

Pregnant women with hemolysis, hepatic dysfunction, and thrombocytopenia who do not have hypertension or proteinuria should undergo diagnostic evaluation to rule out other etiologies and, if negative, the patient is best managed with the presumption that she will eventually show clear evidence of severe preeclampsia complicated by HELLP syndrome (104).

The symptoms, signs, and degree of laboratory test abnormality can be used to assess the risk of adverse outcome (Table 5) (32). The presence at initial diagnosis of HELLP syndrome of nausea/vomiting or epigastric pain in association with LDH >1400 IU/L, AST >150 IU/L, ALT >100 IU/L, uric acid >7.8 mg/dL, serum creatinine >1mg/dL or 4+ urine proteinuria by dipstick are individually and collectively predictive of a higher risk for significant maternal morbidity. Concentrations of total serum LDH, AST, and uric acid above these cutoff points

Table 5 Admission Risk Factors for Severe Preeclampsia

Symptoms and signs	Laboratory investigations
Epigastric pain, nausea, vomiting	Platelets < 50,000/μL
Severe hypertension	LDH > 1400 IU/L
Placental abruption	AST > 150 IU/L
	ALT > 100 IU/L
	Uric acid > 7.8 mg/dl
	CPK > 200 IU/L
	Creatinine > 1.0

have the strongest predictive value and are risk additive with worsening thrombocytopenia (32).

It is worth emphasizing that the clinical manifestations of evolving, progressive HELLP syndrome differ from those of classical preeclampsia in several regards. Firstly, HELLP syndrome occurs before term in most cases. The disease has been described at various times from midgestation to several days following delivery (95,98,105). The majority of HELLP syndrome cases (70%) are encountered between 27 and 37 weeks' gestation, with approximately 10% occurring earlier and 20% later. Presentation in very early gestation has been described in association with fetal triploidy or maternal antiphospholipid syndrome (106–109). Secondly, in contrast to preeclampsia, HELLP syndrome more frequently afflicts multiparous patients. Thirdly, not all patients with HELLP syndrome exhibit hypertension and/or proteinuria at initial diagnosis and some may never have either of these features. Finally, unlike preeclampsia, approximately two-thirds of patients are diagnosed with HELLP syndrome prior to delivery while the other third present soon after delivery (14,98,110,111).

VIII. INITIAL LABORATORY SCREENING

Basic laboratory screening for the patient with suspected HELLP syndrome includes a complete blood count with platelets, total serum LDH, uric acid, serum creatinine, blood urea nitrogen, the serum transaminases AST/ALT, as well as urinalysis (with 24-hour urine collection if possible). Serum haptoglobin may be obtained if available. Coombs testing, bilirubin studies, and antithrombin III levels occasionally may be ordered if the diagnosis is in doubt (112,113). Serum fibrinogen, prothrombin time, partial thromboplastin time, and fibrin split products should be considered when the maternal platelet count is less than 75,000/mL, and it is well advised that these tests be ordered when the platelet count decreases below 50,000/mL. Electrolytes and glucose usually are not helpful. Since amphetamine and cocaine use can be associated with a syndrome similar to HELLP, a toxicology screen is advised when the physician is clinically suspicious of illicit drug use. Severe nutritional and folate deficiency can be associated with a clinical picture suggestive of HELLP syndrome and individuals at risk for these conditions should be appropriately investigated.

Testing for anticardiolipin antibody and lupus anticoagulant is appropriate in patients with very early onset HELLP syndrome in the second trimester (109,114). Similarly, evaluation for fetal chromosomal abnormality may explain the occurrence of HELLP syndrome prior to fetal viability, sometimes in association with abnormal midgestational biochemical screening (106–108,115).

Other evaluations may include screening for pancreatitis. Baseline arterial blood gases, pulse oximetry, chest x-ray, cultures of the urine and cervix, VDRL, hepatitis, and HIV testing are performed if appropriate. Frequent follow-up surveillance of maternal disease status is individualized with serial platelet counts and LDH/liver transaminases assessed every 8 to 24 hours until recovery is assured.

IX. NATURAL HISTORY OF THE DISEASE

Clinically, HELLP syndrome is often characterized by an initial slow phase of progression followed by an accelerated phase (23). A slowly decreasing platelet count is usually the initial abnormality detected, although a decrease in haptoglobin level may precede this (24). Mild thrombocytopenia can persist for a variable period of time before an accelerated phase ensues. The average daily reduction in the platelet count is 40,000/mL (23). The rate of fall may be as important as the actual platelet count (116). Modest elevations of total serum lactate dehydrogenase (LDH) and AST follow the appearance of mild thrombocytopenia, although some patients infrequently exhibit laboratory evidence of hepatic dysfunction out of proportion to the degree of thrombocytopenia. Disease expression worsens as the liver and vascular tree are progressively affected by microangiopathic hemolytic anemia. LDH to some extent reflects hemolysis and hepatic dysfunction, and thus LDH and platelet count are the two basic recommended tests for routine laboratory surveillance of patients with HELLP syndrome (23). Testing is usually undertaken at intervals of 6 to 12 hours during the acute phase of the disease.

In the absence of any pharmacological manipulation with glucocorticoids or transfusion of platelets, the maternal platelet count, total serum LDH, and transaminases usually worsen before improving following parturition. The platelet count in most gravid women with HELLP syndrome usually decreases until 1 to 2 days postpartum, but it rises within 72 hours. Recovery to more than 100,000/mL platelets usually occurs within 6 to 8 days postpartum (23,86,117–121). The average time for the platelet count to rise above 100,000/mL in patients with HELLP syndrome was 60 hours in one study, and nearly all patients had counts above this by 95 hours postpartum (122,123). Total serum LDH usually continues to rise postpartum for the first 24 to 48 hours, with normalization by the fourth postpartum day. The recovery of AST, ALT, and LDH usually follows the platelet count (23,96,124). Nocturnal blood pressure increases during the first week postpartum. This can persist up to 8 weeks and indicates a longer-lasting impact on endothelial and vascular function than suggested by the normalizing laboratory parameters (125).

Failure of an increase in platelets within 96 hours of delivery or the detection of a rapidly decreasing count may signal the development of a very serious, uncompensated disorder with multiorgan dysfunction (126). This condition may be averted by glucocorticoid therapy (to be described further on). Rarely, plasma exchange may arrest and/or reverse persistent postpartum HELLP syndrome.

The presence of laboratory parameters suggestive of concurrent or secondary DIC (prolongation of prothrombin time, and partial thromboplastin time, decrease in fibrinogen, presence of fibin-split products) is more common in severe disease (98). If overt DIC is diagnosed in concert with mild thrombocytopenia, the underlying disorder is probably not HELLP syndrome but more likely placental abruption or liver failure secondary to acute fatty liver of pregnancy (127–129). The most likely disorder to be confused with class 2 or 3 HELLP syndrome is gestational thrombocytopenia in women with a platelet count as low as 50,000/mL but without associated increases in LDH or AST/ALT (130–134). Apart from HELLP syndrome and gestational thrombocytopenia, the differential diagnosis of thrombocytopenia in pregnancy principally includes immune thrombocytopenia, cocaine intoxication, drug reaction, acute fatty liver of pregnancy, systemic lupus erythematosus (SLE), disseminated sepsis, obstetric coagulopathy, and TTP-HUS (Table 6).

X. MATERNAL MORBIDITY

The seriousness of HELLP syndrome is evident from the risk of maternal morbidity and the spectrum of multiple organ system complications. Categories of major maternal morbidity include cardiopulmonary, hematologic-coagulation, central nervous system-visual, renal, hepatic-gastrointestinal, infection, and fluid-related complications. The incidence of all types of morbidity increased from 11% in patients with severe preeclampsia without HELLP syndrome to 21% with patients in class 3, 22% in class 2, and 49% in class 1 HELLP syndrome (Table 7). These values are representative of a review of the almost 17-year experience at the University of Mississippi (94). A similarly high incidence of grave complications prior to routine corticosteroid use was reported for 43 patients with HELLP syndrome treated in Germany between 1980 and 1993 (135) and in France between 1993 and 1998 (136).

Although a rise in LDH, AST and uric acid are usually observed as HELLP syndrome worsens, there is considerable individual patient variation. Inexplicably, some patients with significant laboratory abnormalities will exhibit minimal morbidity, while others with apparently mild laboratory abnormalities can exhibit significant clinical disease (98). Although hepatic hemorrhage and rupture can occur in all classes, cardiopulmonary complications, specifically acute lung injury and acute respiratory distress syndrome, are almost exclusively confined to class 1. Transient renal dysfunction appears to be closely related to cardiopulmonary morbidity (137).

The two most common categories of maternal morbidity are hematological-

Table 6 Usual Signs and Symptoms of HELLP Syndrome Versus Other Disease Processes

	HELLP	TTP	HUS	ITP	AFLP
Major affected site/system	Liver, systemic	CNS/neurologic systemic	Renal	Spleen systemic	Liver
Gestational age	26–36 wks	Second trimester	Postpartum	All trimesters	36 wks +
Hypertension	±	−	++	−	±
Proteinuria	±	−	++	−	±
Fever	−	+	±	−	−
Sensorium changes/CNS findings	−	+	±	−	+
Petechiae	−	±	−	±	−
Hemolysis/MHA	+	−	±	−	−
Platelets	↓	↓	↓	↓	↓
PT/PTT	N	N	N	N	↑↑
Fibrinogen	N	N	N	N	↓↓
Total LDH	↑↑	↑↑	↑↑	N	↑
AST-ALT transaminases	↑↑	N	N	N	↑↑↑
Uric acid	↑	N	↑↑	N	↑
Creatinine	N	N	↑↑	N	↑↑
Glucose	N	N	N	N	↓↓
Platelet antibodies	−	−	−	+	−
Haptoglobin	↓↓	N	N	N	N

Key: TTP, thrombotic thrombocytopenic purpura; ITP, autoimmune thrombocytopenia; HUS, hemolytic uremic syndrome; AFLP, acute fatty liver of pregnancy; LDH, lactic dehydrogenase; N, no increase; AST, aspartate aminotransferase; ALT, alanine aminotransferase; MHA, microangiopathic hemolytic anemia; CNS, central nervous system; Arrows up, increase, down, decrease.

Table 7 Maternal Morbidity (Mississippi HELLP Series)

Category	HELLP syndrome			Severe preeclampsia	p value
	Class 1	Class 2	Class 3		
Hematologic/coagulation	32%	13%	8%	1%	< 0.001
Cardio/pulmonary	22%	10%	14%	10%	< 0.001
Central nervous system/ visual	4.5%	3%	0.36%	1%	0.009
Renal	3%	0%	1.1%	0%	0.003
Hepatic/gastrointestinal	1.5%	0.33%	0.36%	0%	NS
None	51%	78%	79%	89%	< 0.001
1-System	38%	19%	18%	10%	< 0.001
2-Systems	9%	3%	3%	1%	< 0.001
3-Systems	2.5%	0.33%	0%	0%	< 0.001

coagulation and cardiopulmonary, both of which account for more than 90% of problems (Table 8). The hematologic risks of spontaneous and postpartum hemorrhage, need for blood transfusion, and the development of superimposed DIC are foremost. Use of blood products in these patients was more liberal in the 1980s (10–55%) before restrictions were tightened and better therapy became available.

Eclampsia is more likely to be associated with HELLP syndrome at early gestational ages; the outlook for a woman with eclampsia and HELLP syndrome is much worse than with HELLP syndrome alone (138,139). Similar high incidence and variety of maternal morbidity with HELLP syndrome has been reported by Sibai and others (14,15,95).

A small percentage of patients develop renal or hepatic abnormalities including acute renal failure and hepatic rupture. Since the length of time for postpartum diuresis to occur is related to the severity of the HELLP syndrome, some degree of renal dysfunction must be part of the disease process (140). Electrolyte abnormalities are unusual in the absence of exogenous fluid administration, although a patient with unexplained hyponatremia has been reported (141). Approximately 10 to 20% of HELLP syndrome pregnancies are complicated by significant renal compromise in the form of acute renal failure or, less frequently, acute tubular necrosis (reversible) or cortical necrosis (nonreversible) (14,142, 143). Attempts to identify this group of women by level of diastolic hypertension, mean arterial pressure, and degree of microangiopathic hemolytic anemia have been unsuccessful although these complications are most commonly noted in patients with class 1 HELLP syndrome. Temporary or permanent hemodialysis may be required in women with renal failure complicating HELLP syndrome.

A small subset of patients with HELLP syndrome will have continuing renal

Table 8 Significant Maternal Morbidity Was Combined for Consideration into Several Categories

---

Cardiopulmonary
   Cardiogenic or noncardiogenic pulmonary edema
   Cardiac or pulmonary arrest
   Pulmonary embolus
   Indicated invasive central monitoring
   Indicated intubation or continuous positive airway pressure
   Need for mechanical ventilation
   Myocardial ischemia with chest pain
Hematologic and coagulation
   Clinically significant bleeding required transfusion of blood or blood products
   Ecchymoses
   Hematoma formation
   Presence of disseminated intravascular coagulopathy (with PTT time > 40 s)
Central nervous system and visual
   Central venous thrombosis
   Hypertensive encephalopathy
   Change in sensorium
   Cerebral edema
   Serous macular or retinal detachment
   Transient blindness
Renal
   Acute renal failure
   Acute tubular necrosis
   Need for dialysis
Hepatic and gastrointestinal
   Subcapsular hematoma
   Rupture of the liver capsule
   Pancreatitis
Infection
   Endometritis
   Pyelonephritis
   Wound infection
Preeclampsia, fluid-related
   Peripheral edema
   Facial edema
   Ascites

---

deterioration into the puerperium with increasing serum creatinine and BUN (14,143,144). The level of diastolic hypertension, mean arterial pressure, and degree of microangiopathic hemolytic anemia are not predictive of persistent oliguria in postpartum patients with HELLP syndrome. The incidence of acute renal failure (defined as a creatinine clearance of <20 mL/min) in postpartum patients with HELLP syndrome may be as high as 20 to 30% (14,146–148). When conservative medical management and judicious fluid administration fail to correct the renal dysfunction, hemodialysis with or without plasma exchange should be considered (126).

Liver involvement in women with preeclampsia who do not have HELLP syndrome is usually subclinical and is not associated with elevation of total serum LDH or hepatic transaminases. In HELLP syndrome, hepatic sinusoids contain hyaline deposits of a fibrin-like material, reminiscent of the fibrin deposits found in small blood vessels of patients with TTP-HUS. These can obstruct hepatic blood flow, leading to periportal hepatocellular necrosis that coalesces and dissects into the liver capsule. Hepatic necrosis and hemorrhage is a particular risk for patients with antiphospholipid antibodies (115,149). Spotty to widespread hepatic ischemia leading to infarction or hemorrhage could explain the right-upper-quadrant/epigastric pain that affects the majority of patients with advanced HELLP syndrome.

The subject of hepatic hemorrhage and rupture in the pregnant patient with preeclampsia/HELLP syndrome has been reviewed extensively (150,151). If a subcapsular hematoma ruptures, surgical intervention is necessary to prevent maternal exsanguination and death (150–152). This subject is dealt with elsewhere. .

Both CT scan and ultrasonography have been shown to demonstrate abnormal liver findings in HELLP syndrome (153,154). Abnormal sonographic liver findings have been demonstrated at least 24 hours prior to the onset of symptoms associated with severe preeclampsia-HELLP syndrome (155,156). Although CT evaluation of the liver is useful in the diagnosis of subcapsular liver or renal hematoma, it has not been found to reliably predict which patients will develop peripartum HELLP syndrome (157). Nevertheless, imaging of the liver is recommended in any patient with HELLP syndrome having complaints of right upper quadrant pain, neck pain, shoulder pain or relapsing hypotension (158). Hepatic rupture cannot always be averted even when appropriate therapy is instituted following the presumptive diagnosis of a subcapsular liver hematoma (159). Hepatobiliary scintigraphy can assist in the exclusion of acute cholecystitis or may demonstrate focal defects consistent with a hematoma and/or necrosis (160). Abnormalities found on scintigraphy have been alleged to antedate findings later detected by ultrasound (161).

Mild to severe decreases in visual acuity have been reported in women with HELLP syndrome (162). The range of opthalmologic abnormalities includes cortical blindness, retinal detachment, and vitreal hemorrhage (163–166).

XI. MATERNAL MORTALITY

Maternal mortality in HELLP syndrome has been reported to range between 1.1 and 24.2% (95). Until 1996 the average maternal death rate, in a review of six publications involving 746 women, was 4% (167). Death cannot be reliably predicted by the severity of the thrombocytopenia, total serum LDH concentration, or extent of hepatic enzyme abnormalities. In a review of 54 HELLP-related maternal mortalities, Isler and coworkers determined that the presenting complaint in 71.4% of patients who died was nausea/vomiting/right-upper-quadrant pain. In these women the mean gestational age was 33 to 34 weeks, and death occurred by a variety of pathological processes including cardiopulmonary arrest (40%), DIC (39%), ARDS (28%), renal failure (28%), sepsis (23%), and hypoxic ischemic encephalopathy (16%) (167). Hepatic rupture was the primary cause of death in only 7.5% of the patients but was an important contributing factor in 1 of 5 mortalities due to HELLP syndrome.

The most frequent cause of maternal death associated with HELLP syndrome is cerebral catastrophe (45–70%), described as large cerebral and brainstem hemorrhages, extensive thrombosis and infarction, severe cerebral edema with brain herniation, and carotid artery thrombosis associated with reactive thrombosis (167–170). Hemorrhage into the central nervous system has been observed in two patients with HELLP syndrome whose blood pressures were not in the range where antihypertensive therapy was indicated. This suggests that HELLP syndrome is associated with central nervous system pathology but may not be directly causative. Aberrations and differences in cerebral blood flow among patients may become important in disease assessment (171), although in one small patient series no difference in blood flow velocity wave forms in the middle cerebral artery was noted between patients with severe preeclampsia and those with HELLP syndrome (172). The same group has reported an increase in cerebral perfusion pressure (30%) reflective of some loss of cerebral autoregulation (173).

Delayed (174) or incorrect diagnosis of HELLP syndrome has been shown to contribute to 51% of all deaths ascribed to this condition (167,174).

XII. PERINATAL MORBIDITY AND MORTALITY

HELLP syndrome is considered to represent a form of severe preeclampsia or eclampsia; as such, the definitive treatment is pregnancy termination. This includes delivery of the placenta with elimination of most functioning chorionic villi and the factor(s) cytotoxic to endothelial cells, which are somehow responsible for HELLP syndrome.

How quickly to accomplish delivery, and by which method, are dependent upon a number of considerations including maternal disease severity and course, the gestational age of the fetus, an estimation of the fetal condition and reserve, and a determination of whether or not there is evidence of fetal growth retardation. Hospitalization of the gravida in a facility capable of managing high-risk pregnancy is preferable. The more preterm the gestation, the more appropriate the transfer to a hospital center with special capabilities for complicated newborn care. Raval's group at Cook County Hospital in Chicago observed that newborns from HELLP syndrome pregnancies required more resuscitation and experienced a higher incidence of cardiopulmonary instability than babies from matched control preeclamptic pregnancies without HELLP syndrome (175). The presence of growth restriction prior to 32 weeks may further aggravate perinatal condition in HELLP pregnancies (176). Joern reported that fetuses of women with HELLP syndrome were more likely than those of women with severe preeclampsia to have abnormal Doppler velocimetry indicating impaired placental hemodynamics (177).

With rare exception, any pregnancy beyond 34 weeks' gestation (especially in the presence of fetal growth restriction) and all mothers with class 1 HELLP syndrome are usually delivered within 24 hours. In pregnancies ≤34 weeks which are associated with class 2 or 3 HELLP syndrome and in which the mother and fetus are considered to be stable during the first 6 to 12 hours of maternal-fetal monitoring, the mothers are candidates for corticosteroid administration. In standard dosages (as betamethasone or dexamethasone) corticosteroids have been used to enhance fetal lung maturity and reduce the incidence of intraventricular hemorrhage, necrotizing enterocolitis, and fetal death in preterm deliveries. Use of these medications in the acutely or chronically hypertensive gravida has been confirmed to be safe and efficacious. A National Institutes of Health (NIH) consensus panel in March 1994 recommended that all pregnancies between 24 and 34 weeks' gestation at risk for preterm delivery be considered candidates for corticosteroid therapy even if delivery might not be postponed the ideal 24 to 48 hour period of time. The American College of Obstetricians and Gynecologists (ACOG) Committee on Obstetrical Practice has now adopted those recommendations (178).

Neonatal mortality is dependent on fetal maturity at the time of delivery. In the Mississippi series, perinatal mortality in class 1 HELLP syndrome was twice that for severe preeclampsia without HELLP syndrome (Table 9) (98). The difference in perinatal mortality between the groups was primarily influenced

Table 9 Perinatal Data (Mississippi HELLP Series)

Category	HELLP syndrome			Severe preeclampsia	p value
	Class 1	Class 2	Class 3		
Birth weight (g)	1568 ± 829	1762 ± 887	2100 ± 997	2100 ± 978	< 0.001
Stillbirths	14 (7%)	19 (6.3%)	7 (2.5%)	4 (2%)	0.017
Neonatal deaths	10 (5%)	11 (3.6%)	13 (4.7%)	7 (3.6%)	0.840
Perinatal mortality	119:1000	100:1000	73:1000	57:1000	0.104

by the stillbirth rate (98). Several investigators have however demonstrated that perinatal morbidity and mortality are increased in pregnancies complicated by HELLP syndrome, mainly due to preterm delivery (180,181), and not due to the underlying disorder itself (179,181,182,242). The incidence of small for gestational age infants is reported to affect as many as 39% of HELLP syndrome pregnancies, perinatal asphyxia occurs in 5.6%, and very low birth weight infants have a high frequency of leukopenia (21%), neutropenia (33%), and thrombocytopenia (33%) (181). In addition, fetal hemograms demonstrate an increase in red cell mass and anisocytosis (243).

Neonatal thrombocytopenia is no more common in newborns from mothers with HELLP syndrome than in those of preeclamptic patients (183), but basal platelet activation has been reported to be increased (184). Because of the association of low maternal platelet count and an increased risk of intraventricular hemorrhage in the fetus, early routine assessment of the neonatal platelet count is recommended in newborns from mothers with HELLP syndrome. When birthweight is <600 g and gestational age is <25 weeks, intact neonatal survival is poor in pregnancies complicated by HELLP syndrome (185). The long-term prognosis for children of mothers with HELLP syndrome appears to be comparable to controls matched for gestational age (183).

Up to 30% of patients with eclampsia have concurrent HELLP syndrome (138,139). Gestational age and birth weight are lower and perinatal mortality is higher in such patients as compared to pregnancies complicated by eclampsia alone (138).

XIII. DIFFERENTIAL DIAGNOSIS: CONFOUNDERS IN THE DISEASE SPECTRUM

HELLP syndrome has been referred to as the "great imitator" because of its wide spectrum of disease presentation, but other disease processes can also mimic HELLP syndrome (129,186). Acute fatty liver, TTP-HUS, HELLP syndrome, and preeclampsia-eclampsia with liver dysfunction share many clinical and laboratory abnormalities and could be different manifestations of the same, or related diseases. Differentiating HELLP syndrome from its imitators is best accomplished by early assessment of laboratory parameters since late in their disease courses most of the thrombotic microangiopathies assume a common final clinical presentation of multisystem disease (Table 1).

After a prodromal phase that usually lasts 1 to 2 weeks, patients with acute fatty liver typically develop very high conjugated/direct bilirubin concentrations, jaundice, hypoglycemia, hyperuricemia and a very prolonged PT/PTT associated at worst with only a mild thrombocytopenia (129). In contrast, HELLP syndrome patients usually develop severe thrombocytopenia and increased total serum LDH which precede any other coagulation abnormalities (prolonged PT/PTT decreased fibrinogen), increases in bilirubin or other laboratory evidence of hepatic dysfunction. Evidence of preeclampsia may or may not be present in the patient with acute fatty liver (187). The observation that both disease conditions can recur in consecutive pregnancies lends support to the possibility that acute fatty liver and preeclampsia are related disorders. Severe hypoglycemia accompanying HELLP syndrome has been described, similar to that seen with acute fatty liver of pregnancy in apparent response to altered glycogenolysis and gluconeogenesis (188, 189). Like HELLP syndrome, patients with reversible peripartum liver failure (AFLP) may eventually have full recovery of hepatic function (190).

Patients with thrombotic thrombocytopenic purpura (TTP) can exhibit features characteristic of HELLP syndrome including microangiopathic hemolytic anemia, proteinuria, increased serum LDH concentrations, and possibly renal compromise (191–193). They are intermittently febrile with waxing and waning neurologic signs. Unlike HELLP syndrome, patients with TTP usually are not hypertensive and do not exhibit elevated liver transaminases. Exacerbations of TTP can occur at any time in life or during pregnancy and persist into the puerperium long after HELLP syndrome resolution is expected. TTP carries a high mortality rate of over 50% and is best treated with plasma exchange (194).

Hemolytic uremic syndrome (HUS) as a sister disorder to TTP and HELLP syndrome is characterized by microangiopathic hemolysis, hypertension, proteinuria, and renal failure (129,191). Histopathologic lesions characteristic of HUS in the kidney may be required to make the diagnosis in confusing cases (195). The serum creatinine is usually markedly elevated in contrast to that seen in patients with HELLP syndrome. Optimal therapy includes fresh frozen plasma infusions and serial plasma exchange procedures. Unlike HELLP syndrome, patients with HUS usually do not exhibit laboratory evidence of hepatic dysfunction.

The thrombotic microangiopathic process in each of these disorders appears to primarily target the liver in HELLP syndrome, the central nervous system in TTP, and the kidneys in HUS. Even though these disorders are described as unique conditions, they appear to be interrelated with considerable overlap. Thus, a spectrum of disease is seen in which distinctions among the parent diseases become blurred with progression into advanced multiple organ system disease (129). Some patients originally considered to have HELLP syndrome actually may later be discovered to have exhibited "pseudo-HELLP" with complex clinical pictures and atypical stories. An example is a patient reported to have intrahepatic cholangiocarcinoma masquerading as HELLP syndrome in pregnancy (196). Also, Minakami and colleagues have provided evidence that gestational thrombocytopenia in one pregnancy may be a risk factor for the subsequent development of full fledged HELLP syndrome and this may recur in subsequent pregnancies (197).

XIV. INNOVATIVE INTERVENTIONS

A. Glucocorticoids

In our center we consider glucocorticoid therapy fundamental to the management of HELLP syndrome. This followed a serendipitous finding that steroid therapy administered for other indications had a positive effect on maternal outcomes. In an observational study of 454 patients with HELLP syndrome, only 27 received a complete course of steroids administered to improve fetal lung maturation (94). In these women there was a halving of neonatal respiratory complications compared to an equal number of gestational age and HELLP severity-matched controls (198). In addition the platelet count either stabilized or increased in 25 of the 27 patients compared to none of the untreated mothers. Decreases in LDH and AST were also observed in most dexamethasone-treated mothers. It appeared that maternal therapy administered for the benefit of the fetus had arrested or improved the mothers' condition (199).

As a consequence of these observations, two separate randomized, prospective clinical trials were undertaken in patients with HELLP syndrome. A double dose of intravenous dexamethasone was arbitrarily chosen in order to maximize maternal and fetal impact over a short timespan. In the first study, 12 patients were randomly assigned to receive a double dose of intravenous dexamethasone until delivery, and 13 received standard therapy. Compared with standard therapy those given the double dose had an improvement in platelet count, liver function enzymes, urine output and LDH (200). They also had a significantly longer interval from study-entry to delivery (41 hours compared to 15 hours for controls).

In a second study of 40 postpartum HELLP patients randomized to receive intravenous dexamethasone (10 mg for two doses followed by 5 mg for two doses at 12-hour intervals) or general supportive therapy, the steroid-treated patients showed a more rapid improvement in their platelet counts, liver function values, LDH, blood pressure, and urinary output (201). Nevertheless, neither trial was placebo-controlled and the numbers of patients were too small to demonstrate significant differences.

Following these two investigations in 1993, we routinely administered intravenous dexamethasone to all antepartum and postpartum patients with class 1 or 2, and in selected antepartum class 3 "complicated" HELLP syndrome patients (eclampsia, very high transaminases, epigastric pain or significant maternal morbidity of any type). A cohort analysis of our 1994–1995 experience with this practice pattern, compared to the four year 1988–1991 period, demonstrated a higher total steroid use (85% versus 18%), fewer patients with a platelet count below 50,000/mL (30 versus 44%), less use of blood products (8 versus 33%), less need for CPAP or mechanical respiratory support (3 versus 6%), less clinically significant bleeding (3 versus 11%), less infectious morbidity (19 versus 46%), and a lower incidence of neonatal respiratory disease (28 versus 48%) (Table 10)

Table 10 Cohort Study for Antepartum Dexamethasone in HELLP

	Year		
	1988–1991	1994–1995	Significance
Steroids administered	18%	85%	p < 0.001
Platelet nadir	57,000	67,000	p = 0.011
Proportion class 1	44%	30%	p = 0.07
Number transfused	56 (33%)	5 (8%)	p < 0.05
Mechanical ventilation	10 (6%)	2 (3%)	p < 0.01
Wound infection	46%	19%	p < 0.05
I.V. site bleeding	11%	3%	p < 0.05
Hyaline membrane disease	48%	28%	p < 0.05

(202). Similarly, patients treated with intravenous dexamethasone had a shorter disease course, faster recovery with shorter hospitalization, less morbidity and less interventionist therapy than controls (Table 11) (203–205).

Review of the literature published prior to our observations revealed that others had noted similar beneficial effects of steroid therapy in isolated cases (186,204–211). Prospective, randomized clinical trials have suggested that dexamethasone is superior to betamethasone in patients with HELLP syndrome. Postpartum dexamethasone produced greater reductions in mean arterial pressure, need for antihypertensive therapy and number of readmissions to the recovery room for surveillance and intervention (212). Antepartum dexamethasone was associated with improved laboratory results, less hypertension, better urinary output and less need for intervention for increased blood pressure or oliguria (213). Although these data tend to support the concept that dexamethasone may enhance vascular relaxation and renal perfusion while inhibiting the underlying micro-

Table 11 Study of Postpartum Dexamethasone in HELLP

	Control	Steroid treatment	Significance
Apresoline	44%	25%	p < 0.05
Number transfused	31%	5%	p < 0.001
Plasma exchange	11%	0%	p < 0.05
Infection	42%	12%	p < 0.001
Mechanical ventilation	n = 13	n = 1	p < 0.05
Delivery to discharge	6 ± 3 days	4 ± 2 days	p < 0.05

angiopathic hemolytic anemia of HELLP syndrome, larger numbers of patients would need to be studied to determine the clinical impact of this intervention.

In terms of dosage, Barton and coworkers' observed that the impact of corticosteroid therapy upon the laboratory indices is dose-dependent. They concluded that a higher dose of steroids than that used in standard regimens for fetal lung maturity enhancement should be considered for the therapy of HELLP syndrome (214).

Dexamethasone administration has also been shown to ameliorate maternal HELLP syndrome in very preterm pregnancy so that immediate delivery was not required. This is a highly controversial area of obstetrics and a dilemma for the clinician (215). Pregnancy prolongation has been reported in isolated cases for up to 19 days (216–218).

No evidence of fetal adrenal suppression or adverse effect on neural development has been observed in our unit after high dose dexamethasone treatment of HELLP syndrome pregnancy for <7 days. Mothers who receive more than 2 weeks of continuous corticosteroid therapy are candidates for tapering therapy. Shorter treatment duration has not been shown to influence the maternal risks of infection or wound healing, although it is a theoretical risk. A risk of steroid administration is the potential for the misinterpretation of the clinical response to be a sign of disease disappearance. The time obtained by steroid administration should be used to effect transfer of the patient to a tertiary care center or for delivery under controlled conditions.

We believe that the time at which dexamethasone therapy is initiated could be important since the response may be absent once the disease process is too far advanced (219). The "conservative treatment" of HELLP syndrome to prolong gestation beyond 27 to 28 weeks for more than 48 to 72 hours has been associated with increased maternal and perinatal morbidity related to placental abruption (220). The additional risk to the mother must be balanced against the potential gain in neonatal maturation (221–223). Although no adverse neonatal effects have been demonstrated to date, a more complete study of the impact of high-dose short-term dexamethasone therapy upon the fetus and neonate is desirable.

The mechanism of action of dexamethasone in HELLP syndrome remains to be elucidated (224–228).

B. Plasma Exchange

The role for plasmapheresis and fresh frozen plasma infusion in the postpartum HELLP syndrome patient has decreased over the years. In our center, the advent of steroid therapy has significantly reduced the number of patients receiving this therapy (125). Details on the use of plasmapheresis are summarized later in this chapter. It remains an option for the seriously ill patient unresponsive to conservative measures (229–231).

C. Nitric Oxide Donors and Antioxidants

Other therapeutic interventions that have been considered for the interruption, amelioration or prevention of HELLP syndrome are vitamin E and C supplements (232) and nitric oxide donors such as transdermal isosorbide dinitrate (233). Nitric oxide is a potent vasodilator that has been reported to reverse platelet activation and HELLP syndrome progression (233). The theoretical basis for its use lies in its ability to reduce resistance in the spiral arteriole bed beneath the placenta, and to decrease the circulating vasoactive substances, oxygen-free radicals and lipid peroxidase.

D. Volume Expansion/Vasodilation

Two European groups have reported some success in expectantly managing patients with severe preeclampsia and HELLP syndrome (234,235). Only one of these trials was prospective, and neither of the two were randomized or controlled. Van Pampas reported difficulty prolonging gestation when antihypertensive therapy was required (234). Visser and Wallenburg claimed successful prolongation of some pregnancies between 20 to 32 weeks when plasma volume expansion and pharmacologic vasodilation was carried out guided by central hemodynamic monitoring (235). This approach has not been universally accepted due to the increased risk associated with invasive monitoring in a mother with impaired hemostasis and who is at increased risk for placental abruption.

XV. GENERAL MANAGEMENT CONSIDERATIONS: PRACTICE GUIDELINES

Successful management of the patient with HELLP syndrome requires early recognition, institution of appropriate therapy, and collaborative critical care by medical and nursing staff. Since the management of HELLP syndrome is broadly similar to that of severe preeclampsia which is discussed elsewhere, the following section is limited to management issues specific for HELLP syndrome. Detailed practice guidelines have been published and are based on the preceding discussion and the expert opinions of others (236–241).

The goals of therapy are to minimize overall maternal and perinatal morbidity/mortality. This can be partly addressed by due vigilance and early intervention to prevent disease progression into class 1 HELLP syndrome. In those women with HELLP syndrome care must be taken to prevent eclampsia and to this end institution of magnesium sulfate therapy is considered important in the United States, although this approach is still questioned in some parts of Europe. Control of maternal blood pressure is paramount and every effort to limit the MAP <126 mmHg (160/110 mmHg) should be made because of the increased risk of complications seen when this limit is persistently exceeded. As discussed above, we believe that the use of invasive devices should be minimized and confined to those patients where the use of such monitoring is imperative for appropriate care. Likewise, operative intervention should be restricted unless obstetrically indicated. It is important that patients with HELLP syndrome are managed in an appropriate tertiary care facility and in an appropriate site within that facility (such as an intensive care unit).

Eclamptic seizures frequently precede or follow the development of HELLP syndrome (97,134). It is currently recommended in the United States that all HELLP syndrome patients (particularly in labor, postpartum, or whenever epigastric pain is present) receive intravenous magnesium sulfate given as a 4- to 6-g bolus followed by constant infusion of 1.5 to 4.0 g/h individualized to the patient. The dose is monitored by patellar reflexes, urinary output, and serum magnesium levels.

Magnesium sulfate appears to be the ideal anticonvulsant for patients with preeclampsia-eclampsia (244). A second beneficial action is its ability to modestly relax peripheral and central vasculature possibly resulting in less platelet clumping (245,246). In the rare patient in whom magnesium is contraindicated, such as the mother with myasthenia gravis, phenytoin is a second-line drug. The loading dose of phenytoin is 15 mg/kg given at a rate of 40 mg/min with monitoring of the patient's heart rate by an ECG monitor and assessment of the patient's blood pressure every 5 minutes. The therapeutic range of phenytoin is 10 to 20 mg/mL.

The severe systolic and diastolic hypertension which can accompany HELLP syndrome must be treated appropriately. The maternal complications of excessively elevated blood pressure include myocardial infarction and cerebral hemorrhage/infarction, while placental abruption can occur in as many as 20% of pregnancies complicated by HELLP syndrome (247).

In view of the compromised capillary and coagulation systems in patients with HELLP syndrome, we consider treating any patient with a systolic pressure over 150 mmHg or with a diastolic pressure over 100 mmHg so that mean arterial pressure elevations are minimized in the presence of a fragile vascular state. This is especially true during the puerperium when a fetus is no longer present. Prior to delivery, the clinician is severely constrained to prevent underperfusion of the placenta so diastolic pressure should probably not persist below 80 to 90 mmHg.

Hydralazine in intermittent 2.5 to 5 mg intravenous boluses is effective, but care must be taken not to administer hydralazine or any other antihypertensive agents too rapidly and bring about a precipitous fall in blood pressure which could thereby impair uteroplacental blood flow. Diastolic blood pressure should be reduced to 90 mmHg but not below this level prior to delivery. If the initial dose of hydralazine is ineffective, a repeat dose of 5 mg or an increase to 10 mg is attempted 30 minutes later. When using potent peripheral vasodilator drugs, care should be taken to adequately preload the patient, as is standard management prior to regional anesthesia. The judicious use of volume expansion prior to decreasing systemic vascular resistance with potent antihypertensive agents may help prevent precipitous drops in blood pressure and resultant fall in uteroplacental perfusion, which often results in fetal distress. The volume of fluid to be infused depends on the underlying state of hydration and cardiac function but is usually in the range of 500 to 1000 mL of crystalloid given over 30 minutes with appropriate non-invasive monitoring of peripheral oxygen saturation. Intra-arterial blood pressure monitoring should be considered in those cases where potent antihypertensive agents are to be used. If volume status is uncertain, or fluid overload suspected, noninvasive echocardiography may be useful.

Labetalol, in an initial bolus of 10 or 20 mg intravenously, with 40- to 80-mg doses given up to a total of 300 mg, is effective in lowering blood pressure in pregnancy while maintaining placental perfusion. Its antihypertensive efficacy is similar to that of hydralazine, but it may be associated with a lower incidence of fetal distress (248).

An ideal postpartum agent is the long-acting form of the dihydropyridine calcium channel blocker nifedipine which causes peripheral arterial vasodilation with renal and cardiac sparing effects (249). In addition, nifedipine promotes diuresis and appears to inhibit platelet aggregation (250) and red cell aggregation (251).

Agents such as alpha-methyl-dopa, clonidine and prazocin have not been sufficiently researched in patients with HELLP syndrome to recommend first line use. Angiotensin converting enzyme (ACE) inhibitors are contraindicated in pregnancy for fetal reasons and should be avoided antepartum unless there are compelling reasons (for example cardiomyopathy) and the mother gives informed consent. Ketanserin, a serotonin antagonist, does not appear to be an effective antihypertensive therapy for hypertension in HELLP syndrome (252).

Large-volume maternal ascites is frequently found in patients with HELLP syndrome (253). Compared to patients without any apparent ascites at the time of cesarean delivery, those with massive ascites have a sixfold increase in the incidence congestive heart failure and a ninefold increase in the incidence of acute respiratory distress syndrome. These complications usually becomes apparent within the first 24 hours postpartum which mandates close observation for at least this duration after delivery (253).

Pulmonary capillary wedge pressure (PCWP) monitoring with a Swan-Ganz catheter is usually restricted to patients with pulmonary edema, and those with preeclampsia associated with acute lung injury and multiorgan failure. In those patients with oliguria not responsive to fluid boluses, and in patients with resistant severe hypertension, noninvasive echocardiography and Doppler studies may be used to assess the central hemodynamics in order to guide therapy. These women are unlikely to require prolonged hemodynamic monitoring and noninvasive monitoring is safer given the potential for coagulopathy in HELLP syndrome.

In most cases maternal cardiac function is satisfactory and intravascular volume constriction is present. Fluid and antihypertensive therapy can be adjusted using the information gained from a single noninvasive estimation and invasive monitoring is usually not required (253a,b).

If invasive monitoring is required, the antecubital vein should be used to minimize the risk of trauma to large central vessels.

As discussed above, glucocorticoids (dexamethasone 10 mg q 12 h IV) should be considered for maternal benefit in the following patients: class 1, 2, and complicated class 3 HELLP syndrome (eclampsia, epigastric pain, LDH ≥1400 IU/L, AST ≥150 IU/L, uric acid ≥7.8 mg/dL, or significant maternal morbidity). Dexamethasone therapy may be used in order to postpone delivery if gestational age is much less than 26 weeks and/or estimated fetal weight much less than 700 g. The dexamethasone administered for maternal benefit replaces the usual corticosteroids given for fetal benefit. In cases where high-dose dexamethasone is not given, betamethasone (two doses of 12 mg IM, 24 hours apart) is indicated for fetal benefit if the estimated gestational age is between 23 and 34 weeks. Postpartum, dexamethasone 10 mg IV every 12 hours for two doses, followed by 5 mg every 12 hours for an additional two doses, may be given for maternal benefit. Postpartum dexamethasone treatment may be extended if laboratory and/or clinical parameters do not indicate disease resolution.

Clinically significant postpartum bleeding following vaginal or abdominal delivery has not been observed in patients with HELLP syndrome who have a platelet count above 40,000/mL (254). Prophylactic transfusion with 6 units of platelets should be considered in women with HELLP syndrome undergoing cesarean or vaginal delivery if the platelet count is <40,000 or <20,000/mL, respectively. Platelet transfusion is indicated in any patient with evidence of spontaneous, excessive bleeding regardless of platelet count. The postpartum platelet count should be maintained for the first 24 hours postpartum to avert hematoma formation.

Plasma exchange therapy, either by automated IBM Cell Separator apparatus or similar equipment, has been used in patients with HELLP syndrome prior to delivery, during the immediate peripartal period, or postpartum if recovery does not occur within 72 to 96 hours of delivery (255–268). In these rare patients with unremitting and complicated disease, plasma exchange with fresh frozen plasma is a further therapeutic option (126,268). The mechanism(s) of action of plasma exchange may be in part related to removal of the debris resulting from the microangiopathic hemolytic anemic process, and/or the supplementation of deficient factors which have been depleted during the course of the disease.

Vaginal delivery should be attempted whenever possible, with cervical ripening and intensive maternal-fetal surveillance. Without the use of high-dose corticosteroids, the likelihood of vaginal delivery in a preterm case with an unripe cervix is low (269). Use of high-dose corticosteroids in these cases may allow more time for cervical ripening and induction of labor. When cesarean delivery is required, careful attention to hemostasis is emphasized. Utilization of a vertical skin incision rather than a transverse lower abdominal incision is associated with fewer wound complications including wound separation and infection (270). Delayed skin closure does not appear to be more advantageous than primary skin closure (271). Low vertical uterine incisions are used when the lower uterine segment is poorly developed (usually <32 weeks) and the fetal presentation is other than cephalic. Rather than use forceful and precipitous extraction, the placenta should be allowed to spontaneously separate since this decreases blood loss (272). If the uterus can be repaired in situ rather than exteriorizing it, unnecessary uterine and adnexal trauma can be prevented or minimized, and infection may be averted (273). Closure of the vesicouterine peritoneum is not recommended. A mass closure or Smead-Jones fascial closure should be used to complete the abdominal repair. Drainage of the suprafascial space with Jackson-Pratt type drainage is advisable in obese patients. A short course (24 to 48 hours) of broad-spectrum antibiotics is administered, particularly if blood products have been given since higher infectious morbidity has been reported in the transfused patient compared to those who were not given blood products (94,138).

Accelerated recovery from preeclampsia has been reported in women who underwent immediate postpartum uterine curettage of the placental bed (274–277). This finding has recently been challenged in a retrospective, uncontrolled investigation (278). Orally administered (rather than sublingual) nifedipine (10 mg given every 4 hours) for the first 48 hours postpartum has been used in the management of severely preeclamptic women and appears to be as effective as postpartum curettage in lowering the mean arterial pressure and increasing the urinary output (277).

In the presence of hemodynamic instability and/or severe coagulopathy, regional anesthesia is contraindicated. In these situations, maternal analgesia during labor can be provided by intermittent infusion of butorphanol or meperidine with promethazine. Carefully controlled and skillfully executed nonoperative vaginal delivery is recommended with locally infiltrated 1% lidocaine as needed but without pudendal block. The anesthetic management of HELLP syndrome patients undergoing abdominal delivery can be challenging (279–282). The anesthetic of choice for the individual patient depends on the patient's condition, fetal well-being, and the urgency of the situation. Epidural anesthesia can be safely administered in normal patients without adverse hemorrhagic and neurological sequelae if the maternal platelet count exceeds 100,000/mL or if clotting appears normal. Primarily because of the dominant concern of the altered coagulation status of patients with HELLP syndrome (particularly with class 1 and class 2 disease) general anesthesia with intubation remains the anesthesia of choice. Laryngeal edema can render intubation difficult. Moreover, acute hypertension can accompany intubation.

Frequently, HELLP syndrome first becomes apparent during the puerperium, most often during the first 24 to 48 hours postpartum (95–98) It is recommended that all patients with severe preeclampsia-HELLP syndrome be managed in an obstetric recovery room or in an intensive care unit until (a) the maternal platelet count exhibits a consistent upward and the LDH exhibits a consistent downward trend; (b) the patient begins a spontaneous diuresis (100 mL/h over 2 consecutive hours without administration of a fluid bolus or diuretics); (c) the hypertension is well controlled with the systolic pressure <150 mmHg and the diastolic <100 mmHg using orally administered agents (hydralazine 25 to 75 mg every 6 hours or nifedipine XL 30 to 60 mg twice daily); and (d) the clinical improvement is obvious to providers and there are no significant complications. Laboratory assessment is individualized but should include platelet count and LDH determination every 8 to 24 hours as long as the patient remains in the recovery unit. Magnesium sulfate is continued likewise until resolution of the preeclampsia and the HELLP syndrome are well underway. Assessment of prothrombin time (PT), partial thromboplastin time (PTT), fibrinogen, and fibrin split products are not needed routinely unless the maternal platelet count is below 50,000/mL, the patient has an abruption, or there is evidence of a progressive coagulopathy.

The clinician must be particularly vigilant for hepatic hemorrhage and rupture during the peripartal period. The diagnosis and management of hepatic rupture and hemorrhage are reviewed elsewhere (150,151).

XVI. COUNSELING

In a study from Mississippi, where 75% of the patients were African American, the recurrence risk was 42 to 43% for any type of preeclampsia-eclampsia, and 19 to 17% for HELLP syndrome (296). If the index pregnancy was delivered at <32 weeks, then the recurrence risk for another preterm delivery with preeclampsia-eclampsia is 61% (296). Sibai's group in Memphis saw a much lower recurrence risk for HELLP syndrome (3 to 4%) (297). Differences between these studies may be secondary to genetic, ethnic, tertiary care/geographic differences and possibly diagnostic criteria. There is a single case report of a patient who experienced recurrent HELLP syndrome in four successive pregnancies (298).

In a limited number of cases reported to the Food and Drug Administration, a possible association was reported between postpartum progesterone contraceptive use (Norplant system, levonorgestrel, but not Depo-Provera) and HUS-TTP (299). No such association has been reported in postpartum women whose pregnancy was complicated by HELLP syndrome.

The value of low dose aspirin in preventing recurrent HELLP syndrome or preeclampsia remains uncertain but it is possibly efficacious in the rare patient with an occult coagulopathy or vasculopathy. Since calcium supplementation (1.5–2.0 g/day) has not been shown to have significant risk and may benefit some patients by lowering blood pressure and the risk of recurrent preeclampsia, it is reasonable to consider this therapy for patients with prior HELLP syndrome.

REFERENCES

1. Weinstein L. Syndrome of hemolysis, elevated liver enzymes, and plow platelet count: a severe consequence of hypertension in pregnancy. Am J Obstet Gynecol 1982; 142:159–167.
2. Dieckmann WJ. The Toxemias of Pregnancy, 2d ed. St. Louis: Mosby, 1952:362–369.
3. Pritchard JA, Weisman R Jr, Ratnoff OD, Vosburgh GJ. Intravascular hemolysis, thrombocytopenia and other hematologic abnormalities associated with severe toxemia of pregnancy. N Engl J Med 1954; 250:89–98.
4. Brain MC, Kuah K-B, Dixon HG. Heparin treatment of haemolysis and thrombocytopenia in pre-eclampsia. J Obstet Gynaecol Br Commonw 1967; 74:702–711.
5. Scott R, Gordon S, Schatz A, Casella S. Acute hemolysis and thrombocytopenia in eclampsia. Obstet Gynecol 1970; 36:128–131.
6. McKay DG. Hematologic evidence of disseminated intravascular coagulation in eclampsia. Obstet Gynecol Surv 1972; 27:399–407.
7. Vardi J, Fields GA. Microangiopathic hemolytic anemia in severe pre-eclampsia. Am J Obstet Gynecol 1974; 119:617–622.
8. Killam AP, Dillard SH, Patton RC, Pederson PR. Pregnancy-induced hypertension complicated by acute liver disease and disseminated intravascular coagulation. Am J Obstet Gynecol 1975; 123:823–828.
9. Lopez-Llera M, de la Luz Espinosa M, Diaz de Leon M, Linares GR. Abnormal coagulation and fibrinolysis in eclampsia. A clinical and laboratory correlation study. Am J Obstet Gynecol 1976; 124:681–692.
10. Schwartz ML, Brenner WE. The obfuscation of eclampsia by thrombotic thrombocytopenic purpura. Am J Obstet Gynecol 1978; 131:18–24.
11. Goodlin RC, Cotton DB, Haesslein HC. Severe EPH gestosis. Am J Obstet Gynecol 1978; 132:595–598.
12. Chesley L. Disseminated intravascular coagulation. Hypertensive Disorders in Pregnancy. New York: Appleton-Century-Crofts, 1978:103–117.
13. Kitzmiller JL, Lang JE, Telenosky PF, Lucas WE. Hematologic assays in pre-eclampsia. Am J Obstet Gynecol 1974; 118:362–367.
14. Sibai BM, Taslimi MM, el-Nazer A, Amon E, Mabie BC, Ryan GM. Maternal-perinatal outcome associated with the syndrome of hemolysis, elevated liver enzymes, and low platelets in severe preeclampsia-eclampsia. Am J Obstet Gynecol 1986; 155:501–509.
15. Sibai BM. The HELLP syndrome (hemolysis, elevated liver enzymes, and low platelets): much ado about nothing? Am J Obstet Gynecol 1990; 162:311–316.
16. Magann EF, Martin JN Jr. The laboratory evaluation of hypertensive gravidas. Obstet Gynecol Surv 1995; 50:138–145.

17. Sanchez-Ramos L, Adair CD, Todd JC, Mollitt DL, Briones DK. Erythrocyte membrane fluidity in patients with preeclampsia and the HELLP syndrome: a preliminary study. J Matern Fetal Invest 1994; 4:237–239.

18. Hamm W, Richardsen G, Switkowski R. Lactate dehydrogenase isoenzymes in patients with HELLP syndrome. Z Gerburtshilfe Neonatol 1996; 200:115–118.

19. Wilke G, Rath W, Schutz E, Armstrong VW, Kuhn W. Haptoglobin as a sensitive marker of hemolysis in HELLP syndrome. Int J Gynaecol Obstet 1992; 39:29–34.

20. Marchand A, Galen RS, Lonte VF. The predictive value of serum haptoglobin in haemolytic disease. JAMA 1980; 243:1909–1911.

21. Poldre PA. Haptoglobin helps diagnose the HELLP syndrome. Am J Obstet Gynecol 1987; 157:1267.

22. Schröcksnadel H, Sitte B, Steckel-Berger G, Dapunt O. Hemolysis in hypertensive disorders of pregnancy. Gynecol Obstet Invest 1992; 34:211–216.

23. Martin JN Jr, Blake PG, Perry KG Jr, McCaul JF, Hess LW, Martin RW. The natural history of HELLP syndrome: patterns of disease progression and regression. Am J Obstet Gynecol 1991; 164:1500–1513.

24. Burlet G, Ciepluchia V, Routiot T, Bayoumeu F, Schweitzer M. Haemolysis as a early and sensitive parameter in predicting acute evolution of HELLP syndrome (abstr). Hypertension in Pregnancy 2000; 19(suppl 1):150.

25. Kew MC. Serum aminotransferase concentration as evidence of hepatocellular damage. Lancet 2000; 355:591–592.

26. Martin JN Jr. Reply: Letter to the editor (Am J Obstet Gynecol 1999; 180:1373–1384). Am J Obstet Gynecol 2000; 1271–1272.

27. Stubbs TM, Lazarchick J, Horger EO III, Loadholt CB. Schistocytosis, aminotransferase elevation and thrombocytopenia in preeclampsia/eclampsia. J Reprod Med 1987; 32:777–779.

28. Barton JR, Riely CA, Adamec TA, Shanklin DR, Khoury AD, Sibai BM. Hepatic histopathologic condition does not correlate with laboratory abnormalities in HELLP syndrome (hemolysis, elevated liver enzymes, and low platelet count). Am J Obstet Gynecol 1992; 167:1538–1543.

29. Beyer C, Hofland M, Que DG. Lactate dehydrogenase isoenzyme 6 in serum of two patients with severe pre-eclampsia. Clin Chem 1990; 36:411–412.

30. McMahon LP, O'Coigligh S, Redman CWG. Hepatic enzymes and the HELLP syndrome: a long-standing error? Br J Obstet Gynaecol 1993; 100:693–695.

31. Churchill D, Kilby MD, Bignell A, Whittle MJ, Beevers DG. Gamma-glutamyl transferase activity in gestational hypertension. Br J Obstet Gynaecol 1994; 101:251–253.

32. Martin JN Jr, Magann EF, Blake PG, Terrone DA, Rinehart BK, May WL. Early risk assessment of severe preeclampsia: admission battery of symptoms and laboratory tests to predict likelihood of subsequent significant maternal morbidity. Am J Obstet Gynecol 1999; 180:1407–1414.

33. Iioka H. Clinical use of human hepatocyte growth factor in the early detection of HELLP syndrome. Gynecol Obstet Invest 1996; 41:103–105.

34. Friedman SA, Taylor RN, Roberts JM. Pathophysiology of preeclampsia. Clin Perinatol 1991; 18:661–682.

35. Roberts JM, Redman CWG. Pre-eclampsia: more than pregnancy-induced hypertension. Lancet 1993; 341:1447–1454.

36. Roberts JM, Taylor RN, Musci TJ, Rodgers GM, Hubel CA, McLaughlin MK. Preeclampsia: an endothelial cell disorder. Am J Obstet Gynecol 1989; 161:1200–1204.

37. Roberts JM. Objective evidence of endothelial dysfunction in preeclampsia. Am J Kidney Dis 1999; 33:992–997.

38. Lindheimer M, Cunningham G. Hypertension in pregnancy. N Engl J Med 1992; 326:927–932.

39. Zeeman GG, Dekker GA, van Geijn HP, Kraayenbrink AA. Endothelial function in normal and pre-eclamptic pregnancies: a hypothesis. Eur J Obstet Gynecol Reprod Biol 1992; 43:113–122.

40. Stratta P, Canavese C, Vercellone A. HELLP, microangiopathic hemolytic anemia, and preeclampsia. Hypertens Pregn 1993; 12:487–496.

41. Schlembach D, Beinder E. Measurement of microcirculation in normal pregnancy, preeclampsia and HELLP syndrome (abstr). Hypertens Pregn 2000; 19(suppl 1):114.

42. Knapen MFCM, Mulder TPJ, Van Rooij IALM, Peters WHM, Steegers EAP. Low whole blood glutathione levels in pregnancies complicated by preeclampsia or the hemolysis, elevated liver enzymes, low platelets syndrome. Obstet Gynecol 1998; 92:1012–1015.

43. Roes EM, Raijmakers MTM, Zusterzeel PLM, Knapen MFCM, Peters WHM, Steegers EAP. Deficient detoxificating capacity in the pathophysiology of pre-eclampsia (abstr). Hypertens Pregn 2000; 19(suppl 1):172.

44. Groten T, Kreienberg R, Fialka I, Huber L, Wedlich D. Disruption of cadherin-5 membrane targeting by serum of preeclamptic patients (abstr). Hypertens Pregn 2000; 19(suppl 1):71.

45. Haeger M, Bengtsson A, Karlsson K, Heidemann M. Complement activation and anaphylatoxin (C3a and C5a) formation in preeclampsia and by amniotic fluid. Obstet Gynecol 1989; 73:551–556.

46. Haeger M, Unander M, Norder-Hansson B, Tylman M, Bengtsson A. Complement, neutrophil, and macrophage activation in women with severe preeclampsia and the syndrome of hemolysis elevated liver enzymes, and low platelet count. Obstet Gynecol 1992; 79:19–26.

47. Dalmasso AP. Complement in the pathophysiology and diagnosis of human diseases. Crit Rev Clin Lab Sci 1986; 24:123–183.

48. Dudley DJ, Hunter C, Mitchell MD, Varner MW, Gately M. Elevations of serum interleukin-12 concentrations in women with severe pre-eclampsia and HELLP syndrome. J Reprod Immunol 1996; 31:97–107.

49. Bussen S, Sutterlin M, Steck T. Plasma endothelin and big endothelin levels in women with severe preeclampsia or HELLP-syndrome. Arch Gynecol Obstet 1999; 262:113–119.

50. Terrone DA, May WL, Moore A, Magann EF, Martin JN Jr. Does the admission complete blood count reflect evidence of inflammation in patients with HELLP syndrome (abstr)? Society for Maternal-Fetal Medicine, Miami Beach, Florida, 1998.

51. Halim A, Kanayama N, El Maradny E, Maehara K, Takahashi A, Nosaka K, Fukuo S, Amamiya A, Kobayashi T, Terao T. Immunohistological study in cases of HELLP syndrome (hemolysis, elevated liver enzymes and low platelets) and acute fatty liver of pregnancy. Gynecol Obstet Invest 1996; 41:106–112.

52. Riordan SM, Williams R. Acute liver failure: targeted artificial and hepatocyte-based support of liver regeneration and reversal of multiorgan failure. J Hepatol 2000; 32:63–76.

53. Visser W, Beckmann I, Bremer HA, Lim HL, Wallenburg HC. Bioactive tumour necrosis factor a in pre-eclamptic patients with and without the HELLP syndrome. Br J Obstet Gynaecol 1994; 101:1081–1082.

54. Wisdom SJ, Wilson R, McKillop JH, Walker JJ. Antioxidant systems in normal pregnancy and in pregnancy-induced hypertension. Am J Obstet Gynecol 1991; 165: 1701–1704.

55. Davidge ST, Hubel CA, Brayden RD, Capeless EC, McLaughlin MK. Sera antioxidant activity in uncomplicated and preeclamptic pregnancies. Obstet Gynecol 1992; 79:897–901.

56. Raijmakers MTM, Roes EM, Zusterzeel PLM, Steegers EAP, Mulder TPJ, Peters WHM. Oxidised and total free thiol levels in whole blood during preeclampsia. Hypertens Pregn 2000; 19(suppl 1):11.

57. Ibdah JA, Bennett MJ, Rinaldo P, Zhao Y, Gibson B, Sims HF, Strauss AW. A fetal fatty-acid oxidation disorder as a cause of liver disease in pregnant women. N Engl J Med 1999; 340:1723–1731.

58. Zusterzeel PLM, Visser W, Peters WHM, Merkus JMHM, Steegers EAP. Association between polymorphisms in the genes of biotransformation enzymes and pre-eclampsia. Hypertens Pregn 2000; 19(suppl 1):31.

59. Gleicher N. Pregnancy and autoimmunity. Acta Haematol 1986; 76:68–77.

60. Sibai BM. Immunologic aspects of preeclampsia. Clin Obstet Gynecol 1991; 34:27–33.

61. Redman CWG. Immunology of preeclampsia. Semin Perinatol 1991; 15:257–262.

62. Haeger M, Bengtsson A. Humoral immunology in normotensive and hypertensive pregnancy. Fetal Matern Med Rev 1994; 6:95–112.

63. Haeger M, Unander AM, Bengtsson A. Enhanced anaphylatoxin and terminal C5b-9 complement formation in patients with the syndrome of hemolysis, elevated liver enzymes and low platelet count. Obstet Gynecol 1990; 76:698–702.

64. Cunningham DS, Christie TL, Evans EE, McCaul JF. Effect of the HELLP syndrome on maternal immune function. J Reprod Med 1993; 38:459–464.

65. Chesley L, Cooper D. Genetics of hypertension in pregnancy: possible single gene control of preeclampsia in the descendants of eclamptic women. Br J Obstet Gynaecol 1986; 93:644–653.

66. Hutt R, Ogunniyi SO, Sullivan MH, Elder MG. Increased platelet volume and aggregation precede the onset of preeclampsia. Obstet Gynecol 1994; 83:146–149.

67. Ahmed Y, van Iddekinge B, Paul C, Sullivan HF, Elder MG. Retrospective analysis of platelet numbers and volumes in normal pregnancy and in pre-eclampsia. Br J Obstet Gynaecol 1993; 100:216–220.

68. Pekonen F, Rasi V, Ammala M, Viinikka L, Ylikorkala O. Platelet function and coagulation in normal and preeclamptic pregnancy. Thromb Res 1986; 43:553–560.

69. Rakoczi I, Tallian F, Bagdany S, Gati I. Platelet life-span in normal pregnancy and pre-eclampsia as determined by a non-radioisotope technique. Thromb Res 1979; 15: 553–556.

70. Pritchard JA, Cunningham FG, Mason RA. Coagulation changes in eclampsia: their frequency and pathogenesis. Am J Obstet Gynecol 1976; 124:855–864.

71. Garzetti GG, Tranquilli AL, Cugini AM, Mazzanti L, Cester N, Romanini. Altered lipid composition, increased lipid peroxidation, and altered fluidity of the membrane as evidence of platelet damage in preeclampsia. Obstet Gynecol 1993; 81:337–340.

72. Norris LA, Sheppard BL, Bumke G, Bonnar J. Platelet activation in normotensive and hypertensive pregnancies complicated by intrauterine growth retardation. Br J Obstet Gynaecol 1994; 101:209–214.

73. Benedetto C, Massobrio M, Bertini E, Abbondanza M, Enrieu N, Tetta C. Reduced serum inhibition of platelet-activating factor activity in preeclampsia. Am J Obstet Gynecol 1989; 160:100–104.

74. Stubbs TM, Lazarchick J, Van Dorsten JP, Cox J, Loadholt CB. Evidence of accelerated platelet production and consumption in nonthrombocytopenic preeclampsia. Am J Obstet Gynecol 1986; 155:263–265.

75. Rinder HM, Bonan JL, Anandan S, Rinder CS, Rodrigues PA, Smith BR. Noninvasive measurement of platelet kinetics in normal and hypertensive pregnancies. Am J Obstet Gynecol 1994; 170:117–122.

76. Socol ML, Weiner CP, Louis G, Espana F, Aznar J, Galbis M. Platelet activation in preeclampsia. Am J Obstet Gynecol 1985; 151:494–497.

77. Gilabert J, Estellés A, Ridocci F, Espana F, Aznar J, Galbis M. Clinical and haemostatic parameters in the HELLP syndrome: relevance of plasminogen activator inhibitors. Gynecol Obstet Invest 1990; 30:81–86.

78. Ellison J, Sattar N, Greer I. HELLP syndrome: mechanisms and management. Hosp Med 1999; 60(4):243–249.

79. Vedernikov YP, Kravtsov GM, Postnov YV, Saade G, Garfield RE. Effect of red blood cells and hemoglobin on spontaneously hypertensive and normotensive rat aortas. Am J Hypertens 1998; 11:105–112.

80. Kaibara M, Mitsuhashi Y, Watanbe T, Tamiaki F, Nishihira M, Sadatsuki M, Aisaka K. Effects of red blood cells on the coagulation of blood in normal and preeclamptic pregnancies. Am J Obstet Gynecol 1999; 180:402–405.

81. von Templehoff GF, Schneider D, Knirsch KM, Hommel G, Heilmann L. Incidence of the factor V Leiden-mutation, coagulation inhibitor deficiency and elevated antiphospholipid antibodies in patients with preeclampsia or HELLP-Syndrome (abstr). Hypertens Pregn 2000; 19(suppl 1):3.

82. Brenner B, Lanir N, Thaler I. HELLP syndrome associated with factor V R506Q mutation. Br J Haematol 1996; 92:999–1001.

83. Paternoster DM, Rodi J, Santarossa C, Vanin M, Simioni P, Girolami A. Acute pancreatitis and deep vein thrombosis associated with HELLP syndrome. Minerva Ginecol 1999; 51:31–33.

84. Krauss T, Augustin HG, Osmers R, Meden H, Unterhault M, Kuhn W. Activated protein C resistance and factor V Leiden in patients with hemolysis, elevated liver enzymes, low platelets syndrome. Obstet Gynecol 1998; 92:457–460.

85. Schlembach D, Zingsem J, Beinder E, Fischer T. Factor V Leiden-, G20210A prothrombin-mutation and activated protein-C resistance in mothers with HELLP syndrome and their children (abstr). Hypertens Pregn 2000; 19(suppl 1):44.

86. Visser W, Van Vliet H, Debruijn BAH, Wladmiroff JW, Kappers-Klunne M. Hemostatic abnormalities in women with a history of pre-eclampsia with and without the HELLP syndrome (abstr). Hypertens Pregn 2000; 19(suppl 1):24.

87. Sullivan CA, Magann EF, Perry KG Jr. The recurrence risk of HELLP syndrome in subsequent gestations. Am J Obstet Gynecol 1994; 171:940–943.

88. von Steinburg SP, Konrad I, Werner G, Kolben M, Schneider KTM, Lengyel E, Schmitt M. Differential placental gene expression in preeclampsia and HELLP syndrome (abstr). Hypertens Pregn 2000; 19(suppl 1):40.

89. Podolsky V, Vovk I, Latysheva Z. Impact of congenital factors in pregnant women with hypertension form of vascular dystonia on hypertantion in labour (abstr). Hypertens Pregn 2000; 19(suppl 1):109.

90. Williams KP, Wilson S. Ethnic variation in the incidence of HELLP syndrome in a hypertensive pregnant population. J Perinat Med 1997; 25:498–501.

91. Magann EF, Chauhan SP, Morrison JC, Martin JN Jr. Absence of seasonal variation on the frequency of HELLP syndrome. South Med J 1998; 91:731–732.

92. Megier P, Causse X, Hebert C, Desroches A. Gallbladder wall thickening forerunner of a HELLP syndrome (haemolysis, elevated liver enzymes and low platelets) (abstr). Hypertens Pregn 2000; 19(suppl 1):175.

93. Weitgasser R, Spitzer D, Kartnig I, Zajc M, Staudach A, Sandhofer F. Association of HELLP syndrome with autoimmune antibodies and glucose intolerance. Diabetes Care 2000; 23(6):786–790.

94. Martin JN Jr, Magann EF, Blake PG, Martin RW, Perry KG Jr, Roberts WE. Analysis of 454 pregnancies with severe preeclampsia/eclampsia HELLP syndrome using the 3-class system of classification (abstr). Am J Obstet Gynecol 1993; 68:386.

95. Sibai BM, Ramadan MK, Usta I, Salama M, Mercer BM, Friedman SA. Maternal morbidity and mortality in 442 pregnancies with hemolysis, elevated liver enzymes, and low platelets (HELLP syndrome). Am J Obstet Gynecol 1993; 169:1000–1006.

96. Martin JN Jr, Blake PG, Lowry SL, Perry KG Jr, Files JC, Morrison JC. Pregnancy complicated by preeclampsia-eclampsia with the syndrome of hemolysis, elevated liver enzymes, and low platelet count: how rapid is postpartum recovery? Obstet Gynecol 1990; 76:737–741.

97. Sibai BM, Taslimi MM, el-Nazer A, Amon E, Mabie BC, Ryan GM. Maternal-perinatal outcome associated with the syndrome of hemolysis, elevated liver enzymes, and low platelets in severe preeclampsia-eclampsia. Am J Obstet Gynecol 1986; 155:501–509.

98. Martin JN Jr, Rinehart BK, May WL, Magann EF, Terrone DA, Blake PG. The spectrum of severe preeclampsia: comparative analysis by HELLP (hemolysis, elevated liver enzyme levels, and low platelet count) syndrome classification. Am J Obstet Gynecol 1999; 180:1373–1384.

99. Audibert F, Friedman SA, Frangieh AY, Sibai BM. Clinical utility of strict diagnostic criteria for the HELLP (hemolysis, elevated liver enzymes, and low platelets) syndrome. Am J Obstet Gynecol 1996; 175:460–464.

100. Abbade JF, Peracoli JC, Calderon IMP, Borges VTM, Miano FAG, Rudge MVC. The importance of partial HELLP syndrome (abstr). Hypertens Pregn 2000; 19(suppl 1):95.

101. Faridi A, Rath W. Differential HELLP syndrome diagnosis. Z Gerburtshilfe 1996; 200:88–95.

102. Isler CM, Rinehart BK, Terrone DA, May WL, Magann EF, Martin JN Jr. Major maternal morbidity doubles when the parous patient with HELLP syndrome/severe

preeclampsia develops eclampsia (abstr). 67th Annual Meeting of the Central Association of Obstetricians and Gynecologists, Maui, Hawaii, October 25-27, 1999.

103. Martin JN Jr, May WL, Rinehart BK, Martin RW, Magann EF. Increasing maternal weight: a risk factor for preeclampsia/eclampsia but apparently not for HELLP syndrome. South Med J 2000; 93:686-691.

104. Segal S, Shenhav S, Gemer O. Thrombocytopenia with the HELLP syndrome. Report of two cases with reversal in normotensive and nonproteinuric gravidas. J Reprod Med 1998; 43:227-229.

105. Neuhaus W, Crombach G, Hamm W, Bolte A. A case of HELLP syndrome at 23 weeks' gestation. Arch Gynecol Obstet 1994; 255:217-219.

106. Mueller MD, Bruhwiler H. HELLP syndrome and trisomy 18 in a multi-parity patient. Z Geburtshilfe 1996; 200:119-121.

107. Reister F, Heyl W, Emmerich D, Hermanns B, Rath W. HELLP syndrome in the 21st week of pregnancy in mosaic trisomy 9. Zentralbl Gynakol 1996; 118:669-672.

108. Craig K, Pinette MG, Blackstone J, Chard R, Cartin A. Highly abnormal maternal inhibin and b-human chorionic gonadotropin levels along with severe HELLP (hemolysis, elevated liver enzymes, and low platelet count) syndrome at 17 weeks' gestation with triploidy. Am J Obstet Gynecol 2000; 182:737-739.

109. Alsulyman OM, Castro MA, Zuckerman E, McGehee W, Goodwin TM. Preeclampsia and liver infarction in early pregnancy associated with the antiphospholipid syndrome. Obstet Gynecol 1996; 88:644-646.

110. Tilstra JH. Two patients with postpartum HELLP syndrome after normotensive twin pregnancy. Int J Gynecol Obstet 1994; 47:49-51.

111. Yilmaztürk A, Schlüter W. Postpartum HELLP syndrome. Eur J Obstet Gynecol Reprod Biol 1992; 43:243-244.

112. Izumi A, Minakami H, Matsubara S, Sato I. Triplet pregnancy complicated by a gradual decline in antithrombin-III activity and HELLP syndrome: a case report. J Obstet Gynaecol Res 1998; 24:275-279.

113. Minakami H, Watanabe T, Izumi A, Matsubara S, Koike T, Sayama M, Moriyama I, Sato I. Association of a decrease in antithrombin III activity with a perinatal elevation in aspartate aminotransferase in women with twin pregnancies: relevance to the HELLP syndrome. J Hepatol 1999; 30:603-611.

114. Mecacci F, Cioni R, Carignani L, Parretti E, La Torre P, Martini E, Lucchetti R, Piccioli A, Mello G. Early onset HELLP syndrome associated with antiphospholipid antibodies (APA) syndrome: report on two cases (abstr). Hypertens Pregn 2000; 19(suppl 1):154.

115. Morssink LP, Heringa MP, Beekhuis JR, De Wolf BTHM, Mantingh A. The HELLP syndrome: its association with unexplained elevation of MSAFP and MshCG in the second trimester. Prenat Diagn 1997; 17:601-606.

116. Pourrat O, Pierre F. Falling platelet counts should be taken into account far earlier than usual in the course of pregnancy. Hypertens Pregn 2000; 19(suppl 1):176.

117. Stedman CM, Huddleston JF, Quinlan RW, et al. Thrombocytopenia and transaminase elevation associated with preeclampsia: the rapidity of postpartal improvement (abstr). 7th Annual Meeting, Society of Perinatal Obstetricians, Lake Buena Vista, FL, Feb 5-7, 1987.

118. Catanzarite V. The pattern and time course of laboratory abnormalities in HELLP

syndrome (abstr). 9th Annual Meeting, Society of Perinatal Obstetricians, New Orleans, LA, Feb 1–4, 1989;

119. Catanzarite V. HELLP syndrome and its complications. Contemp Ob/Gyn 1991; 36:13–21.

120. Figini E, Za G, Squarcina M, Marras M, Passamonti U, Bocchino G, Mori PG, Gandolfo A, Massone ML, Santi E. Course and regression on HELLP syndrome. Minerva Ginecol 1996; 48:405–408.

121. Makkonen N, Harju M, Kirkinen P. Postpartum recovery after severe pre-eclampsia and HELLP syndrome. J Perinat Med 1996; 24:641–649.

122. Katz VL, Thorp JM Jr, Rozas L, Bowes WA Jr. The natural history of thrombocytopenia associated with preeclampsia. Am J Obstet Gynecol 1990; 163:1142–1143.

123. Neiger R, Contag SA, Coustan DR. The resolution of preeclampsia-related thrombocytopenia. Obstet Gynecol 1991; 77:692–695.

124. Williams KP, Rychel V. Correlation of platelet changes with liver cell destruction in HELLP syndrome (abstr). Hypertens Pregn 2000; 19(suppl 1):149.

125. Ruschitzka F, Schulz E, Kling H, Schrader J, Rath W. Longitudinal study of 24-hour blood pressure behavior in pregnancy and puerperium in patients with normal pregnancy, pre-eclampsia and HELLP syndrome. Z Geburtshilfe 1996; 200: 100–103.

126. Martin JN Jr, Files JC, Blake PG, Perry KG Jr, Morrison JC, Norman PH. Postpartum plasma exchange for atypical preeclampsia-eclampsia as HELLP (hemolysis, elevated liver enzymes, and low platelets) syndrome. Am J Obstet Gynecol 1995; 172:1107–1127.

127. Magann EF, Chauhan SP, Naef RW, Blake PG, Morrison JC, Martin JN Jr. Standard parameters of preeclampsia: can the clinician depend upon them to reliably identify the patient with the HELLP syndrome? Aust NZ J Obstet Gynaecol 1993; 33: 122–126.

128. Ogle M, Sanders AB. Preeclampsia. Ann Emerg Med 1984; 13:368–370.

129. Martin JN Jr, Stedman CM. Imitators of preeclampsia and HELLP syndrome. Obstet Gynecol Clin North Am 1991; 18:181–198.

130. Aster RH. Gestational thrombocytopenia. N Engl J Med 1990; 323:262–266.

131. Burrows RF, Kelton JG. Fetal thrombocytopenia in healthy mothers and their infants. N Engl J Med 1988; 319:142–145.

132. Burrows RF, Kelton JG. Thrombocytopenia at delivery: a prospective survey of 6715 deliveries. Am J Obstet Gynecol 1990; 162:731–734.

133. Burrows RF, Kelton JG. Fetal thrombocytopenia and its relation to maternal thrombocytopenia. N Engl J Med 1993; 329:1463–1466.

134. Sullivan CA, Martin JN Jr. Management of the obstetric patient with thrombocytopenia. Clin Obstet Gynecol. In press.

135. Tanner B, Ohler WG, Hawighorst S, Schaffer U, Knapstein PG. Complications in HELLP syndrome due to peripartal hemostatic disorder. Zentralbl Gynakol 1996; 118:213–220.

136. Roussillon E, Tunon De Lara C, Ekouevi D, Leng JJ, Dallay D, Horovitz J. The significance of thrombocytopenia in the management of the HELLP syndrome: 62 cases report (abstr). Hypertens Pregn 2000; 19(suppl 1):154.

137. Terrone DA, Isler CM, May WL, Magann EF, Norman PF, Martin JN Jr. Cardio-

pulmonary morbidity as a complication of severe preeclampsia HELLP syndrome. J Perinatol 2000; 2:78–81.

138. Martin JN Jr, Perry KG Jr, Miles JF Jr, Blake PG, Magann EF, Roberts WE, Martin RW. The interrelationship of eclampsia, HELLP syndrome, and prematurity: cofactors for significant maternal and perinatal risk. Br J Obstet Gynaecol 1993; 100: 1095–1100.

139. Miles JF, Martin JN Jr, Blake PG, Perry KG Jr, Martin RW, Meeks GR. Postpartum eclampsia: a recurring perinatal dilemma. Obstet Gynecol 1990; 76:328–331.

140. Perry KG Jr, Blake PG, Martin RW, McCaul JF, Martin JN Jr. Severity of HELLP syndrome and hypertension in association with onset of postpartum diuresis (abstr). Tenth Annual Meeting, Society of Perinatal Obstetricians, Houston, TX 1990.

141. Goodlin R, Mostello D. Maternal hyponatremia and the syndrome of hemolysis, elevated liver enzymes, and low platelet count. Am J Obstet Gynecol 1987; 156:910–911.

142. Vigil-de Gracia PE, Tenorio-Maranon FR, Cejudo-Carranza E, Helguera-Martinez A, Garcia-Caceres E. Difference between preeclampsia, HELLP syndrome and eclampsia, maternal evaluation. Ginecol Obstet Mex 1996; 64:377–382.

143. Beller FK, Dame WR, Ebert C. Pregnancy-induced hypertension complicated by thrombocytopenia, haemolysis and elevated liver enzymes (HELLP) syndrome. Renal biopsies and outcome. Aust NZ J Obstet Gynaecol 1985; 25:83–86.

144. Ghosh AK, Vashisht K, Varma S, Khullar D, Sakhuja V. Acute renal failure in a patient with HELLP syndrome—an unusual complication of eclampsia. Ren Fail 1994; 16:295–298.

145. Audibert F, Coffineau A, Edouard D, Brivet F, Ville Y, Frydman R, Fernandez H. Management of HELLP syndrome before 32 weeks of amenorrhea. 22 cases. Presse Med 1996; 25:235–239.

146. Martinez de Ita AL, Garcia CE, Helguera MAM, Cejudo CE. Acute renal insufficiency in HELLP syndrome. Ginecol Obstet Mex 1998; 66:462–468.

147. Rodriguez GD, Godina GM, Hernandez CA, Ramirez GA, Hernandez CR. Severe pre-eclampsia, HELLP syndrome and renal failure. Ginecol Obstet Mex 1998; 66:48–51.

148. Selcuk NY, Odabas AR, Cetinkaya R, Tonbul HZ, San A. Outcome of pregnancies with HELLP syndrome complicated by acute renal failure (1989–1998). Ren Fail 2000; 22:319–327.

149. Amant F, Spitz B, Arnout J, Van Assche FA. Hepatic necrosis and haemorrhage in pregnant patients with antiphospholipid antibodies. Lupus 1997; 6:552–555.

150. Rinehart BK, Terrone DA, Magann EF, Martin RW, May WL, Martin JN Jr. Preeclampsia-associated hepatic hemorrhage and rupture: mode of management related to maternal and perinatal outcome. Obstet Gynecol Surv 1999; 54:196–202.

151. Sheikh RA, Yasmeen S, Riegler JL. Spontaneous intrahepatic hemorrhage and hepatic rupture in the HELLP syndrome. J Clin Gastroenterol 1999; 28:323–328.

152. Cerwenka H, Bacher H, Werkgartner G, El-Shabrawi A, Mischinger HJ. Massive liver haemorrhage and rupture caused by HELLP-syndrome treated by collagen fleeces coated with fibrin glue. Eur J Surg 1998; 164:709–711.

153. Zissin R, Yaffe D, Fejgin M, Olsfanger D, Shapiro-Feinberg M. Hepatic infarction in preeclampsia as part of the HELLP syndrome: CT appearance. Abdom Imaging 1999; 24:594–596.

154. Chan ADS, Gerscovich EO. Imaging of subcapsular hepatic and renal hematomas in pregnancy complicated by preeclampsia and the HELLP syndrome. J Clin Ultrasound 1999; 27:35–40.

155. Benacerraf BR, Frigoletto FD, Martini CA. Sonographic findings in severe preeclampsia twenty-four hours prior to clinical signs. Am J Obstet Gynecol 1985; 152: 684–685.

156. Strauss S, Walden R, Mashiach S, Graif M. Sonographic liver changes prior to clinical signs of preeclampsia. Gynecol Obstet Invest 1991; 31:114–115.

157. Minakami H, Sugimoto H, Manaka C, Takahashi T, Sato I, Tamada T. HELLP syndrome: CT evaluation. Gynecol Obstet Invest 1994; 38:28–30.

158. Barton JR, Sibai BM. Hepatic imaging in HELLP syndrome (hemolysis, elevated liver enzymes, and low platelet count). Am J Obstet Gynecol 1996; 174:1820–1827.

159. Risseeuw JJ, de Vries JE, van Eyck J, Arabin B. Liver rupture postpartum associated with preeclampsia and HELLP syndrome. J Matern Fetal Med 1999; 8:32–35.

160. Rosen JM, Luhmann KC, Tank RA. Hepatobiliary scintigraphy in the evaluation of preeclampsia and HELLP syndrome. Clin Nucl Med 1994; 19:740–741.

161. Davidson RM, Barron BJ, White PA, Fraire AE. Diagnosis by radiocolloid imaging of postpartum hepatic necrosis in the syndrome of hemolysis, elevated liver enzymes, and low platelets. Clin Nucl Med 1992; 17:322–324.

162. Wenzel M, Lehnen H. A case of mild ocular manifestations in pregnancy-induced hypertension with HELLP syndrome. Acta Ophthalmol 1994; 72:391–392.

163. Bumke JP, Whyte I, Macewen CJ. Bilateral serous retinal detachments in the HELLP syndrome. Acta Opthalmol 1989; 67:322–334.

164. Leff SR, Yarian DL, Masciulli L, Green SN, Baldomero RE. Vitreous haemorrhage as a complication of HELLP syndrome. Br J Ophthalmol 1990; 74:498.

165. Levavi H, Neri A, Zoldan J, Segal J, Ovadia J. Preeclampsia, "HELLP" syndrome and postictal cortical blindness. Acta Obstet Gynaecol Scand 1987; 66:91–92.

166. Gupta LY, Mansour SE. Bilateral bullous retinal detachment as a complication of the HELLP syndrome. Can J Ophthalmol 1994; 29:242–245.

167. Isler CM, Rinehart BK, Terrone DA, Martin RW, Magann EF, Martin JN Jr. Maternal mortality associated with HELLP (hemolysis, elevated liver enzymes, and low platelets) syndrome. Am J Obstet Gynecol 1999; 181:924–928.

168. Cardwell MS. Maternal death due to the HELLP syndrome. J Tenn Med Assoc 1987; 80:473–474.

169. Katz VL, Cefalo RC. Maternal death from carotid artery thrombosis associated with the syndrome of hemolysis, elevated liver function, and low platelets. Am J Perinatol 1989; 6:360–362.

170. Helguera-Martinez AM, Tenorio-Maranon R, Vigil-de Gracia PE, Garcia-Caceres E. HELLP syndrome. Analysis of 102 cases. Ginecol Obstet Mex 1996; 64:528–533.

171. Feske SK, Sperling RA, Schwartz RB. Extensive reversible brain magnetic resonance lesions in a patient with HELLP syndrome. J Neuroimaging 1997; 7:247–250.

172. Williams KP, Wilson S. Maternal middle cerebral artery velocity changes in HELLP syndrome versus pre-eclampsia. Ultrasound Obstet Gynecol 1998; 11:195–198.

173. Williams KP, Wilson S. Cerebral perfusion pressure changes in HELLP syndrome. Hypertens Pregn 2000; 19(suppl 1):120.

174. Onrust S, Santema JG, Aarnoudse JG. Pre-eclampsia and the HELLP syndrome still

cause maternal mortality in the Netherlands and other developed countries: can we reduce it? Eur J Obstet Gynecol Reprod Biol 1999; 82:41–46.

175. Raval DS, Co S, Reid MA, Pildes R. Maternal and neonatal outcome of pregnancies complicated with maternal HELLP syndrome. J Perinatol 1997; 17:266–269.

176. Dotsch J, Hohmann M, Kuhl PG. Neonatal morbidity and mortality associated with maternal haemolysis elevated liver enzymes and low platelets syndrome. Eur J Pediatr 1998; 157:439–440.

177. Joern H, Funk A, Rath W. Doppler sonographic findings for hypertension in pregnancy and HELLP syndrome. J Perinat Med 1999; 27:388–394.

178. ACOG Committee Opinion on Obstetric Practice: Antenatal corticosteroid therapy for fetal maturation. No. 147, December 1994.

179. Gortner L, Pohlandt F, Bartmann P, Terinde R, Versmold H, Dorigo O. Short term outcome in infants with birth weights <1750 g born to mothers with HELLP syndrome. J Perinat Med 1992; 20:25–28.

180. Abramovici D, Friedman SA, Mercer BM, Audibert F, Kao L, Sibai BM: Neonatal outcome in severe preeclampsia at 24 to 36 weeks' gestation: does the HELLP (hemolysis, elevated liver enzymes, and low platelet count) syndrome matter? Am J Obstet Gynecol 1999; 180:221–225.

181. Harms K, Rath W, Herting E, Kuhn W. Maternal hemolysis, elevated liver enzymes, low platelet count, and neonatal outcome. Am J Perinatol 1995; 12:1–6.

182. Magann EF, Perry KG Jr, Chauhan SP, Graves GR, Blake PG, Martin JN Jr. Neonatal salvage by weeks' gestation in pregnancy complicated by HELLP syndrome. J Soc Gynecol Invest 1994; 1:206–209.

183. Kandler C, Kevekordes B, Zenker M, Kandler M, Beinder E, Lang N, Harms D. Prognosis of children born to mothers with HELLP syndrome. J Perinat Med 1998; 26:486–490.

184. Klein B, Rath W. Flow-cytometric determination of platelet activation in newborn of preeclamptic mothers compared to newborn of healthy mothers (abstr). Hypertens Pregn 2000; 19(suppl 1):124.

185. Ascarelli MH, Perry KG Jr, Magann EF, May WL, Blake PG, Martin JN Jr. A birthweight of 600 grams: cutpoint on the cusp of perinatal viability in pregnancies delivered very preterm for HELLP syndrome. J Matern Fetal Invest 1997; 7:184–187.

186. Goodlin RC. Severe preeclampsia: another great imitator. Am J Obstet Gynecol 1976; 125:747–753.

187. Brown MA, Passaris G, Carlton MA. Pregnancy-induced hypertension and acute fatty liver of pregnancy: atypical presentations. Am J Obstet Gynecol 1990; 163:1154–1156.

188. Egley GC, Gutliph J, Bowes WA. Severe hypoglycemia associated with HELLP syndrome. Am J Obstet Gynecol 1985; 152:576–577.

189. Neuman M, Ron-El R, Langer R, Bukovsky I, Caspi E. Maternal death caused by HELLP syndrome (with hypoglycemia) complicating mild pregnancy-induced hypertension in a twin gestation. Am J Obstet Gynecol 1990; 162:372–373.

190. Castro MA, Fassett MJ, Reynolds TB, Shaw KJ, Goodwin TM. Reversible peripartum liver failure: a new perspective on the diagnosis, treatment, and cause of acute fatty liver of pregnancy, based on 28 consecutive cases. Am J Obstet Gynecol 1999; 181:389–395.

191. Martin JN Jr, Files JC, Morrison JC. Peripartal adult thrombotic thrombocytopenic purpura and hemolytic-uremic syndrome. In: Clark SL, Cotton DB, Hankins GDV, et al (eds). Critical Care Obstetrics. Boston: Blackwell Scientific, 1991:464–483.

192. Kaiser C, Distler W. Thrombotic thrombocytopenic purpura and HELLP (hemolysis, elevated liver enzymes, and low platelets) syndrome: differential diagnostic problems. Am J Obstet Gynecol 1995; 172:1107–1125.

193. Martin JN Jr, Files J. Reply: Letter to the editor. (Am J Obstet Gynecol 1995; 172:1107–1127.) Am J Obstet Gynecol 1996; 175:507.

194. Shepard KV, Fishleder A, Lucas FV, Goormastic M, Bukowski RM. Thrombotic thrombocytopenic purpura treated with plasma exchange or exchange transfusions. West J Med 1991; 154:410–415.

195. Kahra K, Draganov B, Sund S, Hovig T. Postpartum renal failure: a complex case with probable coexistence of hemolysis, elevated liver enzymes, low platelet count, and hemolytic uremic syndrome. Obstet Gynecol 1998; 92:698–700.

196. Balderston KD, Tewari K, Azizi F, Yu JK. Intrahepatic cholangiocarcinoma masquerading as the HELLP syndrome (hemolysis, elevated liver enzymes, and low platelet count) in pregnancy: case report. Am J Obstet Gynecol 1998; 179:823–824.

197. Minakami H, Kohmura Y, Izumi A, Watanabe T, Matsubara S, Sato I. Relation between gestation thrombocytopenia and the syndrome of hemolysis, elevated liver enzymes, and low platelet count (HELLP syndrome). Gynecol Obstet Invest 1998; 46:41–45.

198. Magann EF, Graves GR, Roberts WE, Blake PG, Morrison JC, Martin JN Jr. Corticosteroids for enhanced fetal lung maturation in patients with HELLP syndrome: impact on neonates. Aust NZ J Obstet Gynaecol 1993; 33:131–135.

199. Magann EF, Martin RW, Isaacs JD, Blake PG, Morrison JC, Martin JN Jr. Corticosteroids for the enhancement of fetal lung maturity: impact on the gravida with preeclampsia and HELLP syndrome. Aust NZ J Obstet Gynaecol 1993; 33:127–130.

200. Magann EF, Bass D, Chauhan SP, Sullivan DL, Martin RW, Martin JN Jr. Antepartum corticosteroids: disease stabilization in patients with HELLP syndrome. Am J Obstet Gynecol 1994; 171:1148–1153.

201. Magann EF, Perry KG Jr, Meydrech EF, Harris RL, Chauhan SP, Martin JN Jr. Postpartum corticosteroids: accelerated recovery from HELLP syndrome. Am J Obstet Gynecol 1994; 171:1154–1158.

202. Perry KG Jr, Martin RW, Magann EF, Blake PG, Robinette L, Martin JN Jr. Expanded implementation of dexamethasone for HELLP syndrome pregnancies improves maternal-perinatal outcomes (abstr). Society of Perinatal Obstetricians, Anaheim, CA, 1997.

203. Martin JN Jr, Perry KG Jr, Blake PG, May WA, Moore A, Robinette L. Better maternal outcomes are achieved with dexamethasone therapy for postpartum HELLP syndrome. Am J Obstet Gynecol 1997; 177:1011–1017.

204. Vigil-de Gracia P, Garcia-Caceres E. Dexamethasone in the postpartum treatment of HELLP syndrome. Int J Gynaecol Obstet 1997; 59:217–221.

205. Yalcin OT, Sener T, Hass H, Ozalp S, Okur A. Effects of postpartum corticosteroids in patients with HELLP syndrome. Int J Gynaecol Obstet 1998; 61:141–148.

206. Thiagarajah S, Bourgeois FS, Harbert GM, Caudle MR. Thrombocytopenia in preeclampsia: associated abnormalities and management principles. Am J Obstet Gynecol 1984; 150:1–7.

207. Clark SL, Phelan JR, Allen SH, Golde SR. Antepartum reversal of hematologic abnormalities associated with the HELLP syndrome. J Reprod Med 1986; 31:70–72.

208. Yeast JD, Coronado S. Hepatic dysfunction, thrombocytopenia and late-onset preeclampsia. J Reprod Med 1987; 32:781–784.

209. Heyborne KD, Burke MS, Porreco RP. Prolongation of premature gestation in women with hemolysis, elevated liver enzymes and low platelets. J Reprod Med 1990; 35:53–57.

210. Heller CS, Elliott JP. High-order multiple pregnancies complicated by HELLP syndrome. A report of four cases with corticosteroid therapy to prolong gestation. J Reprod Med 1997; 42:743–746.

211. Tompkins MJ, Thiagarajah S. HELLP (hemolysis, elevated liver enzymes, and low platelet count) syndrome: the benefit of corticosteroids. Am J Obstet Gynecol 1999; 181:304–309.

212. Isler CM, Magann EF, Rinehart BK, Terrone DA, Bass JD, Martin JN Jr. Dexamethasone versus betamethasone for postpartum HELLP syndrome: a randomized prospective clinical trial of comparative efficacy (abstr). Society for Maternal-Fetal Medicine, Miami Beach, Florida, Jan 31–Feb 5, 2000.

213. Isler CM, Barrilleaux PS, Magann EF, Bass JD, Martin JN Jr. A prospective, randomized trial comparing the efficacy of dexamethasone and betamethasone for the treatment of antepartum HELLP syndrome (abstr). 68th Annual Meeting, Central Association of Obstetricians and Gynecologists, Chicago, IL, Oct 18–21, 2000.

214. Barton JR, Bush K, O'Brien JM, Milligan DA. The impact of high dose corticosteroid on laboratory changes in women with hemolysis, elevated liver enzymes and low platelet count (HELLP syndrome) (abstr). Hypertens Pregn 2000; 19(suppl 1):144.

215. Many A, Kuperminc MJ, Pausner D, Lessing JB. Treatment of severe preeclampsia remote from term: a clinical dilemma. Obstet Gynecol Surv 1999; 54:723–727.

216. Magann EF, Washburne JF, Sullivan CA, Chauhan SP, Morrison JC, Martin JN Jr. Corticosteroid-induced arrest of HELLP syndrome progression in a marginally-viable pregnancy. Eur J Obstet Gynecol Reprod Biol 1995; 59:217–219.

217. O'Boyle JD, Magann EF, Washburne Sullivan CA, Schorr SJ, Morrison JC, Martin JN Jr. Dexamethasone-facilitated postponement of delivery in an extremely preterm pregnancy complicated by HELLP syndrome. Mil Med 1999; 164:316–318.

218. Pourrat O, Sarfati R, Wager I, Demeeus JB, Pierre F, Magnin G. Evidence of efficiency of steroids in an anecdotal case of early-onset preeclampsia complicated by HELLP syndrome (abstr). Hypertens Pregn 2000; 19(suppl 1):158.

219. Martin JN Jr, Magann EF. High-dose dexamethasone: a promising therapeutic option for HELLP. Contemp Ob/Gyn 1999; Nov:55–57.

220. Tsatsaris V, Carbonne B, La Tour MD, Cabrol D, Milliez J. Is conservative treatment of HELLP syndrome safe? Eur J Obstet Gynecol Reprod Biol 1998; 80:139–141.

221. Faridi A, Reister F, Heyl W, Rath W. Preliminary results of the international HELLP-multicenter-study—aggressive versus expectant management (abstr). Hypertens Pregn 2000; 19(suppl 1):140.

222. Tissier I, Langer B, Sebahoune V, David-Montefiore E, Baldauf JJ, Boudier E, Treisser A, Ritter J (abstr). Hypertension in Pregnancy 2000; 19(suppl 1):142.

223. Faridi A, Heyl W, Rath W. Preliminary results of the International HELLP multicenter study. Int J Gynaecol Obstet 2000; 69:279–280.

224. Shima H, Oue T, Taira Y, Miyazaki E, Puri P. Antenatal dexamethasone enhances endothelin receptor β expression in hypoplastic lung in nitrofen-induced diaphragmatic hernia in rats. J Pediatr Surg 2000; 35:203–207.
225. Ziegler JW, Ivy DD, Kinsella JP, Abman SH. The role of nitric oxide, endothelin, and prostaglandins in the transition of the pulmonary circulation. Clin Perinatol 1995; 22:387–403.
226. Stern N, Palant L, Ozaki L, Tuck ML. Dexamethasone enhances active cation transport in cultured aortic smooth muscle cells. Am J Hypertens 1994; 7:146–150.
227. Homuth V, Wallukat G, Fischer T, Lindschau C, Dechend R, Haller H, Dudenhausen JW, Luft FC. Agonistic autoantibodies to the angiotensin AT1 receptor in maternal and neonatal sera in patients with preeclampsia and HELLP syndrome (abstr). Hypertens Pregn 2000; 19(suppl 1):138.
228. Wallace EM, Baker LS. Effect of antenatal betamethasone administration on placental vascular resistance. Lancet 1999; 353:1404–1407.
229. Ulrich S, Piper C, Kalder M, Berle P. Severe HELLP syndrome with temporary kidney and lung failure. Geburtshilfe Frauenheilkd 1996; 56:443–446.
230. Hamada S, Takishita Y, Tamura T, Naka O, Higuchi K, Takahashi H. Plasma exchange in a patient with postpartum HELLP syndrome. J Obstet Gynaecol Res 1996; 22:371–374.
231. Pourrat O, Goujon JM, Hauet TH, Robert R, Bauwens M, Touchard G. Are plasma exchanges useful in severe postpartum HELLP syndrome (abstr)? Hypertens Pregn 2000; 19(suppl 1):152.
232. Chappell LC, Seed PT, Briley AL, Kelly FJ, Lee R, Hunt BJ, Parmar K, Bewley SJ, Shennan AH, Steer PJ, Poston L. Effect of antioxidants on the occurrence of preeclampsia in women at increased risk: a randomised trial. Lancet 1999; 354:810–816.
233. Nakatsuka M, Tada K, Kimura Y, Asagiri K, Kamada Y, Takata M, Nakata T, Inoue N, Kudo T. Clinical experience of long-term transdermal treatment with nitric oxide donor for women with preeclampsia. Gynecol Obstet Invest 1999; 47:13–19.
234. Van Pampus MG, Wolf H, Westenberg SM, can der Post JA, Bonsel GJ, Treffers PE. Maternal and perinatal outcome after expectant management of the HELLP syndrome compared with pre-eclampsia without HELLP syndrome. Eur J Obstet Gynecol Reprod Biol 1998; 76:31–36.
235. Visser W, Wallenburg HCS. Maternal and perinatal outcome of temporizing management in 254 consecutive patients with severe pre-eclampsia remote from term. Eur J Obstet Gynecol Reprod Biol 1995; 63:147–154.
236. Saphier CJ, Repke JT. Hemolysis, elevated liver enzymes, and low platelets (HELLP) syndrome: a review of diagnosis and management. Semin Perinatol 1998; 22:118–133.
237. Geary M. The HELLP syndrome. Br J Obstet Gynaecol 1997; 104:887–891.
238. Curtin WM, Weinstein L. A review of HELLP syndrome. J Perinatol 1999; 19:138–143.
239. Egerman RS, Sibai BM. HELLP syndrome. Clin Obstet Gynecol 1999; 42:381–389.
240. Ellison J, Sattar N, Greer I. HELLP syndrome: mechanisms and management. Hosp Med 1999; 60:243–249.
241. Magann EF, Martin JN Jr. Twelve steps to optimal management of HELLP syndrome. Clin Obstet Gynecol 1999; 42:532–550.

242. Abroug F, Boujdaria R, Nouira S, Abroug S, Souissi M, Najjar MF, Secourgeon JF, Bouchoucha S. HELLP syndrome: incidence and maternal-fetal outcome—a prospective study. Intens Care Med 1992; 18:274–277.

243. Huang S, Chang F. The adverse effect on fetal hemogram by preeclampsia: marked anisocytosis with normocytic, normochromic erythrocythemia as well as thrombocytopenia. Early Hum Dev 1994; 37:91–98.

244. Sibai BM. Magnesium sulfate is the ideal anticonvulsant in preeclampsia-eclampsia. Am J Obstet Gynecol 1990; 162:1141–1145.

245. Vliegen JHR, Muskens E, Keunen RW, Smith SJ, Godfried WH, Gerretsen G. Abnormal cerebral hemodynamics in pregnancy-related hypertensive encephalopathy. Eur J Obstet Gynecol Reprod Biol 1993; 49:198–200.

246. Belfort MA, Saade GR, Moise KJ Jr. The effect of magnesium sulfate on maternal and fetal blood flow in pregnancy-induced hypertension. Acta Obstet Gynaecol Scand 1993; 72:526–530.

247. Reubinoff BE, Schenker JG. HELLP syndrome: a syndrome of hemolysis, elevated liver enzymes and low platelet count complicating preeclampsia-eclampsia. Int J Gynecol Obstet 1991; 36:95–102.

248. Mabie WC, Gonzalez AR, Sibai BM, Amon E. A comparative trial of labetalol and hydralazine in the acute management of severe hypertension complicating pregnancy. Obstet Gynecol 1987; 70:328–333.

249. Childress CH, Katz VL. Nifedipine and its indications in obstetrics and gynecology. Obstet Gynecol 1994; 83:616–624.

250. Rubin PC, Butters L, McCabe R. Nifedipine and platelets in preeclampsia. Am J Hypertens 1988; 1:175–177.

251. Tranquilli AL, Garzetti GG, De Tommaso G, Boemi M, Lucino E, Fumelli P, Romanini C. Nifedipine treatment in preeclampsia reverts the increased erythrocyte aggregation to normal. Am J Obstet Gynecol 1992; 167:942–945.

252. Visser W, Senden IPM, Wladimiroff JW. Intravenous ketanserin in the treatment of severe pre-eclampsia (abstr). Hypertens Pregn 2000; 19(suppl 1):140.

253. Woods JB, Blake PG, Perry KG Jr, Magann EF, Martin RW, Martin JN Jr. Ascites: A portent of cardiopulmonary complications in the preeclamptic patient with the syndrome of hemolysis, elevated liver enzymes, and low platelets. Obstet Gynecol 1992; 80:87–91.

253a. Belfort MA, Rokey R, Saade GR, Moise KJ. Rapid echocardiographic assessment of left and right heart hemodynamics in critically ill obstetric patients. Am J Obstet Gynecol 1994; 171(4):884–892.

253b. Belfort MA, Mares A, Saade GR, Wen T, Rokey R. Two-dimensional echocardiography and Doppler ultrasound in managing obstetric patients. Obstet Gynecol 1997; 90(3):326–330.

254. Roberts WE, Perry KG, Woods JB, Files JC, Blake PG, Martin JN Jr. The intrapartum platelet count in patients with HELLP (hemolysis, elevated liver enzymes, and low platelets) syndrome: is it predictive of later hemorrhagic complications? Am J Obstet Gynecol 1994; 171:799–804.

255. Kris M, White DA. Treatment of eclampsia by plasma exchange. Plasma Ther 1981; 2:143–147.

256. Lusvarghi E, Vandelli L, Baldini E, Montagnani G. Plasma exchange in late gestosis. Nephron 1981; 28:258.

257. Spencer CD, Crane FM, Kumar JR, Alving BM. Treatment of postpartum hemolytic uremic syndrome with plasma exchange. JAMA 1982; 247:2808–2809.

258. Caggiano V, Fernando LP, Schneider JM, Haesslein HC, Watson-Williams EJ. Thrombotic thrombocytopenic purpura: report of fourteen cases—occurrence during pregnancy and response to plasma exchange. J Clin Apheresis 1983; 1:71–85.

259. Gordon BR, Saal SD. Post-partum hemolytic uremic syndrome: treatment with plasma exchange. Clin Exp Dialysis Apheresis 1983; 7:169–176.

260. Vandekerckhove F, Noens L, Colardyn F, Thiery M, Delbarge W. Thrombotic thrombocytopenic purpura mimicking toxemia of pregnancy. Am J Obstet Gynecol 1984; 150:320–322.

261. Hakim RM, Schulman G, Churchill WH Jr, Lazarus JM. Successful management of thrombocytopenia, microangiopathic anemia, and acute renal failure by plasmapheresis. Am J Kidney Dis 1985; 5:170–176.

262. Schwartz ML, Brenner W. Severe preeclampsia with persistent postpartum hemolysis and thrombocytopenia treated by plasmapheresis. Obstet Gynecol 1985; 65:53S–55S.

263. Schwartz ML. Possible role for exchange plasmapheresis with fresh frozen plasma for maternal indications in selected cases of preeclampsia and eclampsia. Obstet Gynecol 1986; 67:136–139.

264. Martin JN Jr, Files JC, Blake PG, Norman PH, Martin RW, Hess LW, Morrison JC, Wiser WL. Plasma exchange for preeclampsia: I. Postpartum use for persistently severe preeclampsia-eclampsia with HELLP syndrome. Am J Obstet Gynecol 1990; 162:126–137.

265. Martin JN Jr, Perry KG Jr, Roberts WE, Norman PF, Files JC, Blake PG, Morrison JC, Wiser WL. Plasma exchange for preeclampsia: II. Unsuccessful antepartum utilization for severe preeclampsia with or without HELLP syndrome. J Clin Apheresis 1994; 9:155–161.

266. Martin JN Jr, Perry KG Jr, Roberts WE, Files JC, Norman PF, Morrison JC, Blake PG. Plasma exchange for preeclampsia: III. Immediate peripartal utilization for selected patients with HELLP syndrome. J Clin Apheresis 1994; 9:162–165.

267. Stricker RB, Main EK, Kronfield J, Kallas GS, Gerson LB, Autry AM, Kiprov DD. Severe postpartum eclampsia: response to plasma exchange. J Clin Apheresis 1992; 7:1–3.

268. Katz VL, Watson WJ, Thorp JM Jr, Hansen W, Bowes WA Jr. Treatment of persistent postpartum HELLP syndrome with plasmapheresis. Am J Perinatol 1992; 9:120–122.

269. Magann EF, Roberts WE, Perry KG Jr, Chauhan SP, Blake PG, Martin JN Jr. Factors relevant to mode of preterm delivery with syndrome of HELLP (hemolysis, elevated liver enzymes, and low platelets). Am J Obstet Gynecol 1994; 170:1828–1834.

270. Schorr SJ, Sullivan CA, Calfee EF, Blake PG, Pickett RA, Martin JN Jr. A comparison of Pfannenstiel and vertical skin incisions in patients with severe preeclampsia/HELLP syndrome (abstr). J Soc Gynecol Invest 1995; 2:319.

271. Briggs R, Chari RS, Mercer B, Sibai B. Postoperative incision complications after cesarean section in patients with antepartum syndrome of hemolysis, elevated liver

enzymes, and low platelets (HELLP): does delayed primary closure make a difference? Am J Obstet Gynecol 1996; 175:893–896.

272. Magann EF, Dodson MK, Allbert JR, McCurdy CM, Martin RW, Morrison JC. Blood loss at time of cesarean section by method of placental removal and exteriorization versus in situ repair of the uterine incision. Surg Gynecol Obstet 1993; 177:389–392.

273. Magann EF, Dodson MK, Harris RL, Floyd RC, Martin JN Jr, Morrison JC. Does placental removal or site of uterine incision repair alter endometritis after cesarean delivery? Infect Dis Obstet Gynecol 1993; 1:65–70.

274. Hunter CA Jr, Howard WF, McCormick CO Jr. Amelioration of the hypertension of toxemia by postpartum curettage. Am J Obstet Gynecol 1961; 81:884–889.

275. Harer WB Jr, McIndoe DW. Postpartum eclampsia treated by curettage. Am J Obstet Gynecol 1962; 83:1349–1350.

276. Magann EF, Martin JN Jr, Isaacs JD, Perry KG Jr, Martin RW, Meydrech EF. Immediate postpartum curettage: accelerated recovery from severe preeclampsia. Obstet Gynecol 1993; 81:502–506.

277. Magann EF, Bass JD, Chauhan SP, Perry KG Jr, Morrison JC, Martin JN Jr. Accelerated recovery from severe preeclampsia: uterine curettage versus nifedipine. J Soc Gynecol Invest 1994; 1:206–209.

278. Schlenzig C, Maurer S, Goppelt M, Ulm K, Kolben M. Postpartum curettage in patients with HELLP-syndrome does not result in accelerated recovery. Eur J Obstet Gynecol Reprod Biol 2000; 91:25–28.

279. Rolbin SH, Abbott D, Musclow E, Papsin F, Lie LM, Freedman J. Epidural anesthesia in pregnant patients with low platelet counts. Obstet Gynecol 1988; 71:918–920.

280. Duffy BL. HELLP syndrome and the anaesthetist. Anaesthesia 1988; 43:223–225.

281. Crosby ET, Preston R. Obstetrical anaesthesia for a parturient with preeclampsia, HELLP: anesthesia syndrome and acute cortical blindness. Can J Anaesth 1998; 45:452–459.

282. Portis R, Jacobs MA, Skerman JH, Skerman EB. HELLP syndrome (hemolysis, elevated liver enzymes, and low platelets) pathophysiology and anesthetic considerations. J Am Assoc Nurse Anesth 1997; 65:37–47.

283. Nelson EW, Archibald L, Albo D. Spontaneous hepatic rupture in pregnancy. Am J Surg 1977; 134:817–820.

284. Henry CP, Lim AE, Brummelkamp WH, Buller HR, Ten Cate JW. A review of the importance of acute multidisciplinary treatment following spontaneous rupture of the liver capsule during pregnancy. Surg Gynecol Obstet 1983; 156:593–598.

285. Goodlin RC, Anderson JC, Hodgson PE. Conservative treatment of liver hematoma in the postpartum period. A report of two cases. J Reprod Med 1985; 30:368–370.

286. Smith LG, Moise KJ, Dildy GA, Carpenter RJ. Spontaneous rupture of liver during pregnancy: current therapy. Obstet Gynecol 1991; 77:171–175.

287. Golan A, White RG. Spontaneous rupture of the liver associated with pregnancy. A report of 5 cases. S Afr Med J 1979; 56:133–136.

288. Loevinger EH, Vujic I, Lee WM, Anderson MC. Hepatic rupture associated with pregnancy: treatment with transcatheter embolotherapy. Obstet Gynecol 1985; 65: 281–284.

289. Herbert WN, Brenner WE. Improving survival with liver rupture complicating pregnancy. Am J Obstet Gynecol 1982; 142:530–534.

290. Neerhof MG, Zelman W, Sullivan T. Hepatic rupture in pregnancy. Obstet Gynecol Surv 1989; 44:407–409.

291. Rittenberry AB, Arnold CL, Taslimi MM. Hemostatic wrapping of ruptured liver in two postpartum patients. Am J Obstet Gynecol 1991; 165:705–707.

292. Mays ET, Conti S, Fallahzadeh H, Rosenblatt M. Hepatic artery ligation. Surgery 1979; 86:536–543.

293. Gonzalez GD, Rubel HR, Giep NN, Bottsford JE Jr. Spontaneous hepatic rupture in pregnancy: management with hepatic artery ligation. South Med J 1984; 77: 242–245.

294. Erhard J, Lange R, Niebel W, Scherer R, Kox WH, Philipp T, Eigler FW. Acute liver necrosis in the HELLP syndrome: successful outcome after orthotopic liver transplantation. A case report. Transplant Int 1993; 6:179–181.

295. Hunter SK, Martin M, Benda JA, Zlatnik FJ. Liver transplant after massive spontaneous hepatic rupture in pregnancy complicated by preeclampsia. Obstet Gynecol 1995; 85:819–822.

296. Sullivan CA, Magann EF, Perry KG Jr, Roberts WE, Blake PG, Martin JN Jr. The recurrence risk of the syndrome of hemolysis, elevated liver enzymes, and low platelets (HELLP) in subsequent gestations. Am J Obstet Gynecol 1994; 171: 940–943.

297. Sibai BM, Ramadan MK, Chari RS, Friedman SA. Pregnancies complicated by HELLP syndrome (hemolysis, elevated liver enzymes, and low platelets): subsequent pregnancy outcome and long-term prognosis. Am J Obstet Gynecol 1995; 172: 125–129.

298. Beinder E, Hirschmann A, Wildt L, Junker H. HELLP syndrome: recurrence in 4 consecutive pregnancies. Geburtshilfe Frauendgeulkd 1996; 56:501–503.

299. Fraser JL, Millenson M, Malynn ER, Uhl L, Kruskall MS. Possible association between the Norplant contraceptive system and thrombotic thrombocytopenia purpura. Obstet Gynecol 1996; 87:860–863.

8

Gestational Hypertension: How Much Should We Worry?

Robyn A. North
University of Auckland, Auckland, New Zealand

Mark A. Brown
St. George Hospital and University of New South Wales, Sydney, New South Wales, Australia

I. INTRODUCTION

Pregnant women have serial blood pressure measurements throughout pregnancy, with the aim of identifying those with hypertension. The intrinsic assumption of this practice is that hypertension is a marker for increased risk of an adverse pregnancy outcome. This is a valid assumption if the woman has preeclampsia, but it is more controversial if she has gestational hypertension. Opinion varies from gestational hypertension being merely an exaggeration of the normal physiological rise in blood pressure that ensures adequate placental perfusion toward term to it being a distinct disease that confers significant risk of maternal or fetal complications (1). If we consider it to be a specific condition, a number of issues are raised. Is gestational hypertension an early sign of preeclampsia or is it a separate disease entity with different pathology? What are the risks, if any, conferred by gestational hypertension to the mother and baby in the current and in future pregnancies? How should these women be managed during pregnancy and are there any long-term health implications? Before these issues can be addressed, we should first consider what is meant by gestational hypertension.

II. UNDERSTANDING THE DEFINITION OF GESTATIONAL HYPERTENSION

The diagnostic criteria utilized will determine which women are included under the cloak of gestational hypertension, thus influencing associated maternal and fetal risks. Use of different definitions modifies the perception of the significance of gestational hypertension. Pregnant women with de novo hypertension are considered to have either gestational hypertension or, in the presence of significant proteinuria, preeclampsia. Several other terms—such as *transient hypertension* or *pregnancy-induced hypertension*—have been used, further confusing the classification of hypertensive disorders in pregnancy (see Chapter 1) (2,3). In our chapter, we shall confine terminology to gestational hypertension and preeclampsia.

At the start of this new millennium, there are two main approaches to defining gestational hypertension. In the first, gestational hypertension is the presence of elevated blood pressure detected for the first time after midpregnancy in the absence of proteinuria (4–6). An alternative definition is the presence of isolated elevated blood pressure developing after 20 weeks gestation, with no other features of preeclampsia (2,7,8). At first glance these groups may appear identical, but they are not. The first definition comprises women with de novo hypertension after exclusion of women with associated proteinuria. Such women may still develop complications, such as eclamptic seizures or thrombocytopenia, but they remain under the diagnostic label of gestational hypertension. The second definition includes women with de novo hypertension alone, and if any multisystem complication ensues, by definition the woman is then considered to have preeclampsia (2,7,8). This latter definition recognizes the multisystem nature of preeclampsia and acknowledges that although proteinuria is often the next sign to develop after hypertension, not all women with multisystem complications of preeclampsia have proteinuria.

The impact of these two different approaches was highlighted in an analysis of 1183 consecutive women with hypertensive disorders (9). Sixty one percent were considered to have gestational hypertension by the first definition (de novo hypertension in the absence of proteinuria), whereas after applying the second definition (an isolated de novo elevation in blood pressure), only 43% had gestational hypertension. This decrease resulted from the reclassification of all women with multisystem complications as preeclamptic in the latter definition. Thus gestational hypertension can become a benign condition simply by modifying the classification criteria.

The criteria for defining de novo hypertension and significant proteinuria in pregnancy will also influence the associated risk of an adverse outcome. In a normal pregnant population, blood pressure greater than 140/90 mmHg is more than two standard deviations above the mean blood pressure range from 20 to 34 weeks' gestation, and approximately two standard deviations above the mean from 35 weeks to term (4,10). The criteria for hypertension usually includes sustained systolic blood pressure of at least 140 mmHg or diastolic blood pressure of at least 90 mmHg in a woman who was normotensive before 20 weeks' gestation or is normotensive 6 weeks postpartum (2,6–8). Two classification systems rely only on diastolic blood pressure of at least 90 mmHg (4,5).

A rise in blood pressure of at least 25 mmHg systolic or 15 mmHg diastolic during pregnancy, even if the absolute blood pressure level was less than 140/90 mmHg, was included in past definitions (2,7). Between 27 and 67% of women whose blood pressure remains less than 140/90 mmHg have such a rise in blood pressure during pregnancy (11,12). These women appear to have no increase in adverse pregnancy outcomes except possibly an increase in cesarean section rate (12–14). Inclusion of this group within a gestational hypertension cohort will significantly dilute any inherent maternal or fetal risks associated with a blood pressure >140/90 mmHg. Recent American, Canadian, and Australasian definitions have not included an isolated rise in blood pressure in the definition of gestational hypertension (3,5,6,8).

The definition of significant proteinuria will also impact on which women are classified as having gestational hypertension. In the absence of a 24-h urinary protein measurement, if "1+" or more is considered significant proteinuria, then only women with de novo hypertension and negative or trace proteinuria will be diagnosed with gestational hypertension. The high false-positive rate of 26 to 83% with "1+" proteinuria (15–18). has led to the use of "2+" on urinary dipstick testing as the cutoff for proteinuria (4,7,19). This results in women with "1+" proteinuria and no 24-h urinary protein measurement being included in the gestational hypertension group. Women with gestational hypertension and "1+" proteinuria are more likely to develop severe hypertension or severe maternal disease than those women with negative or trace proteinuria on dipstick (12). This is expected, as this group must include some (about half) with true proteinuria—i.e., preeclampsia. Thus interpretation of data on the outcome of pregnancies complicated by gestational hypertension should take into consideration the diagnostic criteria.

In clinical practice, diagnosis of women with gestational hypertension may be seen as a post hoc process, only possible after systematic, serial assessment of a woman with new onset hypertension in the second half of pregnancy. Often the final diagnosis is not possible until after delivery. In practical terms, the clinician wishes to know how much should he or she worry about a pregnant woman presenting with de novo hypertension in the absence of proteinuria on dipstick after 20 weeks of gestation. A woman presenting with gestational hypertension may progress down one of several paths over the remainder of her pregnancy (Figure 1). The possibility of severe complications underlies the obstetrician's concern associated with the development of gestational hypertension.

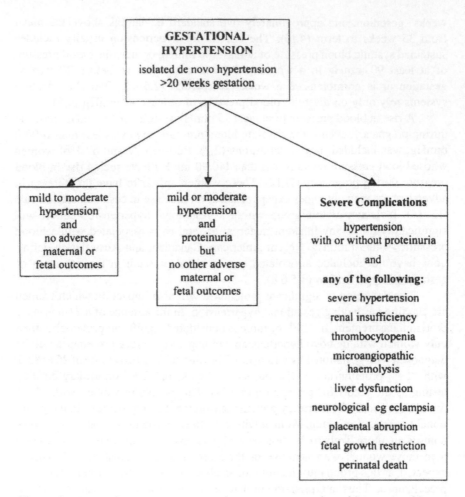

Figure 1   Range of pregnancy outcomes for a woman presenting with gestational hypertension.

III. PREVALENCE AND RISK FACTORS FOR GESTATIONAL HYPERTENSION

Gestational hypertension has been reported to complicate between 4.4 and 17.5% of pregnancies, with a weighted mean of 14.6% (10,12,20–28). Many of these are epidemiological studies utilizing large databases. Recent prospective studies, where the diagnosis was confirmed in every woman, report a similar variation in the prevalence of gestational hypertension in nulliparous women, ranging from

5.6 to 17.3% (12,20,21,24). The differences in prevalence of gestational hypertension cannot easily be explained by systematic differences in study design, definitions, or populations.

The prevalence of gestational hypertension steadily increases with advancing gestation up to 40 weeks. Among the 15,812 women who were entered into the 1997–1999 database at our tertiary referral obstetric hospital, 1128 (7.1%) developed gestational hypertension. The prevalence of gestational hypertension according to gestational age at delivery is shown in Figure 2.

A number of clinical characteristics in early pregnancy are associated with an increased risk of gestational hypertension (Table 1).

A. Race and Ethnic Background

Race does not appear to be an important determinant for the development of gestational hypertension (10,22,23,28–31). In a large study using national databases, gestational hypertension occurred in 13.1% of pregnancies in African-American women and 14.8% of pregnancies in other American women (22).

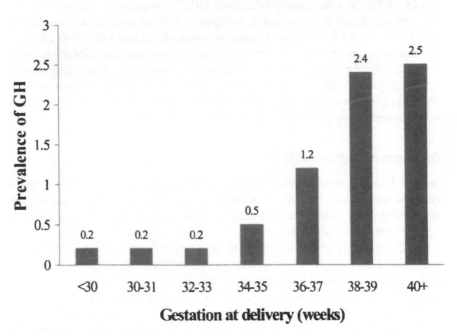

Figure 2 The prevalence of gestational hypertension (GH) in 15,812 women according to gestational age at delivery.

Table 1   Risk Factors in Early Pregnancy Associated
with Gestational Hypertension

Nulliparity
Shorter duration of sexual cohabitation preconception
Donor egg, sperm, or embryo pregnancies
Twins
Age > 35 years
Obesity (BMI > 29)
Nonsmoker
Higher blood pressure < 20 weeks (MAP ≥ 85 mmHg)
Previous gestational hypertension or preeclampsia
Job stress
Reduced leisure time exercise

B. Parity

Gestational hypertension is more common in nulliparous than multiparous women
(1.6- to 2-fold), but the relationship is less striking than that seen in preeclampsia
(23,26,27,32). In a Scottish study of over 130,000 pregnancies, the relative risk
(RR) of gestational hypertension in nulliparous women compared to multiparas
was 1.98 (95% CI 1.94–2.03) in singleton pregnancies and 1.85 (95% CI 1.55–
2.21) in twin pregnancies (27). Among nulliparous women, gestational hypertension was more common in the first pregnancy compared to subsequent pregnancies, [odds ratio (OR) 2.29 (95% CI 1.65-3.20)], and a history of two or more
abortions (spontaneous or induced) was associated with a reduced risk of gestational hypertension [OR 0.42 (95% CI 0.16–0.94)] (30).

C. Immunological Factors

Several lines of circumstantial evidence suggest repeated exposure to paternal
antigens may reduce the risk of gestational hypertension. Multiparous women
who change their partners have a slightly higher risk of developing gestational
hypertension than multiparous women with the same partner [OR 1.3 (95% CI 1.1–
1.6)] (23). The risk of developing gestational hypertension or preeclampsia was
increased 12-fold if the duration of sexual cohabitation before conception was less
than 4 months compared to more than 12 months (33). This paper was criticized
for combining hypertensive groups, and the authors subsequently reported that
primigravid women with gestational hypertension had a significantly shorter
median duration of sexual cohabitation before conception than controls (4.7
versus 17.6 months) (34). Similar findings were seen in multigravid women with a
new partner (34). In keeping with the proposal that immune tolerance following

repeated paternal antigen exposure is protective (35) is the increased rate of gestational hypertension with donor spermatozoa, donor oocytes, or embryo donation (36). The similarity of these findings in gestational hypertension and preeclampsia provides support for common pathological mechanisms for these two conditions, at least in some women.

D. Multiple Pregnancy

Gestational hypertension is more common in twin pregnancies (12.9%) than singleton pregnancies (6.3%) [adjusted OR 1.6 (95% CI 1.32–2.37)] (19). Although the overall incidence of gestational hypertension was higher in the large Scottish study, a similar increase in gestational hypertension in twin pregnancies compared with singleton pregnancies was found (27). This held true in both nulliparous [twins 32.4%, singletons 24.4%, RR 1.33 (95% CI 1.18–1.49)] and multiparous women [twins 17.5%, singletons 12.3%, RR 1.42 (95% CI 1.24–1.63)] (27). Zygosity did not influence the prevalence of gestational hypertension (27).

E. Age and Body Mass Index (BMI)

As in preeclampsia, older age and increasing BMI are associated with an increased risk of gestational hypertension (10,26,28,30,37). Compared with underweight women with BMI <19.8, obese women with a BMI >29 had an increased risk of gestation hypertension [OR 4.85 (95% CI 1.97–11.92)] (25). Other studies have reported a similar association between increasing BMI and increased risk (1.7- to 3-fold) of developing gestational hypertension (26,28,30,37). Smoking is associated with a reduced risk of gestational hypertension in most (25,26,28,38–40), but not all studies (30). The protective effect of smoking is particularly evident if more than 10 cigarettes are smoked each day during pregnancy (25,28).

F. Early Pregnancy Blood Pressure

Women destined to develop gestational hypertension have higher clinic and 24-hour blood pressure measurements in the first and second trimesters than women who remain normotensive (41,42). Among women with a mean arterial pressure of at least 85 mmHg at 20 weeks' gestation, 7.3% developed gestational hypertension, compared to 0.17% of those with a mean arterial pressure less than 85 mmHg (43).

G. Prior Hypertension in Pregnancy

Multigravid women whose first pregnancy was complicated by gestational hypertension or preeclampsia are at increased risk of developing gestational hyperten-

Table 2 Outcome of Second Pregnancy According to Whether First Pregnancy Was Normal or Complicated by Gestational Hypertension or Preeclampsia

First pregnancy	Second pregnancy[a]		
	Normotensive	Gestational hypertension	Preeclampsia
Normotensive (44) (n = 3507)	90%	9.3%	0.7%
Gestational hypertension (44,45) (n = 1460)	68 (52–69)%	30 (29–44)%	2 (2–2)%
Preeclampsia (44,45,133) (n = 435)	50 (28–62)%	36 (30–53%)	8 (5–8)%

[a]Expressed as weighted mean % (range %).

sion in their next pregnancy (Table 2) (44,45). One-third of women with gestational hypertension or preeclampsia in their first pregnancy developed gestational hypertension in their second pregnancy.

H. Job Stress

Two studies have reported that high job stress (high demand with low latitude in job) have a modest association with gestational hypertension (46,47). Lower levels of physical exercise have also been associated with the development of gestational hypertension (47,48). Women who performed regular leisure time physical activity, compared with those who did not, had a trend to a reduced risk of developing gestational hypertension [adjusted RR 0.75 (95% CI 0.54–1.05)] (48).

IV. ARE GESTATIONAL HYPERTENSION AND PREECLAMPSIA SEPARATE DISEASE ENTITIES?

Gestational hypertension is simply a sign in pregnant women of a range of possible conditions including an apparently normal physiological event, a predisposition for essential hypertension unmasked by pregnancy, or an early manifestation of preeclampsia. Few studies have reported the proportion of women with gestational hypertension who progress to preeclampsia (49–51). Saudan determined the rate of progression from a database of women with hypertensive complications in pregnancy as well as in a prospective cohort (50). Among women with isolated mild to moderate hypertension developing after 20 weeks of gestation, 6% in the retrospective study and 18% in the prospective study subsequently developed preeclampsia defined as development of proteinuria or HELLP (hemolysis, elevated liver enzymes, low platelets) syndrome. If preeclampsia was defined as de novo hypertension with any of the following: proteinuria, renal impairment, hepatic dysfunction, thrombocytopenia, cerebral involvement or severe hypertension, 15% in the retrospective study and 26% in the prospective study developed preeclampsia. A recent American study reported 46% of 748 women who presented with gestational hypertension between 24 and 35 weeks progressed to preeclampsia, with 9.6% developing severe disease (51).

The earlier gestational hypertension occurs, the greater the likelihood of disease progression. In the Australian study, preeclampsia developed in 42% of women who presented with gestational hypertension before 30 weeks, 36% of those presenting between 30 and 33 weeks, 20% at 34 to 35 weeks, 16% at 36 to 37 weeks, and 7% of women who presented after 37 weeks' gestation. (50). The Rotterdam group reported similar findings (49). One-third of women in their cohort who presented with gestational hypertension at or before 32 weeks gestation eventually developed preeclampsia, whereas only 3% of those diagnosed after 37 weeks progressed to preeclampsia (49). In the American study, half the cases of gestational hypertension presenting before 32 weeks progressed to preeclampsia (51). By 34 to 35 weeks' gestation, the rate of progression had decreased to 37%.

Therefore between one-third to one-half of the women presenting with early-onset gestational hypertension have progressive disease and develop preeclampsia. In some cases of early onset gestational hypertension, the condition may be curtailed when delivery is expedited for fetal indications. The disease progresses in less than 10% of women who develop gestational hypertension after 37 weeks. Progression to preeclampsia may be less frequent at term either because delivery interrupts the natural history before preeclampsia supervenes, or because the disease process was never actually that of preeclampsia.

Before exploring further the differences and similarities between gestational hypertension and preeclampsia, one should appreciate an intrinsic bias in most cross-sectional cohorts of women with gestational hypertension. The majority of women with gestational hypertension develop the condition close to term (Figure 3). Consequently an unselected study population of women with gestational hypertension will usually be biased toward term disease. It is probable that the pathology of early-onset gestational hypertension is different from that at term, but this difference may be obscured in most studies.

Many of the clinical risk factors associated with preeclampsia are also associated with an increased risk of developing gestational hypertension, as outlined in Table 1. A recent study of twins suggests that, like preeclampsia, genetic factors may contribute to the development of gestational hypertension (52).

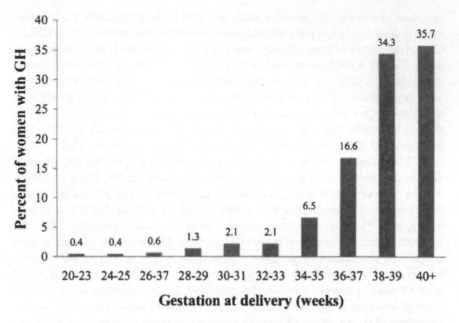

Figure 3 The distribution of women with gestational hypertension ($n = 1128$) according to gestational age at delivery.

A. Placental Factors

Preeclampsia is characterized by impaired uteroplacental perfusion secondary to shallow trophoblast invasion and restricted remodeling of the maternal spiral arteries, activation of maternal endothelial cells and leukocytes, vasoconstriction, reduced plasma volume, and activated coagulation (53–55). Release of placental factors, such as syncytiotrophoblast microvillous membrane fragments or lipid peroxides, into the maternal circulation or modification of components in maternal blood as it passes through the intervillous space appear to trigger the maternal response (54,55). Some but not all of these phenomena also occur in gestational hypertension.

Failure of the normal physiological changes in the spiral arteries may occur in gestational hypertension (56,57). As data on placental bed biopsy histology in gestational hypertension are very limited, it is not possible to determine how common or important defective trophoblast invasion is in this condition. Uterine artery Doppler studies at 24 weeks' gestation suggest that the majority (95%) of women ($n = 134$) with gestational hypertension have normal uteroplacental blood flow (58). Women with preeclampsia are more likely to have abnormal uterine artery waveforms than those with gestational hypertension (58), but several studies also report that only a minority of unselected preeclamptic women have abnormal uterine artery Doppler studies (59–61). Further studies are required to determine the true prevalence of abnormal uteroplacental blood flow in early- and late-onset gestational hypertension.

B. Markers of Endothelial and Inflammatory Cell Activation

In preeclampsia, several circulating markers indicate endothelial cell and leukocyte activation. Activated endothelial cells express fibronectin, a high-molecular-weight glycoprotein with procoagulant and adhesion properties. Endothelial cell derived isoforms of fibronectin are increased in preeclampsia, but not gestational hypertension (62). On the other hand, total plasma fibronectin, which may be derived from endothelial cells, platelets, or trophoblast, has been found to be increased throughout pregnancy in both gestational hypertension and preeclampsia (63). Vascular cell adhesion molecule 1 is expressed on endothelial cells and plays a role in mononuclear leukocyte adhesion to endothelium. Soluble forms may be released into the circulation with endothelial cell activation. Vascular cell adhesion molecule 1 is increased in preeclampsia, but unchanged in gestational hypertension (64). These data suggest that activation of maternal endothelial cells does not occur to the same degree in gestational hypertension as it occurs in preeclampsia. Further research is required to clarify whether vascular changes similar to those seen in preeclampsia occur in women with early onset gestational hypertension.

C. Hemodynamic Changes

Vasoconstriction with increased peripheral resistance is typical of preeclampsia (65), but not gestational hypertension (66). Consistent with this peripheral vasoconstriction in preeclampsia is a redistribution of the circulating blood volume away from smaller vessels, whereas this is not evident in gestational hypertension (67). In gestational hypertension, the cardiac output steadily increases throughout gestation, whereas in preeclampsia the cardiac output increases before the hypertension is apparent and falls with the onset of clinical disease (66). These data suggest that the pathophysiological processes resulting in hypertension in these two conditions may be different.

It is well established that preeclampsia is associated with a reduction in total blood volume and plasma volume (67). Some investigators report no reduction in total blood volume or plasma volume in gestational hypertension (67), whereas others found a small, but significant reduction in plasma volume (68,69). Again, these findings generally support pathophysiological differences between gestational hypertension and preeclampsia.

C. Renin-Aldosterone-Angiotensin System

Women with gestational hypertension have reduced plasma renin and aldosterone concentrations, which are intermediate between those of normal pregnant women and women with established preeclampsia. Further, the plasma aldosterone:renin ratio is significantly elevated compared with that in normal pregnant women, but again not to the same levels as seen in women with preeclampsia (70). The mechanism(s) producing this apparent enhanced adrenal sensitivity have not yet been elucidated. These data imply that there is either enhanced adrenal responsiveness to angiotensin II (perhaps in keeping with apparent enhanced vascular responsiveness to angiotensin II in preeclampsia /gestational hypertension) or else adrenal resistance to factors that usually suppress aldosterone release, such as dopamine or atrial natriuretic peptide.

D. Uric Acid

Plasma uric acid, produced in purine catabolism, is elevated in preeclampsia and to a lesser degree in gestational hypertension. In gestational hypertension, serum uric acid levels are intermediate between normotensive pregnant women and women with preeclampsia (71). Again there is wide scatter, with about half the uric acid values being higher than those found in normotensive women, and uric acid was not useful in differentiating preeclampsia from gestational hypertension (71).

E. Coagulation and Thrombophilias

Increased platelet aggregation and activated coagulation is a key feature of preeclampsia but not gestational hypertension. Circulating levels of thrombin-antithrombin complexes, thrombomodulin, and plasminogen activator inhibitor are increased in preeclampsia, whereas they are unchanged in gestational hypertension (72–75). Recently thrombophilias—in particular acquired resistance to activated protein C, factor V Leiden, and hyperhomocysteinemia—have been associated with preeclampsia (76). Grandone et al. reported a fivefold increase in the prevalence of factor V Leiden mutation in gestational hypertension [OR 5.96 (95% CI 1.69–21.0)], but the prevalence of either the prothrombin G20210A mutation or the C677T 5-10 methylenetetrahydrofolate reductase polymorphism was not increased (77). Further studies are required to define any changes in coagulation or underlying thrombophilias in women with gestational hypertension, particularly those with early-onset disease.

F. Metabolic Differences

There is increasing evidence that many women with preeclampsia have underlying metabolic differences compared with normotensive pregnant women. These include hypertriglyceridemia, elevated free fatty acids, reduced high-density-lipoprotein (HDL) cholesterol, and reduced insulin sensitivity (78–80). This dyslipidemia may predispose women to the endothelial cell activation seen in preeclampsia (79). Elevated serum triglycerides and nonesterified fatty acids have also been reported in gestational hypertension (81,82). Others found that serum triglycerides and lipid peroxides were elevated only in women with severe gestational hypertension (diastolic blood pressure >110 mmHg or multisystem complications in the absence of proteinuria) and not in women with mild gestational hypertension (83). In addition, serum triglyceride levels appear to be elevated in the second trimester in women destined to develop severe—but not mild—gestational hypertension (83). There are conflicting data as to whether HDL cholesterol is unchanged or reduced in gestational hypertension (81,82). Serum total cholesterol, low-density lipoprotein (LDL) cholesterol, very low density lipoprotein (VLDL) cholesterol, and apolipoprotein B levels are unchanged prior to and during gestational hypertension (37,81–84).

Women with gestational hypertension may have hyperinsulinemia (81,85), reduced glucose tolerance following an oral glucose load (85), and reduced insulin sensitivity (82). Similar findings are reported in preeclampsia (80), although some authors have postulated that insulin resistance is a feature of gestational hypertension and not preeclampsia (82,86). One-third of women with gestational hypertension had an abnormal 50-g oral glucose loading test earlier in pregnancy (24–32 weeks) compared with 9% in normotensive controls, ($p > 0.0001$) (87). Among nondiabetic women, hemoglobin $A1_C$ levels at 28 weeks were higher in those who subsequently developed gestational hypertension than in normotensive women (88). A larger study found an increased risk of gestational hypertension only in overt gestational diabetes [RR 1.48 (95% CI 0.99–2.22)] (89). Further research is needed to clarify the precise nature of any underlying metabolic disturbance in gestational hypertension, particularly as this may have long-term health implications.

G. Calcium Metabolism

Compared with controls, basal platelet intracellular free calcium is similar in gestational hypertension but reduced in preeclamptic women (90). Hypocalciuria has been described in preeclampsia but does not appear to occur in gestational hypertension (85). Women with gestational hypertension who later develop preeclampsia have lower urinary calcium/creatinine ratios than those women who remain as gestational hypertensives (91).

H. Activin A and Inhibin A

Activin A and inhibin A are glycoprotein hormones belonging to the transforming growth factor superfamily. Women with preeclampsia, particularly those with early-onset severe disease, have markedly elevated serum total activin A and inhibin A (92,93). Serum concentrations of total activin A, but not inhibin A, are elevated in gestational hypertension compared with normotensive pregnant controls (92). Total activin A is increased from early in the third trimester and before the onset of clinical disease in women who later develop gestational hypertension (93). The precise role, if any, of these hormones in the pathogenesis of preeclampsia and gestational hypertension is currently unknown.

I. Summary of Pathophysiological Changes in Gestational Hypertension

In summary, gestational hypertension shares a number of clinical and pathological characteristics with preeclampsia, but usually to a lesser degree. There are also clear differences in pathological events associated between these two forms of hypertension. In particular, there does not appear to be the same degree of activation of the endothelium or coagulation in gestational hypertension as with preeclampsia. Until the subgroups of gestational hypertension are mapped with greater clarity, we are unlikely to progress in our understanding of the pathophysiology of this heterogeneous group, held together by the common sign of hypertension in late pregnancy.

V. MATERNAL AND FETAL COMPLICATIONS ASSOCIATED WITH GESTATIONAL HYPERTENSION

Maternal and fetal complications in women who develop hypertension after 20 weeks' gestation in the absence of proteinuria are shown in Table 3 (12,19,31, 94,95). Three of these studies used "2+" proteinuria to define significant proteinuria when a 24-hour urinary protein was not available (12,19,94). Two studies, one a prospective screening study of 1496 healthy nulliparous women (12) and the other a prospectively established database of women with hypertensive complications developing during pregnancy (96), reported very similar rates of severe hypertension (22 and 13%) and multisystem disease (5 and 7%) in gestational hypertension (Figure 4). The rate of severe hypertension and multisystem complications was significantly lower in gestational hypertension than that occurring in women with preeclampsia.

The incidence of placental abruption does not appear to be increased in women with gestational hypertension (19,31). Induction of labor was increased in gestational hypertension (25%) compared with normotensive pregnancies (12%) (31). One-third of the singleton babies born to mothers with gestational hypertension are delivered by cesarean section (12,19,31,95).

Preterm birth was lower in singleton or twin pregnancies complicated by gestational hypertension compared with those in normotensive controls (12,27, 31,95). SGA infants were more common in women with gestational hypertension

Table 3 Maternal and Fetal Complications in Gestational Hypertension—Defined as Isolated De Novo Hypertension Without Proteinuria

Complication	Number	Weighted mean % (range (%)
Maternal		
Severe hypertension (12,31,94)	1529	9.4 (4.3–22.2)
Renal insufficiency (12,31,94)	1529	1.3 (1.0–2.6)
Thrombocytopenia (12,31,94)	1529	4.3 (0.9–8)
Liver involvement (12,31,94)	1529	3.9 (1.3–7)
Imminent eclampsia[a] (12,94)	782	6.0 (0–7)
Placental abruption (19,31)	933	0.4 (0.4–0.54)
Caesarean section (12,19,31,95)	1830	30.3 (29.0–31.3)
Fetal		
Preterm birth		
< 37 weeks (12,19)	303	3.3 (1.6–6.0)
< 34–35 weeks (19,31)	933	2.1 (1.1–5.9)
Small for gestational age infant (12,19, 31,94,95)	2495	10.8 (7.0–20.5)
Perinatal mortality (12,31,94)	1529	0.9 (0.7–1.1)

[a]None had eclamptic seizures.

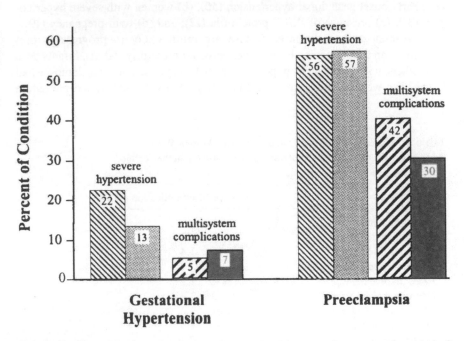

Figure 4 The proportion of women with gestational hypertension or preeclampsia in 2 studies (12,96) who developed (a) severe hypertension (≋North et al.;   Brown et al.) and (b) multisystem complications (≋ North et al.; ■ Brown et al.).

than in normotensive controls (12,31,95). Perinatal mortality and neonatal morbidity—such as respiratory distress syndrome, intraventricular haemorrhage and necrotizing enterocolitis, do not appear to be increased, although published studies do not have enough power to be certain (12,31,94,97).

All these studies report the maternal and fetal risks in women in whom the diagnosis of gestational hypertension is confirmed at or following delivery. Hence women who presented with gestational hypertension and later developed preeclampsia were excluded. The complication rate in all women presenting with gestational hypertension, including the subset of women who later developed preeclampsia, is shown in Table 4 (50). Interestingly, maternal and fetal complications in this cohort were not materially different from those in studies examining only the outcomes of women who remained as having gestational hypertension until delivery. Barton and coworkers found that 9.6% of women ($n = 748$) presenting with gestational hypertension between 24 and 35 weeks developed either severe preeclampsia or severe hypertension (51). In their study, 2.4% developed either thrombocytopenia or HELLP syndrome.

Thus the majority of women with gestational hypertension will have an excellent pregnancy outcome and will not develop any severe maternal or fetal morbidity. There are, however, subgroups of women with gestational hypertension that appear to be at greater risk of maternal or fetal morbidity, including those (a) women with early-onset gestational hypertension (50); (b) women with severe hypertension (31); (c) presence of "1+" proteinuria (12); and (d) twin pregnancy (19).

Women with early-onset disease are more likely to progress to preeclampsia, and such women have higher perinatal morbidity (50,51). Infants born to mothers with gestational hypertension that progressed to preeclampsia had lower birth weights and were more likely to be SGA (25–27%) and premature

Table 4 Maternal and Fetal Outcome of All Women Who Presented with Gestational Hypertension ($n = 416$) Whether or Not They Progressed to Preeclampsia

	Prevalence of complication (%)
Maternal outcome	
Severe hypertension	8.2
Renal insufficiency	1.4
Hematological abnormalities	2.4
Liver involvement	1.9
Neurological features	3.8
Fetal outcome	
Small for gestational age infant	14.9
Perinatal mortality	0.49

From Ref. 50.

compared with those who remained as having gestational hypertension. Further research is needed to accurately ascertain maternal and fetal complications in very early onset gestational hypertension.

Women with severe gestational hypertension were more likely to have renal dysfunction, induction of labor and premature delivery (31). Among women with gestational hypertension, those with "1+" proteinuria ($n = 48$) compared with negative or trace proteinuria ($n = 69$) were more likely to have severe hypertension (33 versus 14.5%) or multisystem disease (10.4 versus 1.5%) (12). This implies either that there is a subgroup of women who have clinically worrisome gestational hypertension or that this group also includes women with true proteinuria (i.e., preeclampsia).

Women with gestational hypertension who have a twin pregnancy are more likely to develop pregnancy complications than are women with singleton pregnancies. Among women with gestational hypertension and twin pregnancies, 48% were delivered by cesarean section, 18% were delivered by 34 weeks, and half were delivered before 37 weeks (19). In comparison, women with gestational hypertension and singleton pregnancies had a cesarean section rate of 31%; preterm deliveries occurred in 5.9%, with only 1.6% born before 35 weeks. Of interest, premature delivery was more common in normotensive twin pregnancies than in twin pregnancies complicated by gestational hypertension or preeclampsia (19,27). This raises the question as to whether gestational hypertension and preeclampsia may, by an unknown mechanism, protect against spontaneous preterm birth. An alternative explanation is that the occurrence of spontaneous preterm birth prevents the later development of gestational hypertension. Among women with gestational hypertension, the proportion of SGA infants was increased twofold in twin pregnancies (14.8%) compared with singleton pregnancies (7%) (19). However, the rate of SGA infants was the same in twin pregnancies whether the mother had gestational hypertension or was normotensive, suggesting that the number of fetuses is the main factor affecting the rate of SGA infants (19).

On first principles, women with gestational hypertension and significant uteroplacental perfusion abnormalities as diagnosed with Doppler ultrasound or with a growth restricted fetus may also represent a group at higher risk of adverse outcomes, but there are no data available to support or refute this.

VI. APPROACH TO MANAGEMENT OF WOMEN WITH GESTATIONAL HYPERTENSION

Although the majority of women with gestational hypertension develop no serious maternal or fetal complications, hypertension in pregnancy is still considered a marker for increased maternal and fetal surveillance. Within the group of women presenting with hypertension after 20 weeks' gestation, there is a small subset that develops serious maternal and fetal pathology. Currently there is no reliable

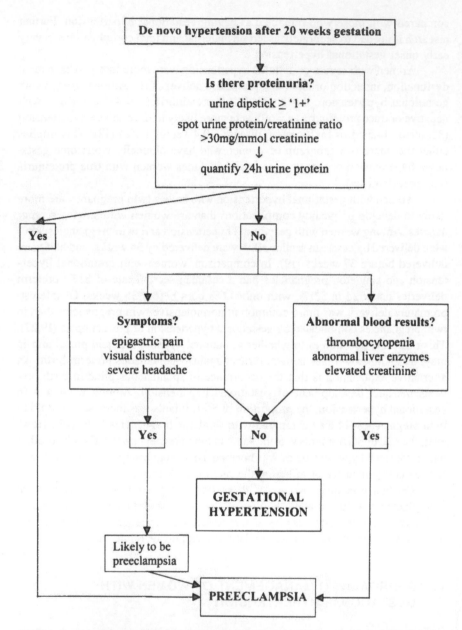

Figure 5 A schematic diagram outlining an approach to diagnosis of gestational hypertension and preeclampsia in women presenting with de novo hypertension after 20 weeks' gestation. In addition, fetal well-being should be assessed.

method of identifying this subset of women when they present with gestational hypertension.

Before considering clinical management, let us review the process of diagnosing gestational hypertension (Figure 5). At the time new hypertension is identified, the usual practice is to classify the woman's condition as either gestational hypertension or preeclampsia according to the presence or absence of proteinuria on dipstick testing of the urine. Understanding the limitations of urinary dipstick testing is essential, as discussed previously. The false-positive rate at "1+" is high and can be considerably lowered with the use of "≥2+" proteinuria (15–18). In addition, a "negative/trace" urinary dipstick on a spot urine sample may be recorded despite significant proteinuria by 24-hour urine collection, resulting in failure to recognize up to one-third of women with significant proteinuria (15). This high false-negative rate has been confirmed in two other studies formally evaluating dipstick assessment of proteinuric solutions (18,98).

The accuracy of urinary dipstick testing can be improved if proteinuria is measured by a trained observer or by automated methodology (17,18), but the deficiencies in urinary dipstick testing have led to the recommendation that the 24-hour urinary protein measurement continue to be used as the "gold standard" (99). This does not fill the clinical need for a rapid, reliable method of measuring proteinuria on a spot urine; a protein:creatinine ratio has been shown to be useful as an alternative test (8,17,100,101). In the future, this may become the screening test of choice. The protein:creatinine ratio should not be confused with the (micro)albumin:creatinine ratio.

Current management of women with gestational hypertension usually consists of more intensive outpatient monitoring. Studies in both the United States and Britain have demonstrated that such women can be safely managed in a structured outpatient setting, with a significant reduction in antenatal hospitalization (102–104). Prior to outpatient management, women presenting with gestational hypertension require systematic review for any clinical symptoms or signs of preeclampsia. Baseline investigations are performed to confirm the diagnosis, exclude multisystem complications, and evaluate the fetus. These include hemoglobin, hematocrit, platelet count, serum creatinine, urate, urinary protein:creatinine ratio or 24 h urinary protein, and possibly liver transaminases and lactic acid dehydrogenase (6). Fetal growth is assessed by clinical examination and often with ultrasound examination. If the fetus is small for gestational age, further tests of fetal well-being such as umbilical Doppler studies, nonstress testing, or biophysical profile should be considered (105).

The type and intensity of ongoing care depend on this evaluation. If the woman has mild to moderate hypertension and no features of preeclampsia, standard care in most centers is outpatient assessment on two or more occasions each week (6,8). Women at higher risk, such as those with early-onset disease, "1+" proteinuria awaiting the results of 24-hour urine protein, twin pregnancy, or fetal growth restriction require closer surveillance, in some cases as inpatients. The woman should be fully informed about the condition, the warning symptoms she should watch for, and the indications for seeking immediate medical attention. Development of severe hypertension, evidence of preeclampsia, and concerns about fetal well-being are indications for hospital admission.

Day-stay facilities, if available, will enable repeated blood pressure measurements to be performed over several hours. To date, no self-initiated home blood pressure monitor has been shown to measure blood pressure in hypertensive pregnant women with sufficient accuracy to endorse their use in clinical practice (106,107). Certain 24-hour blood pressure monitors have been studied but are too expensive for routine clinical use in this setting (108).

Overall, randomized trials have not demonstrated that bed rest clearly improves pregnancy outcome in women with gestational hypertension (104,109,110). The largest randomized trial, from Zimbabwe, reported that hospital bed rest reduced severe hypertension in multigravid but not primigravid women with gestational hypertension (110). Preterm delivery was reduced with bed rest in the Zimbabwe study, but the reason for this is unclear (110).

Lowering of blood pressure to prevent cerebral sequelae of severe hypertension in pregnancy is universally accepted as beneficial (6,8). Whether mild to moderate hypertension should be treated with antihypertensive medication is controversial. There is polarization of thought into those who believe that there is minimal risk of maternal complications with mild to moderate hypertension and no proven fetal benefits of lowering blood pressure in this context (6,111), versus others who consider that treatment of mild to moderate hypertension reduces episodes of severe hypertension (112) and protects the mother from cerebral complications (8). Recent data support the notion that many women with severe preeclampsia have abnormal cerebral autoregulation, with overperfusion of the middle cerebral artery circulation that may result in hypertensive encephalopathy (113). Lowering of blood pressure may be crucial in some women to prevent hypertensive encephalopathy, and this may decrease eclamptic seizures (114).

Published antihypertensive trials of mild to moderate hypertension in pregnancy are too small for definitive answers and often include mixed populations, such as women with gestational hypertension and preeclampsia or chronic hypertension. An overview of trials of mild to moderate hypertension presenting later in pregnancy found that antihypertensive treatment prevents severe hypertension and reduces the prevalence of proteinuria at delivery (112). Whether the reduced prevalence of proteinuria reflected a reduction in preeclampsia was not clear. Neonatal respiratory distress syndrome was reduced despite no reduction in preterm birth. There were no other definite perinatal benefits with antihypertensive therapy and there was a suggestion that the rate of SGA infants may be increased. Similar findings were reported in a systematic review of randomized trials of beta blockers used to treat mild to moderate hypertension in pregnancy (115). These authors concluded that beta blockers reduced the incidence of severe hypertension but did not prevent preeclampsia or offer other substantive benefits to the baby. They and others have raised concern over the possible increase in SGA infants with antihypertensive therapy, especially beta blockers (115–117). No specific type of antihypertensive medication appears to be advantageous (112), but angiotensin converting enzyme inhibitors and probably atenolol should be avoided (118,119). Large randomized trials are required to ascertain whether antihypertensive treatment in mild to moderate hypertension is beneficial or harmful (115).

Following delivery, gestational hypertension does not resolve immediately. The mean time before women with gestational hypertension ($n = 159$) became normotensive was reported as 6 (SD 5.5) days postpartum (120). At 5 days postdelivery, approximately 45% of women with gestational hypertension were still hypertensive. By day 10, a total of 32% were still hypertensive, but by day 20 postpartum this situation had significantly resolved and less than 5% had elevated blood pressure. Therefore it is important not to cease antihypertensive medication automatically at delivery and to continue monitoring women with gestational hypertension in the postpartum period. The disease process may continue in some women despite delivery, resulting in the postpartum development of multisystem complications, including eclampsia (121). Monitoring of patients with gestational hypertension must continue following delivery, and these women should be instructed to seek medical attention for any of the warning symptoms of impending cerebrovascular complications.

Many women with gestational hypertension will, in retrospect, have a normal pregnancy outcome. With hindsight, this more intensive surveillance will have seemed unnecessary. Further diagnosis of gestational hypertension may create considerable anxiety for the woman, consume additional medical resources, and appears to be associated with an increased induction and cesarean section rate. It is not valid, however, to assume it is safe to reduce the level of care to women with gestational hypertension. Until we are able to effectively separate those women with gestational hypertension who will have uncomplicated pregnancies from the subgroup at risk of maternal and fetal morbidity, the judicious approach is to continue increased monitoring of all women with gestational hypertension.

VII. PREDICTION OF GESTATIONAL HYPERTENSION AND THE SUBGROUP WHO LATER DEVELOP PREECLAMPSIA

Few studies have investigated early pregnancy prediction of gestational hypertension separately from preeclampsia. Although mean arterial pressure is higher at 20 weeks' gestation in women who subsequently develop gestational hypertension, it is not sufficiently discriminating to be a useful predictor for an individual woman. In a study of 580 women, of whom 10.8% developed gestational hypertension, a mean arterial pressure >85 mmHg in the second half of pregnancy had a sensitivity of 72%, specificity of 79%, and a positive predictive value of 30% for the later development of gestational hypertension (41). Uterine artery Doppler waveforms at 20 to 24 weeks had low sensitivity (16–40%) and positive predictive values (<10%) when used as a screening method for gestational hypertension (58,59).

Neither human chorionic gonadotropin (122–124), α-fetoprotein (124), inhibin A (93,124), activin A (93), total renin (124), platelet angiotensin II binding (125), albumin:creatinine ratio, or calcium:creatinine ratio (126) were useful predictors of gestational hypertension before 20 weeks of gestation. Total plasma fibronectin is significantly increased in the first and second trimesters in women destined to develop gestational hypertension compared with those who remained normotensive. However the poor performance of total fibronectin as a predictor for gestational hypertension precludes its use as a clinical screening test (63). Neither first- nor second-trimester plasma endothelin, urinary thromboxane B2, or 6-keto PGF1α were different in women who subsequently developed gestational hypertension compared with controls (127). Hence, to date, no single biochemical marker in early pregnancy has proved to be a useful predictor of later gestational hypertension. As the majority of women with gestational hypertension have a normal pregnancy outcome, it would be more useful to focus on prediction of the subgroup who develop significant maternal or fetal morbidity. To our knowledge this has not been addressed in early pregnancy screening studies.

An alternative approach is to develop screening tests that predict which women with gestational hypertension will later develop preeclampsia or adverse fetal outcomes. The first clinical clue is that women presenting with gestational hypertension before 34 weeks are more likely to develop preeclampsia than women presenting at term, but none of the usual laboratory markers have been found to be useful in identifying those in whom preeclampsia will supervene (50). Women presenting with gestational hypertension who later develop preeclampsia have lower urinary calcium/creatinine ratios than those who remain as gestational hypertensives, but the urinary calcium:creatinine ratio was not sufficiently sensitive to be used as a screening test (91). Hence, currently there is no effective screening test to determine which women with gestational hypertension will subsequently develop preeclampsia. Future research in this area is required.

VIII. WHAT ARE THE RISKS OF RECURRENCE IN FUTURE PREGNANCIES?

The risk of developing gestational hypertension or preeclampsia in the second pregnancy faced by women who were either normotensive or who had gestational hypertension or preeclampsia in the first pregnancy are shown in Table 2. Among the women with gestational hypertension in the first pregnancy, 30% developed gestational hypertension again and 2% developed preeclampsia in their second pregnancy.

IX. WHAT ARE THE LONG-TERM HEALTH IMPLICATIONS OF GESTATIONAL HYPERTENSION?

The risk for essential hypertension in later life is increased in women with a history of gestational hypertension as compared with women who were normotensive in pregnancy or the expected prevalence of essential hypertension in the general population (128–130). In a Spanish study where women were followed up for a mean of 13 years, 54% of those with gestational hypertension developed essential hypertension (128). This was significantly higher than the rate in the controls (14%) or in women in Spanish general population studies (14 to 23%).

Other studies have also reported an increase in essential hypertension following gestational hypertension (129–131). At 3 to 80 months postpartum, 14% of 99 women with gestational hypertension had essential hypertension and two women had renal disease (130). Nissell and coworkers followed up 49 women with gestational hypertension 7 years after the index pregnancy (129). At follow-up, the gestational hypertension group had higher blood pressure, 37% being hypertensive, versus 2% of women who had been normotensive in pregnancy. Another study reported very similar rates of hypertension (39%) 15 years after a diagnosis of gestational hypertension (131). Microalbuminuria, a potential marker of renal endothelial cell dysfunction, was also more common (14 versus 2%) in women with a history of gestational hypertension compared with controls (129).

Further studies are required to elucidate the long-term risks of hypertension, ischemic heart disease, and type 2 diabetes in women who develop gestational hypertension. There are important public health implications if gestational hypertension is shown to be a forerunner of future cardiovascular disease (132).

X. CONCLUSIONS AND AREAS OF FUTURE RESEARCH

Gestational hypertension is a diagnosis that groups women with divergent pathophysiology. Some women appear to have a normal rise in blood pressure at term, presumably to maintain placental perfusion. In others, pregnancy either unmasks a predisposition to essential hypertension or the hypertension may be an early manifestation of preeclampsia. Gestational hypertension and preeclampsia share a number of common clinical risk factors and biochemical features, but there are also distinct differences in their pathophysiology. The majority of women with gestational hypertension will have an uncomplicated pregnancy with an excellent perinatal outcome. A small subset will, however, develop significant maternal or perinatal morbidity. It is this group that should be the focus of more intensive antenatal care. Unfortunately, we currently have no method of identifying such women before complications supervene. Hence increased outpatient surveillance of all women with gestational hypertension continues to be appropriate management.

Key areas for further research on gestational hypertension include the following:

1. Pathogenesis, in particular of early-onset gestational hypertension.
2. Prediction of the subgroup of women with gestational hypertension who will progress to preeclampsia or develop major maternal or fetal sequelae. An effective screening test may allow rationalization of antenatal surveillance of women with gestational hypertension.
3. Large randomized trials to demonstrate that less intensive surveillance of women with gestational hypertension is not associated with an increase in maternal or fetal morbidity. The entry criteria for such studies would require careful consideration.
4. Large randomized trials of antihypertensive treatment of mild to moderate hypertension with sufficient power to determine benefits and risks for clinically important maternal and fetal endpoints.
5. Prospective long-term studies to clarify the health implications for women with a history of gestational hypertension.

ACKNOWLEDGMENT

We wish to thank Mrs. Rennae Taylor for her assistance with the data analysis and the preparation of this manuscript.

REFERENCES

1. Broughton Pipkin F. The hypertensive disorders of pregnancy. Br Med J 1995; 311: 609–613.
2. National High Blood Pressure Education Program Working Group Report on High Blood Pressure in Pregnancy. Am J Obstet Gynecol 1990; 163:1691–1712.
3. Hypertension in Pregnancy. Washington DC. American College of Obstetrics and Gynecology, 1996.
4. Davey DA, MacGillivray I. The classification and definition of the hypertensive disorders of pregnancy. Am J Obstet Gynecol 1988; 158:892–898.
5. Helewa M, Burrows R, Smith J, Williams K, Brain P, Rabkin S. Report of the Canadian Hypertension Society consensus conference: 1. Definitions, evaluation and classification of hypertensive disorders in pregnancy. Can Med Assoc J 1997; 157: 715–725.
6. Working Group Report on High Blood Pressure in Pregnancy. National High Blood Pressure Education Program. NIH Publication No. 00–3029. Washington, DC: NIH, 2000.
7. Anonymous. Management of hypertension in pregnancy: executive summary. Aus-

tralasian Society for the Study of Hypertension in Pregnancy. Med J Aust 1993; 158: 700–702.

8. Brown M, Hague W, Higgins J, et al. The detection, investigation and management of hypertension in pregnancy: executive summary and full consensus statement. Aust NZ J Obstet Gynaecol 2000; 40:133–155.

9. Brown M, de Swiet M. Classification of hypertension in pregnancy. Ballieres Clin Obstet Gynaecol 1999; 13:27–39.

10. Stone P, Cook D, Hutton J, Purdie G, Murray H, Harcourt L. Measurements of blood pressure, oedema and proteinuria in a pregnant population of New Zealand. Aust NZ J Obstet Gynaecol 1995; 35:32–37.

11. Villar MA, Sibai BM. Clinical significance of elevated mean arterial blood pressure in second trimester and threshold increase in systolic or diastolic blood pressure during third trimester. Am J Obstet Gynecol 1989; 160:419–423.

12. North RA, Taylor RS, Schellenberg JC. Evaluation of a definition of pre-eclampsia. Br J Obstet Gynaecol 1999; 106:767–773.

13. Levine R. Should the definition of preeclampsia include a rise in diastolic blood pressure of ≥15 mmHg? Am J Obstet Gynecol 2000; 182:S84.

14. Zhang J, Klebanoff MA, Roberts JM. Prediction of adverse outcomes by common definitions of hypertension in pregnancy. Obstet Gynecol. 2001; 97:261–267.

15. Meyer N, Mercer B, Friedman S, Sibai B. Urinary dipstick protein: a poor predictor of absent or severe proteinuria. Am J Obstet Gynecol 1994; 170:137–141.

16. Brown M, Buddle M. Inadequacy of dipstick proteinuria in hypertensive pregnancy. Aust NZ J Obstet Gynaecol 1995; 35:366–369.

17. Saudan P, Brown M, Farrell T, Shaw L. Improved methods of assessing proteinuria in hypertensive pregnancy. Br J Obstet Gynaecol 1997; 104:1159–1164.

18. Bell S, Halligan A, Martin A, et al. The role of observer error in antenatal dipstick proteinuria analysis. Br J Obstet Gynaecol 1999; 106:1177–1180.

19. Sibai BM, Hauth J, Caritis S, et al. Hypertensive disorders in twin versus singleton pregnancies. Am J Obstet Gynecol 2000; 182:938–942.

20. Sibai BM, Caritis SN, Thom E, et al. Prevention of preeclampsia with low-dose aspirin in healthy, nulliparous pregnant women. The National Institute of Child Health and Human Development Network of Maternal-Fetal Medicine Units. N Engl J Med 1993; 329:1213–1218.

21. Hauth JC, Goldenberg RL, Parker CR Jr et al. Low-dose aspirin therapy to prevent preeclampsia. Am J Obst Gynecol 1993; 168:1083–1091.

22. Samadi AR, Mayberry RM, Zaidi AA, Pleasant JC, McGhee N Jr, Rice RJ. Maternal hypertension and associated pregnancy complications among African-American and other women in the United States. Obstet Gynecol 1996; 87:557–563.

23. Trupin LS, Simon LP, Eskenazi B. Change in paternity: a risk factor for preeclampsia in multiparas. Epidemiology 1996; 7:240–244.

24. Levine RJ, Hauth JC, Curet LB, et al. Trial of calcium to prevent preeclampsia. N Engl J Med 1997; 337:69–76.

25. Ros HS, Cnattingius S, Lipworth L. Comparison of risk factors for preeclampsia and gestational hypertension in a population-based cohort study. Am J Epidemiol 1998; 147:1062–1070.

26. Hartikainen A-L, Aliharmi R, Rantakallio P. A cohort study of epidemiological

associations and outcomes of pregnancies with hypertensive disorders. Hypertens Pregn 1998; 17:31–41.

27. Campbell DM, MacGillivray I. Preeclampsia in twin pregnancies: incidence and outcome. Hypertens Pregn 1999; 18:197–207.

28. Zhang J, Klebanoff MA, Levine RJ, Puri M, Moyer P. The puzzling association between smoking and hypertension during pregnancy. Am J Obstet Gynecol 1999; 181:1407–1413.

29. Irwin D, Savitz D, Hertz-Picciotto I, St Andre K. The risk of pregnancy-induced hypertension: black and white differences in a military population. Am J Public Health 1994; 84:1508–1510.

30. Eras JL, Saftlas AF, Triche E, Hsu CD, Risch HA, Bracken MB. Abortion and its effect on risk of preeclampsia and transient hypertension. Epidemiology 2000; 11: 36–43.

31. Hauth JC, Ewell MG, Levine RJ, et al. Pregnancy outcomes in healthy nulliparas who developed hypertension. Obstet Gynecol 2000; 95:24–28.

32. Misra DP, Kiely JL. The association between nulliparity and gestational hypertension. J Clin Epidemiol 1997; 50:851–855.

33. Robillard PY, Hulsey TC, Perianin J, Janky E, Miri EH, Papiernik E. Association of pregnancy-induced hypertension with duration of sexual cohabitation before conception. Lancet 1994; 344:973–975.

34. Robillard PY, Hulsey TC. Association of pregnancy-induced-hypertension, pre-eclampsia, and eclampsia with duration of sexual cohabitation before conception. Lancet 1996; 347:619.

35. Dekker G, Sibai B. Etiology and pathogenesis of preeclampsia: current concepts. Am J Obstet Gynecol 1998; 179:1359–1375.

36. Salha O, Sharma V, Dada T, et al. The influence of donated gametes on the incidence of hypertensive disorders of pregnancy. Hum Reprod 1999; 14:2268–2273.

37. Thadhani R, Stampfer MJ, Hunter DJ, Manson JE, Solomon CG, Curhan GC. High body mass index and hypercholesterolemia: risk of hypertensive disorders of pregnancy. Obstet Gynecol 1999; 94:543–550.

38. Marcoux S, Brisson J, Fabia J. The effect of cigarette smoking on the risk of preeclampsia and gestational hypertension. Am J Epidemiol 1989; 130:950–957.

39. Misra D, Kiely J. The effect of smoking on the risk of gestational hypertension. Early Hum Dev 1995; 40:95–107.

40. Rasmussen S, Oian P. Smoking, haemoglobin concentration and pregnancy-induced hypertension. Gynecol Obstet Invest 1998; 46:225–231.

41. Conde-Agudelo A, Belizan JM, Lede R, Bergel EF. What does an elevated mean arterial pressure in the second half of pregnancy predict—gestational hypertension or preeclampsia? Am J Obstet Gynecol 1993; 169:509–514.

42. Hermida RC, Ayala DE. Diagnosing gestational hypertension and preeclampsia with the 24-hour mean of blood pressure. Hypertension 1997; 30:1531–1537.

43. Ales K, Norton M, Druzin M. Early prediction of antepartum hypertension. Obstet Gynecol 1989; 73:928–933.

44. Campbell DM, MacGillivray I, Carr-Hill R. Pre-eclampsia in second pregnancy. Br J Obstet Gynaecol 1985; 92:131–140.

45. Hargood JL, Brown MA. Pregnancy-induced hypertension: recurrence rate in second pregnancies. Med J Aust 1991; 154:376–377.
46. Landsbergis P, Hatch M. Psychological work stress and pregnancy-induced hypertension. Epidemiology 1996; 7:346–351.
47. Marcoux S, Berube S, Brisson C, Mondor M. Job strain and pregnancy-induced hypertension. Epidemiology 1999; 10:376–382.
48. Marcoux S, Brisson J, Fabia J. The effect of leisure time physical activity on the risk of pre-eclampsia and gestational hypertension. J Epidemiol Commun Health 1989; 43:147–152.
49. Collins R, Wallenburg H. Pharmacological prevention and treatment of hypertensive disorders in pregnancy. In: Chalmers I, Enkin M, Kierse M, eds. Effective Care in Pregnancy and Childbirth, Vol 1. Oxford, UK: Oxford University Press, 1992.
50. Saudan P, Brown M, Buddle M, Jones M. Does gestational hypertension become pre-eclampsia? Br J Obstet Gynaecol 1998; 105:1177–1184.
51. Barton JR, O'Brien JM, Berguauer NK, Jacques DL, Sibai BM. Mild gestational hypertension remote from term: progression and outcome. Am J Obstet Gynecol 2001; 184:979–983.
52. Ros H, Lichenstein P, Lipworth L, Cnattingius S. Genetic effects on the liability of developing preeclampsia and gestational hypertension. Am J Med Genet 2000; 91: 256–260.
53. Lim KH, Zhou Y, Janatpour M, et al. Human cytotrophoblast differentiation/invasion is abnormal in pre-eclampsia. Am J Pathol 1997; 151:1809–1818.
54. Taylor RN, de Groot CJ, Cho YK, Lim KH. Circulating factors as markers and mediators of endothelial cell dysfunction in preeclampsia. Semin Reprod Endocrinol 1998; 16:17–31.
55. Redman CW, Sacks GP, Sargent IL. Preeclampsia: an excessive maternal inflammatory response to pregnancy. Am J Obstet Gynecol 1999; 180:499–506.
56. Pijnenborg R, Anthony J, Davey DA, et al. Placental bed spiral arteries in the hypertensive disorders of pregnancy. Br J Obstet Gynaecol 1991; 98:648–655.
57. Olofsson P, Laurini R, Marsal K. A high uterine artery pulsatility index reflects a defective development of placental bed spiral arteries in pregnancies complicated by hypertension and fetal growth retardation. Eur J Obstet Gynecol Repr Biol 1993; 49:161–168.
58. Bower S, Bewley S, Campbell S. Improved prediction of preeclampsia by two-stage screening of uterine arteries using the early diastolic notch and color Doppler imaging. Obstet Gynecol 1993; 82:78–83.
59. North RA, Ferrier C, Long D, Townend K, Kincaid-Smith P. Uterine artery Doppler flow velocity waveforms in the second trimester for the prediction of preeclampsia and fetal growth retardation. Obstet Gynecol 1994; 83:378–386.
60. Irion O, Masse J, Forest JC, Moutquin JM. Prediction of pre-eclampsia, low birthweight for gestation and prematurity by uterine artery blood flow velocity waveforms analysis in low risk nulliparous women. Br J Obstet Gynaecol 1998; 105: 422–429.
61. van Asselt K, Gudmundsson S, Lindqvist P, Marsal K. Uterine and umbilical artery velocimetry in pre-eclampsia. Acta Obstet Gynaecol Scand 1998; 77:614–619.

62. Taylor RN, Crombleholme WR, Friedman SA, Jones LA, Casal DC, Roberts JM. High plasma cellular fibronectin levels correlate with biochemical and clinical features of preeclampsia but cannot be attributed to hypertension alone. Am J Obstet Gynecol 1991; 165:895–901.

63. Paarlberg K, De Jong C, Van Geijn H, Van Kamp G, Heinen A, Dekker G. Total plasma fibronectin as a marker of pregnancy-induced hypertensive disorders: a longitudinal study. Obstet Gynecol 1998; 91:383–388.

64. Higgins JR, Papayianni A, Brady HR, Darling MR, Walshe JJ. Circulating vascular cell adhesion molecule-1 in pre-eclampsia, gestational hypertension, and normal pregnancy: evidence of selective dysregulation of vascular cell adhesion molecule-1 homeostasis in pre-eclampsia. Am J Obstet Gynecol 1998; 179:464–469.

65. Visser W, Wallenburg HC. Central hemodynamic observations in untreated pre-eclamptic patients. Hypertension 1991; 17:1072–1077.

66. Bosio PM, McKenna PJ, Conroy R, O'Herlihy C. Maternal central hemodynamics in hypertensive disorders of pregnancy. Obstet Gynecol 1999; 94:978–984.

67. Silver HM, Seebeck M, Carlson R. Comparison of total blood volume in normal, preeclamptic, and nonproteinuric gestational hypertensive pregnancy by simultaneous measurement of red blood cell and plasma volumes. Am J Obstet Gynecol 1998; 179:87–93.

68. Fievet P, Fournier A, de Bold A, et al. Atrial natriuretic factor in pregnancy-induced hypertension and preeclampsia: increased plasma concentrations possibly explaining these hypovolemic states with paradoxical hyporeninism. Am J Hypertens 1988; 1:16–21.

69. Brown M, Zammit V, Mitar D. Extracellular fluid volumes in pregnancy-induced hypertension. J Hypertens 1992; 10:61–68.

70. Brown MA, Wang J, Whitworth JA. The renin-angiotensin-aldosterone system in pre-eclampsia. Clin Exp Hypertens 1997; 19:713–726.

71. Lim KH, Friedman SA, Ecker JL, Kao L, Kilpatrick SJ. The clinical utility of serum uric acid measurements in hypertensive diseases of pregnancy. Am J Obstet Gynecol 1998; 178:1067–1071.

72. de Boer K, ten Cate JW, Sturk A, Borm JJ, Treffers PE. Enhanced thrombin generation in normal and hypertensive pregnancy. Am J Obstet Gynecol 1989; 160: 95–100.

73. Hsu CD, Copel JA, Hong SF, Chan DW. Thrombomodulin levels in preeclampsia, gestational hypertension, and chronic hypertension. Obstet Gynecol 1995; 86: 897–899.

74. Schjetlein R, Abdelnoor M, Haugen G, Husby H, Sandset PM, Wisloff F. Hemostatic variables as independent predictors for fetal growth retardation in preeclampsia. Acta Obstet Gynaecol Scand 1999; 78:191–197.

75. Cadroy Y, Grandjean H, Pichon J, et al. Evaluation of six markers of haemostatic system in normal pregnancy and pregnancy complicated by hypertension or preeclampsia. Br J Obstet Gynaecol 1993; 100:416–420.

76. McLintock C, North RA, Dekker G. Inherited thrombophilias: Implications for pregnancy-associated venous thromboembolism and obstetric complications. Curr Probl Obstet Gynecol Fertil 2001; 24:109–152.

77. Grandone E, Margaglione M, Colaizzo D, et al. Prothrombotic genetic risk factors

and the occurrence of gestational hypertension with or without proteinuria. Thromb Haemost 1999; 81:349–352.

78. Sattar N, Bendomir A, Berry C, Shepherd J, Greer IA, Packard CJ. Lipoprotein subfraction concentrations in preeclampsia: pathogenic parallels to atherosclerosis. Obstet Gynecol 1997; 89:403–408.

79. Lorentzen B, Henriksen T. Plasma lipids and vascular dysfunction in preeclampsia. Semin Reprod Endocrinol 1998; 16:33–39.

80. Kaaja R, Laivuori H, Laakso M, Tikkanen MJ, Ylikorkala O. Evidence of a state of increased insulin resistance in preeclampsia. Metabolism 1999; 48:892–896.

81. Kaaja R, Tikkanen M, Viinikka L, Ylikorkala O. Serum lipoproteins, insulin, and urinary prostanoid metabolites in normal and hypertensive pregnant women. Obstet Gynecol 1995; 85:353–356.

82. Caruso A, Ferrazzani S, De Carolis S, et al. Gestational hypertension but not pre-eclampsia is associated with insulin resistance syndrome characteristics. Hum Reprod 1999; 14:219–223.

83. Gratacos E, Casals E, Sanllehy C, Cararach V, Alonso PL, Fortuny A. Variation in lipid levels during pregnancy in women with different types of hypertension. Acta Obstet Gynaecol Scand 1996; 75:896–901.

84. van den Elzen HJ, Wladimiroff JW, Cohen-Overbeek TE, de Bruijn AJ, Grobbee DE. Serum lipids in early pregnancy and risk of pre-eclampsia. Br J Obstet Gynaecol 1996; 103:117–122.

85. Bartha JL, Comino-Delgado R. Carbohydrate metabolism. Evaluation in women with de novo hypertension in late pregnancy. J Reprod Med 1997; 42:489–496.

86. Roberts R. Hypertension in women with gestational diabetes. Diabetes Care 1998; 21:B27–B32.

87. Solomon CG, Graves SW, Greene MF, Seely EW. Glucose intolerance as a predictor of hypertension in pregnancy. Hypertension 1994; 23:717–721.

88. Roberts RN, Traub A, Kennedy A, Hadden DR. Glycosylated haemoglobin and hypertension arising in pregnancy. Br J Obstet Gynaecol 1998; 105:1122–1124.

89. Joffe GM, Esterlitz JR, Levine RJ, et al. The relationship between abnormal glucose tolerance and hypertensive disorders of pregnancy in healthy nulliparous women. Calcium for Preeclampsia Prevention (CPEP) Study Group. Am J Obstet Gynecol 1998; 179:1032–1037.

90. Kilby MD, Pipkin FB, Cockbill S, Heptinstall S, Symonds EM. A cross-sectional study of basal platelet intracellular free calcium concentration in normotensive and hypertensive primigravid pregnancies. Clin Sci 1990; 78:75–80.

91. Saudan P, Shaw L, Brown M. Urinary calcium/creatinine ratio as a predictor of preeclampsia. Am J Hypertens 1998; 11:839–843.

92. Silver HM, Lambert-Messerlian GM, Star JA, Hogan J, Canick JA. Comparison of maternal serum total activin A and inhibin A in normal, preeclamptic, and nonproteinuric gestationally hypertensive pregnancies. Am J Obstet Gynecol 1999; 180: 1131–1137.

93. Muttukrishna S, North R, Morris J, et al. Serum inhibin A and activin A are elevated prior to the onset of preeclampsia. Hum Reprod 2000; 15:1640–1645.

94. Brown MA, Buddle ML. What's in a name? Problems with the classification of hypertension in pregnancy. J Hypertens 1997; 15:1049–1054.

95. Xiong X, Mayes D, Demianczuk N, et al. Impact of pregnancy-induced hypertension on fetal growth. Am J Obstet Gynecol 1999; 180:207–213.
96. Brown M, Buddle M. The importance of nonproteinuric hypertension in pregnancy. Hypertens Pregn 1995; 14:57–65.
97. Peek MJ, Horvath JS, Child AG, Henderson-Smart DJ, Peat B, Gillin A. Maternal and neonatal outcome of patients classified according to the Australasian Society for the Study of Hypertension in Pregnancy Consensus Statement. Med J Aust 1995; 162:186–189.
98. Kuo V, Koumantakis G, Gallery E. Proteinuria and its assessment in normal and hypertensive pregnancy. Am J Obstet Gynecol 1992; 167:723–728.
99. Halligan A, Bell S, Taylor D. Dipstick proteinuria: caveat emptor. Br J Obstet Gynaecol 1999; 106:1113–1115.
100. Jaschevatzky OE, Rosenberg RP, Shalit A, Zonder HB, Grunstein S. Protein/creatinine ratio in random urine specimens for quantitation of proteinuria in preeclampsia. Obstet Gynecol 1990; 75:604–606.
101. Young R, Buchanan R, Kinch R. Use of the protein/creatinine ratio of a single voided urine specimen in the evaluation of suspected pregnancy-induced hypertension. J Fam Pract 1996; 42:385–389.
102. Barton JR, Stanziano GJ, Sibai BM. Monitored outpatient management of mild gestational hypertension remote from term. Am J Obstet Gynecol 1994; 170:765–769.
103. Rosenberg K, Twaddle S. Screening and surveillance of pregnancy hypertension—an economic approach to the use of daycare. Bailliere's Clin Obstet Gynaecol 1990; 4:89–107.
104. Tuffnell D, Lilford R, Buchan P, et al. Randomised controlled trial of day care for hypertension in pregnancy. Lancet 1992; 339:224–227.
105. Neilson J, Alfirevic Z. Doppler ultrasound for fetal assessment in high risk pregnancies. (Cochrane Review). In: The Cochrane Library, Issue 4 2000; Oxford, UK: Update Software.
106. Gupta M, Shennan AH, Halligan A, Taylor DJ, de Swiet M. Accuracy of oscillometric blood pressure monitoring in pregnancy and pre-eclampsia. Br J Obstet Gynaecol 1997; 104:350–355.
107. Brown M, Robinson A, Buddle M. Accuracy of automated blood pressure recorders in pregnancy. Aust NZ J Obstet Gynaecol 1998; 38:262–265.
108. Penny JA, Halligan AW, Shennan AH, et al. Automated, ambulatory, or conventional blood pressure measurement in pregnancy: which is the better predictor of severe hypertension? Am J Obstet Gynecol 1998; 178:521–526.
109. Mathews D. A randomized controlled trial of bed rest and sedation or normal activity and non-sedation in the management of non-albumin-uric hypertension in late pregnancy. Br J Obstet Gynaecol 1977; 84:108–114.
110. Crowther C, Bouwmeester A, Ashurst H. Does admission to hospital for bed rest prevent disease progression or improve fetal outcome in pregnancy complicated by non-proteinuric hypertension. Br J Obstet Gynaecol 1992; 99:13–17.
111. Sibai BM. Treatment of hypertension in pregnant women. N Engl J Med 1996; 335: 257–265.
112. Magee L, Onstein M, von Dadelszen P. Management of hypertension in pregnancy. Br Med J 1999; 318:1332–1336.

113. Belfort MA, Grunewald C, Saade GR, Varner M, Nisell H. Preeclampsia may cause both overperfusion and underperfusion of the brain: a cerebral perfusion based model. Acta Obstet Gynaecol Scand 1999; 78:586–591.

114. Belfort MA, Anthony J, Saade GR. Prevention of eclampsia. Semin Perinatol 1999; 23:65–78.

115. Magee L, Duley L. Oral beta-blockers for mild to moderate hypertension during pregnancy (Cochrane Review). In: The Cochrane Library 2000; 4: Oxford, UK: Update Software.

116. von Dadelszen P, Ornstein M, Bull S, Logan A, Koren G, Magee L. Fall in mean arterial pressure and fetal growth restriction in pregnancy hypertension: a meta-analysis. Lancet 2000; 355:87–92.

117. de Swiet M. Maternal blood pressure and birthweight. Lancet 2000; 355:81–82.

118. Mastrobattista JM. Angiotensin converting enzyme inhibitors in pregnancy. Semin Perinatol 1997; 21:124–134.

119. Lydakis C, Lip G, Beevers M, Beevers D. Atenolol and fetal growth in pregnancies complicated by hypertension. Am J Hypertens 1999; 12:541–547.

120. Ferrazzani S, De Carolis S, Pomini F, Testa AC, Mastromarino C, Caruso A. The duration of hypertension in the puerperium of preeclamptic women: relationship with renal impairment and week of delivery. Am J Obstet Gynecol 1994; 171: 506–512.

121. Douglas K, Redman C. Eclampsia in the United Kingdom. Br Med J 1992; 309: 1395–1400.

122. Muller F, Savey L, Le Fiblec B, et al. Maternal serum human chorionic gonadotropin level at fifteen weeks is a predictor for preeclampsia. Am J Obstet Gynecol 1996; 175:37–40.

123. Morssink LP, Heringa MP, Beekhuis JR, De Wolf BT, Mantingh A. The association between hypertensive disorders of pregnancy and abnormal second-trimester maternal serum levels of hCG and alpha-fetoprotein. Obstet Gynecol 1997; 89:666–670.

124. Raty R, Koskinen P, Alanen A, Irjala K, Matinlauri I, Ekblad U. Prediction of pre-eclampsia with maternal mid-trimester total renin, inhibin A, AFP and free beta-hCG levels. Prenat Diagn 1999; 19:122–127.

125. O'Brien PM, Walker TJ, Singh PK, Kilby MD, Jones PW. Failure of platelet angiotensin II binding to predict pregnancy-induced hypertension. Obstet Gynecol 1999; 93:203–206.

126. Baker PN, Hackett GA. The use of urinary albumin-creatinine ratios and calcium-creatinine ratios as screening tests for pregnancy-induced hypertension. Obstet Gynecol 1994; 83:745–749.

127. Paarlberg K, De Jong C, Van Geijn H, Van Kamp G, Heinen A, Dekker G. Vaso-active mediators in pregnancy-induced hypertensive disorders: A longitudinal study. Am J Obstet Gynecol 1998; 179:1559–1564.

128. Marin R, Gorostidi M, Portal C, Sanchez M, Sanchez E, Alvarez J. Long-term prognosis of hypertension in pregnancy. Hypertens Pregn 2000; 19:199–209.

129. Nisell H, Lintu H, Lunell NO, Mollerstrom G, Pettersson E. Blood pressure and renal function seven years after pregnancy complicated by hypertension. Br J Obstet Gynaecol 1995; 102:876–881.

130. Reiter L, Brown MA, Whitworth JA. Hypertension in pregnancy: the incidence of

underlying renal disease and essential hypertension. Am J Kidney Dis 1994; 24: 883–887.

131. Lindeberg S, Hanson U. Hypertension and factors associated with metabolic syndrome at follow-up at 15 years in women with hypertensive disease during first pregnancy. Hypertens Pregn 2000; 19:191–198.

132. Seely E. Hypertension in pregnancy: a potential window into long-term cardiovascular risk in women. J Clin Endocrinol Metab 1999; 84:1858–1861.

133. Safai M, Beaufils M, Uzan S. The pregnancies following preeclampsia. Am J Hypertens 1992; 5:99A.

9

Eclampsia—What's New?

Andrea G. Witlin
University of Texas Medical Branch, Galveston, Texas, U.S.A.

Approximately 5–7% of all pregnancies are complicated by preeclampsia. The incidence of eclamptic seizures in women with preeclampsia is <1%. In the United States, magnesium sulfate is used for seizure prophylaxis in women with preeclampsia and for therapy of eclamptic convulsions. Over the past 10 years, alternatives to magnesium sulfate treatment for women with eclampsia and seizure prophylaxis in women with severe preeclampsia have been suggested. These include phenytoin (1), diazepam (1,2), nimodipine (3), or aggressive antihypertensive therapy (4). Nonetheless, these alternative therapies have not provided equivalent results to magnesium sulfate therapy (1,2). An evidence-based approach to the treatment and prophylaxis of eclamptic seizures is presented, including the MagPie Trial (5). The mechanism(s) of action of magnesium sulfate are also discussed (6,7).

I. HISTORICAL PERSPECTIVE

The use of magnesium sulfate was first reported in the early 1900s for control of tetanic convulsions (8). Shortly thereafter, Lazard reported the use of magnesium sulfate for the control of eclamptic convulsions with an associated fivefold (30 to 5.8%) reduction of maternal mortality (9). Magnesium sulfate therapy was adopted for treatment of eclamptic convulsions based upon observational studies and anecdotal experience. As a natural extension to its use for therapy of eclamptic seizures, magnesium sulfate was then adapted for prophylaxis of seizures in women with severe preeclampsia and subsequently mild preeclampsia. The linking of an orderly progression from gestational hypertension to mild preeclampsia to severe preeclampsia to eclampsia has never been established. Moreover, the prediction or prevention of the development of severe preeclampsia or progression from mild to severe disease cannot be anticipated (10). Several authors (11,12) have suggested that progression from mild to severe preeclampsia is related to gestational age at diagnosis. The earlier in pregnancy that gestational hypertension or preeclampsia is diagnosed, the greater the chance of development of severe disease. Overall approximately 15 to 25% of women initially diagnosed with gestational hypertension will develop preeclampsia, with only 10% risk of disease progression when gestational hypertension is diagnosed after 36 weeks gestation (11,12). In a study undertaken during labor by Witlin et al. (13), 10% of women with mild preeclampsia subsequently developed criteria for severe disease despite magnesium sulfate administration.

The modern obstetric use of magnesium sulfate therapy for preeclampsia and eclampsia has been credited to Pritchard, who popularized the intramuscular route of administration (10 g IM load followed by 5 g IM every 4 hours) (14). Continuous intravenous infusion was recommended by Zuspan (4g IV load followed by 1g/h) (15) and subsequently modified by Sibai (6 g IV load followed by 2g/h) (16,17). According to Pritchard, appropriate serum levels of magnesium for treatment of eclamptic convulsions were 3.5 to 7 mEq/L (4.2–8.4 mg/dL) (14). However, the serum levels of magnesium have not been correlated to the abolition of seizure activity. The concept of appropriate magnesium levels was based upon the clinical experience of Pritchard, that most eclamptic seizures were successfully treated when the above magnesium levels were attained (14).

If one compares the dose of magnesium sulfate (2g/h) used in the United States, as recommended by Sibai et al. (16) to the lower dose (1g/h) of magnesium sulfate used in the Collaborative (2) and MagPie Trials (5), a quandary is raised. The study by Sibai et al. (16) correlated the failure of magnesium sulfate therapy to the hourly infusion rate and serum magnesium level. The Collaborative Trial (2) suggested that magnesium sulfate is the preferred therapy for eclampsia with an infusion rate of 1g/hour. This raises two questions: Is the efficacy dependent on the serum levels? And what is the mechanism of action of magnesium? The latter has been addressed in the cardiology and neurology literature (18–24); however, the exact mechanism remains elusive.

II. CURRENT USE OF MAGNESIUM SULFATE

There are five randomized trials comparing the prophylactic effect of magnesium sulfate to either phenytoin or placebo for inpatients with hypertensive disorders of pregnancy (1,13,25–27). Only one of these trials (1) had an adequate sample size to evaluate the effects of seizure prophylaxis in these women. The remaining trials primarily evaluated side effects of magnesium sulfate therapy (Table 1).

The largest randomized trial conducted in the United States was reported by

Table 1 Randomized Trials of Magnesium Sulfate Versus
Phenytoin or Placebo in Hypertensive Disorders in Pregnancy

		Convulsions	
Authors	Control group	MgSO$_4$	Control
Appleton et al. (25)	Phenytoin	0/24	0/23
Friedman et al. (26)	Phenytoin	0/60	0/43
Atkinson et al. (27)	Phenytoin	0/28	0/26
Lucas et al. (1)	Phenytoin	0/1049	10/1089
Witlin et al. (13)	Placebo	0/67	0/68
All authors		0/1228[a]	10/1249 (0.8%)[a]

[a]$p < 0.001$.

Lucas et al. (1). In it, over 2000 women with various hypertensive disorders of pregnancy were randomized to either intramuscular magnesium sulfate or phenytoin administered during labor and postpartum. The authors found no seizures among 1049 patients receiving magnesium sulfate and 10 cases of eclampsia (0.1%) among 1089 patients assigned to phenytoin (p = 0.004) (1). This trial indicated that magnesium sulfate was superior to phenytoin for seizure prophylaxis in such patients. The MagPie Trial (5) has enrolled in excess of 10,000 women (in developing countries) with both mild and severe preeclampsia. The magnesium sulfate dose in the MagPie Trial is a 4g IV loading dose followed by 1g/h continuous infusion. The current medicolegal situation in the United States has precluded participation in such a trial (especially in women with severe preeclampsia).

Witlin et al. (13) studied women with mild preeclampsia at (>37 weeks' gestation in a randomized, placebo-controlled trial of magnesium sulfate seizure prophylaxis. The authors noted that 10% of women progressed to a clinical diagnosis of severe preeclampsia despite use of magnesium sulfate prophylaxis. The proportion of women progressing to severe preeclampsia was similar in the placebo control group. The mean magnesium level in the magnesium-treated women was 4.7 ± 1.0 mg/dL (13). For those women in the placebo cohort progressing to severe preeclampsia, it was felt that there was sufficient time to safely initiate magnesium sulfate therapy for therapy of severe preeclampsia. This assumed "safety net" must be further evaluated in a larger trial. This trial to date has enrolled in excess of 300 women with mild preeclampsia; none of the women experienced seizures. Further participation has been limited by Institutional Review Board restrictions, willingness of providers and patients to participate in such a trial, and the current medicolegal climate. Selective seizure prophylaxis is not likely to become a standard of care in the United States, although it has been practiced in some settings.

Table 2 Randomized Trials of Magnesium Sulfate Versus Comparator in Severe Preeclampsia

Authors	Antihypertensive therapy (if needed)	Convulsions MgSO$_4$ n (%)	Control n (%)	RR (95% CI)
Moodley and Moodley (4)	Dihydralazine, nifedipine	1/112 (0.9)	0/116 (0)	N/A
Chen et al. (28)	Hydralazine, methyldopa, nifedipine	0/34	0/34	N/A
Belfort et al. (29)	Nimodipine, hydralazine	5/324 (1.5)	11/303 (3.6)	0.43 (0.15–1.21)
Coetzee et al. (30)	Hydralazine, labetalol	1/345 (0.3)	11/340 (3.2)[a]	0.09 (0.01–0.69)
All studies		7/815 (0.86)	22/793 (2.8)	0.31 (0.13–0.72)

[a]Placebo-controlled.

There are four randomized trials comparing the use of magnesium sulfate with placebo and/or antihypertensive drugs (Table 2) (3,28–30). One of these trials had an inadequate sample size (28), whereas the other three were adequate. The trial by Belfort et al. (29) compared the use of magnesium sulfate to nimodipine (a calcium channel blocker with cerebral vasodilatory effects). The authors found a significantly lower incidence of eclampsia in the magnesium sulfate group [7/871 (0.8%) vs. 21/862 (2.4%)]. Twelve patients in the nimodipine group had antepartum and 9 had postpartum seizures. None of the magnesium-treated patients had postpartum seizures. The trial by Coetzee et al. (30) was double-blind and compared IV magnesium sulfate to IV saline in 685 patients with severe preeclampsia. The authors found a significant reduction in development of eclampsia in the magnesium group (Table 2). Therefore, it is apparent that magnesium sulfate prophylaxis should be used in all patients with severe preeclampsia during labor and postpartum. Despite the data presented above, our colleagues in the United Kingdom and South Africa (31,32) believe that the use of magnesium sulfate seizure prophylaxis is still debatable even in women with severe preeclampsia. The opinion of these authors (31,32) is that the efficacy and safety of magnesium sulfate prophylaxis in women with severe preeclampsia remains to be proven.

Moodley and Moodley (4) are among several authors advocating the use of aggressive antihypertensive therapy in women with severe preeclampsia as an alternative to seizure prophylaxis. They explored this hypothesis in a randomized controlled trial using the rapid acting antihypertensive agents dihydralazine and nifedipine. Although the conclusions are limited by the small sample size, the authors (4) suggested that aggressive use of antihypertensive medication alone might be sufficient therapy for severe preeclampsia. In the future this recommendation may be enhanced by selection of agents with combined antihypertensive, cerebrovasodilator, and decreased platelet aggregation action.

Magnesium sulfate does not prevent recurrent seizures in all eclamptic patients. There are six observational studies describing the rate of subsequent seizures in eclamptic women receiving magnesium sulfate (Table 3) (33–38). The overall rate of recurrent seizures among these studies was 10%.

During recent years, several randomized trials have been reported comparing the efficacy of magnesium sulfate to other anticonvulsants in eclamptic women (Table 4) (2,38–41). Four of these trials (38–41) had limited sample size and only one multicenter trial (2) had an adequate sample size. The Collaborative Eclampsia Trial (2) was conducted in several international centers. It included 1680 eclamptic women who were randomized to either magnesium sulfate, phenytoin, or diazepam in two different randomization schemes. The trial demonstrated that magnesium sulfate was superior to both phenytoin and diazepam for the prevention of *recurrent* seizures in eclamptic women (Table 4). In addition, magnesium sulfate reduced the risk of maternal death by one-quarter over those

Table 3 Observational Studies on Subsequent Convulsions in
Eclamptic Women Receiving Magnesium Sulfate

Authors	Number (n) eclampsia	Recurrent convulsions n	(%)
Pritchard et al. (1975) (33)	85	3	3.5
Gedekoh et al. (1981) (34)	52	1	1.9
Pritchard et al. (1984) (35)	83	10	12.0
Dunn et al. (1986) (36)	13	5	38.5
Sibai (1991) (37)	315	41	13.0
Dommisse (1990) (38)	100	3	3.0
All studies	648	63	9.7

treated with diazepam, RR 0.7 (95% CI 0.4–1.4), and it reduced the risk of maternal death by half over those treated with phenytoin, RR 0.5 (95% CI 0.2–2.0). Furthermore, there was a decreased incidence of pneumonia, need for mechanical ventilation, and ICU admission in the magnesium-treated women.

In addition, the data by Bhalla et al. (40) indicated that magnesium sulfate was superior to a lytic cocktail in eclamptic women. Crowther (39) identified a trend toward lower maternal morbidity (recurrent convulsions, cardiopulmonary problems, DIC, and acute renal failure) in the magnesium-treated cohort, RR 0.6 (95% CI 0.3-1.2). In addition, there was a trend toward improved neonatal outcome in the magnesium-treated group with regards to 5-minute Apgar <7, need for intubation, positive-pressure ventilation and NICU admission.

The randomized trials noted above also had adequate information to compare the rate of maternal death between those receiving magnesium sulfate and those receiving other agents (Table 5) (2,39–41) Magnesium sulfate in eclamptic women was associated with a significantly lower maternal mortality compared with other anticonvulsants (3.8% vs. 5.1%, $p < 0.05$).

The baseline risk of eclampsia in an untreated population in the United States is unknown. Recently, Mattar et al. (42) reviewed the experience in women treated for eclampsia at the University of Tennessee in Memphis. The incidence of death (two total) has remained unchanged (42) over the past 20 years despite the change in dosage of magnesium sulfate alluded to earlier. This raises a question regarding the appropriate dose of magnesium sulfate. Furthermore, has the overall care of women with eclampsia in the United States improved? Has earlier delivery precluded development of the most severe disease and respective complications? Alternatively, are we treating more women with mild disease and causing complications or death from overdose?

Table 4 Randomized Trials Performed Prior to the MagPie Trial Comparing Magnesium Sulfate with Other Anticonvulsants in Eclampsia

Authors	Antihypertensive therapy	Recurrent seizures		RR (95% CI)
		MgSO$_4$ n (%)	Other n (%)	
Dommisse (38)	Dihydralazine	0/11 (0)	4/11 (36.7)[a]	0.8 (0.29–2.2)
Crowther (39)	Dihydralazine	5/24 (20.8)	7/27 (26)[b]	
Bhalla et al. (40)	Nifedipine	1/45 (2.2)	11/45 (24.4)[c]	0.09 (0.01–0.68)
Friedman et al. (41)	Nifedipine, labetalol	0/11 (0)	2/13 (15.4)[a]	
Collaborative Trial (2)	NR[d]	60/453 (13.2)	126/452 (27.9)[b]	0.48 (0.36–0.63)
Collaborative Trial (2)	NR	22/388 (5.7)	66/387 (17.1)[a]	0.33 (0.21–0.53)
All studies		88/932 (9.4)	216/935 (23.1)	0.41 (0.32–0.51)

[a]Phenytoin
[b]Diazepam.
[c]Lytic cocktail.
[d]Not reported.

Table 5 Maternal Deaths in Trials Comparing Magnesium Sulfate with Other Anticonvulsants in Eclampsia

Authors	Comparison group	Maternal deaths		RR (95% CI)
		$MgSO_4$ n (%)	Other n (%)	
Dommisse (38)	Phenytoin	0/11	0/11 (0)	
Crowther (39)	Diazepam	1/24 (4.2)	0/27 (0)	
Bhalla et al. (40)	Lytic cocktail	0/45	2/45 (4.4)	
Friedman et al. (41)	Phenytoin	0/11	0/13 (0)	
Collaborative Trial (2)	Phenytoin	10/388 (2.6)	20/387 (5.2)	0.50 (0.24–1.00)
Collaborative Trial (2)	Diazepam	17/453 (3.8)	23/452 (5.1)	0.74 (0.40–1.36)
All studies		28/932 (3.0)	45/935 (4.8)	0.62 (0.39–0.99)

There are a few retrospective studies (43–47) evaluating the frequency of eclampsia in women not receiving seizure prophylaxis (Table 6). The incidence of eclampsia ranges from 1 in 555 for women with hypertension (45) to 1 in 78 in women with severe preeclampsia (43). The heterogeneity of these patients, ranging from nonproteinuric hypertension (45) to severe preeclampsia (43), warrants cautious interpretation of the data. Walker (45) limited evaluation to women with hypertension (without preeclampsia) only, Chua and Redman (43) limited investigation to women with severe preeclampsia only, and the conclusions of Olah et al.

Table 6 Observational Studies Regarding the Incidence and Relevance of Eclampsia in Women with Hypertensive Disorders Without Magnesium Sulfate Prophylaxis

Authors	Classification of disease on presentation	Number of patients	Eclampsia n	(%)
Chua and Redman (1987–1990) (43)	Severe preeclampsia	78	1	1.3
Nelson (1951–1953) (44)	Gestational hypertension	527	2	0.38
Nelson (1951–1953) (44)	Preeclampsia[a]	216	6	2.8
Walker (1981–1989) (45)	Hypertensive disorders	3885	7	0.18
Burrows (1986–1993) (46)	Gestational hypertension	745	1	0.13
Burrows (1986–1993) (46)	Preeclampsia[a]	372	16[b]	4.3
Odendaal and Hall (1983–1993) (47)	Severe preeclampsia	491	3	0.6

[a]Includes mild and severe preeclampsia.
[b]Includes convulsion only intrapartum and postpartum.

(48) are limited by small sample size ($n = 56$). The two largest studies are reviewed below in greater detail.

Odendaal and Hall (47) from South Africa prospectively studied 1001 women with severe preeclampsia treated with magnesium sulfate seizure prophylaxis based upon the clinical presentation suggestive of "impending eclampsia." A total of 510 women received magnesium sulfate seizure prophylaxis and 491 women did not. A total of 5 women developed eclampsia, 2 prior to delivery (both receiving magnesium sulfate therapy) and 3 postpartum (none of whom received magnesium sulfate therapy). Two of the three postpartum seizures occurred greater than 48 hours postpartum. It is not known whether the magnesium-treated cohort represented a group of "higher risk" women who were appropriately treated with magnesium sulfate or whether "impending eclampsia" could not be reliably anticipated. It is this concept of impending eclampsia that is used by those that advocate selective treatment.

Burrows and Burrows (46) performed an 8-year retrospective, single institution, cross-sectional study of 1559 hypertensive gravidas (over half of the women had severe disease) managed without seizure prophylaxis. Seizures occurred in 4.3% of gravidas with preeclampsia and 2.1% of those with chronic hypertension and superimposed preeclampsia. The likelihood of seizures was 17.4 times greater in women with preeclampsia (95% CI 5.2–60.2) and 8.1 times greater for women with chronic hypertension and superimposed preeclampsia (95% CI 1.3–49.4) as compared with women with gestational hypertension or chronic hypertension. This incidence of seizure is markedly higher than that noted previously in women with severe preeclampsia (Table 3). It appears that the authors have either reported upon a cohort of patients at exceedingly high risk for seizure or that their results confirm the utility of magnesium sulfate seizure prophylaxis in a population of women with severe preeclampsia (49).

In summary, a review of randomized trials indicate that magnesium sulfate is the ideal agent to use as a prophylaxis in women with preeclampsia and for the treatment of eclamptic convulsions. There is limited information regarding the need of magnesium sulfate as a prophylaxis in women with mild hypertension without superimposed preeclampsia.

III. CONCLUSIONS

It is important to maintain perspective and contrast the associated incidence and morbidity from eclamptic seizures when comparing studies in developed and developing countries. Both maternal and fetal morbidity and mortality will be worse with unattended seizures at home compared to seizures in hospital in a developed nation with modern health care facilities.

Magnesium sulfate seizure prophylaxis and therapy exemplify current obstetric care in the United States for women with preeclampsia and eclampsia respectively. As reviewed earlier, magnesium sulfate therapy for eclampsia appears to be well supported by level I evidence (49). There appears to be strong support (from levels I, II-1, and II-2) (49) for seizure prophylaxis with magnesium sulfate and antihypertensive/cerebrovasodilator agents for women with severe preeclampsia when the data of Coetzee et al. (30) and Belfort et al. (29) are examined collectively.

Although magnesium sulfate seizure prophylaxis is deemed advantageous, its potential for diminishing the morbidity associated with eclampsia is limited (42). Up to 40% of all eclamptic seizures occur antepartum (prehospitalization), before women receive close medical attention (50,51). In addition, up to 49.2% of seizures occur at a gestational age less than 36 weeks, when there is the greatest incidence of fetal morbidity and mortality (50,51). An additional 16% of eclamptic seizures occur more than 48 hours postpartum (52). Therefore magnesium sulfate seizure prophylaxis can only be expected to have a potential impact for reduction of seizures that occur intrapartum and within 12 to 24 hours postpartum. This represents only about 45 to 50% of all eclamptic seizures.

The obstetric use of magnesium sulfate in the early part of this century appears to have been a serendipitous discovery that we are only now beginning to comprehend. Magnesium sulfate has been shown recently to ameliorate endothelial cell dysfunction and decrease platelet adhesiveness (presumed to be partially responsible for the pathophysiology of preeclampsia) (18,19). Through further understanding of the pathophysiology of preeclampsia and role of magnesium sulfate therapy and its mechanism(s) of action, we may be able to improve upon our current therapy.

Magnesium sulfate is the drug of choice for all women with preeclampsia and eclampsia. The MagPie trial (5) indicates that magnesium sulfate (4g IV load, 1g/h) is appropriate for use in developing countries. The standard of care in the United States remains magnesium sulfate (4–6g IV load, 2g/h). Further basic science studies addressing the actual mechanism of action of magnesium sulfate for seizure prophylaxis will be helpful to determine the proper dosing regimen. *Continued close intrapartum and postpartum surveillance is crucial for optimal maternal/perinatal outcome.* Irrespective of magnesium sulfate therapy, progression from mild to severe disease cannot be prevented. Although the duration of postpartum magnesium sulfate seizure prophylaxis has never been studied in a randomized clinical trial, current opinion is that magnesium sulfate therapy should be continued for up to 12 to 24 hours postpartum, depending upon the severity of the disease. Recently, Ascarelli et al. (53) advocated adjusting the length of postpartum magnesium sulfate depending upon the four clinical parameters of persistent headache, blood pressure levels, initiation of spontaneous diuresis, and level of urinary protein excretion. Furthermore, a presumptive diagnosis of eclampsia not responsive to magnesium sulfate therapy should raise the suspicion of an underlying central nervous system lesion and prompt neuroimaging studies should be performed (54).

REFERENCES

1. Lucas MJ, Leveno KJ, Cunningham FG. A comparison of magnesium sulfate with phenytoin for the prevention of eclampsia. N Engl J Med 1995; 333:201–205.
2. Which anticonvulsant for women with eclampsia? Evidence from the Collaborative Eclampsia Trial. Lancet 1995; 345:1455–1463.
3. Belfort MA, Saade GR, Moise KJ, Cruz A, Adam K, Kramer W, Kirshon B. Nimodipine in the management of preeclampsia: maternal and fetal effects. Am J Obstet Gynecol 1994; 171:417–424.
4. Moodley J, Moodley VV. Prophylactic anticonvulsant therapy in hypertensive crises of pregnancy—the need for a large randomized trial. Hypertens Pregn 1994; 13: 245–252.
5. Duley L. The Magpie Trial: magnesium sulphate versus placebo for women with preeclampsia. Hypertens Pregn 2000; 19:63.
6. Mauskop A, Altura BM. Role of magnesium in the pathogenesis and treatment of migraines. Clin Neurosci 1998; 5:24–27.
7. Altura BM, Altura BT. New perspectives on the role of magnesium in the pathophysiology of the cardiovascular system. Magnesium 1985; 4:226–244.
8. Alton BH, Lincoln GC. The control of eclampsia convulsions by intraspinal injections of magnesium sulphate. Am J Obstet Gynecol 1925; 9:167–177.
9. Lazard EM. A preliminary report on the intravenous use of magnesium sulphate in puerperal eclampsia. Am J Obstet Gynecol 1925; 9:178–188.
10. Katz VL, Farmer R, Kuller JA. Preeclampsia into eclampsia: toward a new paradigm. Am J Obstet Gynecol 2000; 182:1389–1396.
11. Saudan P, Brown MA, Buddle ML, Jones M. Does gestational hypertension become pre-eclampsia? Br J Obstet Gynaecol 1998; 105(11):1177–1184.
12. Barton JR, O'Brien JM, Bergauer NK, Jacques DL, Sibai BM. Mild gestational hypertension remote from term: Progression and outcome. Abstract 136. Poster presented at 19th Annual Meeting of the Society for Maternal-Fetal Medicine, San Francisco, January 1999. Am J Obstet Gynecol 2001; 184:979–983.
13. Witlin AG, Friedman SA, Sibai BM. The effect of magnesium sulfate therapy on the duration of labor in women with mild preeclampsia at term: a randomized, double-blind, placebo-controlled trial. Am J Obstet Gynecol 1997; 176:623–627.
14. Pritchard JA. The use of the magnesium ion in the management of eclamptogenic toxemias. Surg Gynecol Obstet 1955; 100:131–140.
15. Zuspan FP. Treatment of severe preeclampsia and eclampsia. Clin Obstet Gynecol 1966; 9:954–972.
16. Sibai BM, Lipshitz J, Anderson GD, Dilts PV. Reassessment of intravenous MgSO4 therapy in preeclampsia-eclampsia. Obstet Gynecol 1981; 57:199–202.

17. Sibai BM. Magnesium sulfate is the ideal anticonvulsant in preeclampsia-eclampsia. Am J Obstet Gynecol 1990; 162:1141–1145.

18. Ravn HB, Vissinger H, Kristensen SD, Wennmalm A, Thygesen K, Husted SE. Magnesium inhibits platelet activity—an infusion study in healthy volunteers. Thromb Haemostas 1996; 75:939–944.

19. Gawaz M, Ott I, Reininger AJ, Neumann FJ. Effects of magnesium on platelet aggregation and adhesion. Thromb Haemostas 1994; 72:912–918.

20. Komori S, Li B, Matsumura K, Takusagawa M, Sano S, Kohno I, Osada M, Sawanobori T, Ishihara T, Umetani K, Ijiri H, Tamura K. Antiarrhythmic effect of magnesium sulfate against occlusion-induced arrhythmias and reperfusion-induced arrhythmias in anesthetized rats. Mol Cell Biochem 1999; 199:201–208.

21. Perales AJ, Torregrosa G, Salom JB, Barbera MD, Jover T, Alborch E. Effects of magnesium sulphate on the noradrenaline-induced cerebral vasoconstrictor and pressor responses in the goat. Br J Obstet Gynaecol 1997; 104:898–903.

22. Sirin BH, Coskun E, Yilik L, Ortac R, Sirin H, Tetik C. Neuroprotective effects of preischemia subcutaneous magnesium sulfate in transient cerebral ischemia. Eur J Cardiothorrac Surg 1998; 14:82–88.

23. Chahal H, D'Souza SW, Barson AJ, Slater P. Modulation by magnesium of N-methyl-D-asparate receptors in developing human brain. Arch Dis Child Fetal Neonatal Ed 1998; 78:F116–F120.

24. Ravn HB, Moeldrup U, Brookes CIO, Ilkjaer LB, White P, Chew M, Jensen L, Johnsen S, Birk-Soerensen L, Hjortdal VE. Intravenous magnesium reduces infarct size after ischemia/reperfusion injury combined with a thrombogenic lesion in the left anterior descending artery. Arter Thromb Vasc Biol 1999; 19:569–574.

25. Appleton MP, Kuehl TJ, Raebel MA, Adams HR, Knight AB, Gold WR. Magnesium sulfate versus phenytoin for seizure prophylaxis in pregnancy-induced hypertension. Am J Obstet Gynecol 1991; 165:907–913.

26. Friedman SA, Lim KH, Baker CA, Repke JT. Phenytoin versus magnesium sulfate in preeclampsia: a pilot study. Am J Perinatal 1993; 10:233–238.

27. Atkinson MW, Guinn D, Owen J, Hauth JC. Does magnesium sulfate affect the length of labor induction in women with pregnancy-associated hypertension? Am J Obstet Gynecol 1995; 173:1219–1222.

28. Chen F, Chang S, Chu K. Expectant management in severe preeclampsia: does magnesium sulfate prevent the development of eclampsia? Acta Obstet Gynaecol Scand 1995; 74:181–185.

29. Belfort M, Anthony J, Allen J and the Nimodipine Study Group. Magnesium sulfate is more effective at preventing eclampsia than the selective cerebral vasodilator nimodipine. J Soc Gynecol Invest 2001; 8:73A.

30. Coetzee EJ, Dommisse J, Anthony J. A randomized controlled trial of intravenous magnesium sulphate versus placebo in the management of women with severe pre-eclampsia. Br J Obstet Gynaecol 1998; 105:300–303.

31. Thornton JG. Prophylactic anticonvulsants for pre-eclampsia? Br J Obstet Gynaecol 2000; 107:839–840.

32. Hall DR, Odendaal HJ, Smith M. Is the prophylactic administration of magnesium sulphate in women with pre-eclampsia indicated prior to labour? Br J Obstet Gynaecol 2000; 107:903–908.

33. Pritchard JA, Pritchard SA. Standardized treatment of 154 consecutive cases of eclampsia. Am J Obstet Gynecol 1975; 123:543–552.

34. Gedekoh RH, Hayashi TT, MacDonald HMM. Eclampsia at Magee-Women's Hospital 1970 to 1980. Am J Obstet Gynecol 1981; 140:860–866.

35. Pritchard JA, Cunningham FG, Pritchard SA. The Parkland Memorial Hospital protocol for treatment of eclampsia: Evaluation of 245 cases. Am J Obstet Gynecol 1984; 148:951–963.

36. Dunn R, Lee W, Cotton DB. Evaluation of computerized axial tomography of eclamptic women with seizures refractory to magnesium sulfate therapy. Am J Obstet Gynecol 1986; 155:267–268.

37. Sibai BM, Ramanathan J. The case for magnesium sulfate in preeclampsia-eclampsia. Int J Obstet Anesth 1992; 1:167–175.

38. Dommisse J. Phenytoin sodium and magnesium sulphate in the management of eclampsia. Br J Obstet Gynaecol 1990; 97:104–109.

39. Crowther C. Magnesium sulphate versus diazepam in the management of eclampsia: a randomized controlled trial. Br J Obstet Gynaecol 1990; 97:110–117.

40. Bhalla AK, Dhall GI, Dhall K. A safer and more effective treatment regimen for eclampsia. Aust NZ J Obstet Gynaecol 1994; 34:144–148.

41. Friedman SA, Schiff E, Kao L, Sibai BM. Phenytoin versus magnesium sulfate in patients with eclampsia: preliminary results from a randomized trial. Abstract 452. Poster presented at 15th Annual Meeting of the Society of Perinatal Obstetricians, Atlanta, GA, January 23–28, 1995. Am J Obstet Gynecol 1995; 175(1pt2):384.

42. Mattar F, Sibai BM. Risk factors for maternal morbidity. Am J Obstet Gynecol 2000; 182(2):307–312.

43. Chua S, Redman CWG. Are prophylactic anticonvulsants required in severe preeclampsia? Lancet 1991; 337:250–251.

44. Nelson TR. A clinical study of preeclampsia. Part II. J Obstet Gynaecol Br Emp 1955; 62:58–66.

45. Walker JJ. Hypertensive drugs in pregnancy. Hypertens Pregn 1991; 18:845–872.

46. Burrows RF, Burrows EA. The feasibility of a control population for a randomized control trial of seizure prophylaxis in the hypertensive disorders of pregnancy. Am J Obstet Gynecol 1995; 173:929–935.

47. Odendaal HJ, Hall DR. Is magnesium sulfate prophylaxis really necessary in patients with severe preeclampsia? J Mat Fet Inv 1996; 6:14–18.

48. Olah KS, Redman CWG, Gee H. Management of severe, early pre-eclampsia: is conservative management justified? Eur J Obstet Gynaecol Reprod Biol 1993; 51:175–180.

49. Fisher M, ed. Guide to clinical preventive services: an assessment of the effectiveness of 169 interventions. Report of the US Preventive Services Task Force. Baltimore, MD: Williams & Wilkins: 1989:388–389.

50. Douglas KA, Redman CWG. Eclampsia in the United Kingdom. Br Med J 1994; 309:1395–1400.

51. Sibai BM. Eclampsia. VI. Maternal-perinatal outcome in 254 consecutive cases. Am J Obstet Gynecol 1990; 1049–1055.

52. Lubarsky SL, Barton JR, Friedman SA, Nasreddine S, Ramadan MK, Sibai BM. Late postpartum eclampsia revisited. Obstet Gynecol 1994; 83:502–505.

53. Ascarelli MH, Johnson V, May WL, Martin RW, Martin JN. Individually determined postpartum magnesium sulfate therapy with clinical parameters to safely and cost-effectively shorten treatment for pre-eclampsia. Am J Obstet Gynecol 1998; 179(4): 952–956.
54. Witlin AG, Friedman SA, Egerman RE, Frangieh AY, Sibai BM. Cerebrovascular disorders complicating pregnancy—beyond eclampsia. Am J Obstet Gynecol 1997; 176:1139–1148.

10
Antenatal Surveillance in Preeclampsia and Chronic Hypertension

Gary A. Dildy III
Louisiana State University School of Medicine, New Orleans,
Louisiana, U.S.A.

I. INTRODUCTION

A. Purpose of Antepartum Fetal Surveillance

The primary goal of antepartum fetal assessment is to prevent fetal death (1). An ideal secondary goal would be to prevent intrauterine asphyxia (2,3). In both animals and humans, fetal physiological parameters such as the heart rate pattern and level of physical activity are sensitive to the effects of hypoxemia and acidemia (4–7). Hypoxemia may lead to redistribution of fetal blood flow to the brain and myocardium, and away from the renal circulation, leading to oligohydramnios (8). Identification of suboptimal oxygenation or frank acidosis in the fetus may allow for delivery, thus preventing fetal neurological injury or death. The clinical technologies available to assess fetal condition in high-risk pregnancies primarily include maternal perception of fetal movement, various forms of ultrasonography, and electronic fetal heart rate monitoring (EFM). Ultrasound has become an integral component of contemporary obstetrical practice, and EFM has become ubiquitous since its introduction in the late 1960s.

B. Incidence and Classification of the Hypertensive Disorders of Pregnancy

Hypertensive disorders complicate 6 to 8% of pregnancies and remain significant contributors to neonatal morbidity and perinatal mortality rates (9). Classification systems of hypertensive diseases during pregnancy are multiple, are overlapping, and tend to be confusing (see Chapter 1). A 2000 National Institutes of Health (NIH) sponsored working group (9) proposed a modified classification system (Table 1) for the purpose of providing guidance to clinicians in managing hypertensive patients during pregnancy. In this system, *chronic hypertension* is defined as hypertension that is present before pregnancy or diagnosed before the twentieth week of gestation. *Preeclampsia* is defined as the appearance of hypertension plus proteinuria, usually occurring after 20 weeks of gestation. Chronic hypertension may be complicated by superimposed preeclampsia or eclampsia. In this classification system, gestational hypertension is subdivided retrospectively after pregnancy into transient hypertension of pregnancy or chronic hypertension.

C. Perinatal Morbidity and Mortality of Preeclampsia

In the United States, preeclampsia complicates approximately 5% of pregnancies and is the second most common cause of maternal mortality in advanced gestations (10–12). Pathological changes associated with hypertension and preeclampsia, which commonly affect the maternal cardiovascular, renal, hematological, neurological, and hepatic systems (13), may adversely affect the uteroplacental-

Table 1 Classification of Hypertensive Diseases During Pregnancy

Chronic hypertension	Hypertension that is present before pregnancy or diagnosed before the 20th week gestation
Preeclampsia–eclampsia	Hypertension plus proteinuria, usually occuring after 20 weeks of gestation (or earlier with trophoblastic diseases such as hydatidiform mole or hydrops)
Preeclampsia superimposed on chronic hypertension	Chronic hypertension with signs and symptoms of preeclampsia such as BP $\geq$ 160/110 mmHg, proteinuria $\geq$ 2.0 g/24 h, increased serum creatinine > 1.2 mg/dL unless previously elevated, thrombocytopenia, elevated AST or ALT, persistent neurological disturbances, or persistent epigastric pain
Gestational hypertension	
Transient hypertension of pregnancy	If preeclampsia not present at the time of delivery and blood pressure returns to normal by 12 weeks post partum (a retrospective diagnosis)
Chronic hypertension	If preeclampsia not present at the time of delivery and blood pressure persists beyond 12 weeks post partum (a retrospective diagnosis)

BP = blood pressure; AST = aspartate aminotransferase; ALT = alanine aminotransferase.
Source: Modified from Ref. 135.

fetal unit and result in a variety of fetal and neonatal complications. Uteroplacental blood flow can be significantly decreased, leading to intrauterine growth restriction (IUGR), fetal distress, or fetal death (14–16). The degrees of hypertension and proteinuria correlate with perinatal morbidity and mortality rates (17), and the majority of fetal deaths in hypertensive women are thought to be due to placental abnormality, including infarcts, small placental size, and abruption (18).

Hypertensive patients are at higher risk for placental abruption, as illustrated in a series of 265 cases (19). The overall incidence of abruption in the general obstetrical population was approximately 1%, and hypertensive disorders were present in 27% of abruption cases. Preeclamptic, chronic hypertensive, and eclamptic patients were found to have a 2%, 10%, and 24% incidence of abruption, respectively (19,20).

Severe preeclampsia, in general, portends greater maternal and perinatal morbidity and mortality rates (21). Perinatal mortality rates for eclamptic individuals range from 7% to 16% in contemporary American and British series (Table 2). Mortality was secondary to placental abruption, prematurity, and perinatal asphyxia. Antenatal deaths accounted for a significant proportion of the overall perinatal mortality rates. The HELLP (*H*emolysis, *E*levated *L*iver enzymes, *L*ow *P*latelets) syndrome, a variant of severe preeclampsia (22,23), affects up to 12% of patients who have preeclampsia-eclampsia and is associated with a remarkably high perinatal mortality rate (Table 3).

Table 2 Maternal and Perinatal Mortality in Eclampsia

Series	Years	Cases (*n*)	Maternal mortality	Perinatal mortality
Cincinnati, OH (120)	1930–1940	120	1.7%	29%[a]
Cincinnati, OH (121)	1940–1960	133	1.5%	28%[b]
Augusta, GA (122)	1956–1965	69	2.9%	32%[a]
Charlottesville, VA (123)	1939–1963	168	4.8%	22%[a]
Dallas, TX (124)	1955–1975	154	0%	15%[c]
Mexico City, Mexico (125)	1963–1979	704	14%	27%
Dallas, TC (108)	1975–1983	91	1.1%	16%[c]
Ilorin, Nigeria (126)	1972–1987	651	14%	N/A[d]
Memphis, TN (127)	1977–1989	254	0.4%	12%[a]
United Kingdom (128)	1992	383	1.8%	7%[a]

[a]All cases.
[b]Includes 1930–1940 series.
[c]Antepartum and intrapartum cases only.
[d]Not available.
Source: Modified from Ref. 21.

Table 3 Perinatal Outcomes in HELLP Syndrome

Series	Years	Cases (*n*)	Perinatal mortality	SGA	RDS
Greenville, NC (129)	1978–1982	27	11%	N/A	8%
Tucson, AZ (130)	1980–1984	57	8%	N/A	16%
Memphis, TN (131)	1977–1985	112	33%	32%	
New Haven, CT (132)	1981–1984	58	7%	41%	31%

SGA = small for gestational age; RDS = respiratory distress syndrome; N/A not available.
Source: Modified from Ref. 21.

Early-onset preeclampsia, which by its nature is more likely to evolve into the severe form, is associated with a higher rate of perinatal morbidity and mortality than preeclampsia at or near term. In a retrospective series of 49,812 births at a teaching hospital in the United Kingdom between 1986 and 1997, early-onset (less than 30 completed weeks of gestation) preeclampsia complicated 1 in 682 births (24). The intrauterine and neonatal death rates in this group of patients were 16% and 12%, respectively. Thus it can be appreciated that preeclampsia poses a significant potential risk to the fetus, especially when early in onset or complicated by severe manifestations of the clinical disease.

D. Perinatal Morbidity and Mortality of Chronic Hypertension

Chronic hypertension complicates 1 to 5% of U.S. births (25). A systematic review of mild chronic hypertension during pregnancy showed that chronic hypertension triples the risk for perinatal mortality and doubles the risk for placental abruption, when compared to risk in normotensive women or the general population (26). Chronic hypertension is associated with higher rates of perinatal morbidity when complicated by superimposed preeclampsia and/or IUGR (9). In a study of 211 mildly chronic hypertensive women (diastolic blood pressure 90–110 mmHg), the perinatal mortality rate was 28 per 1000 and the majority of perinatal deaths occurred in the group with superimposed preeclampsia (27). The superimposed preeclampsia group also had a higher rate of IUGR (32% versus 5%) than the chronic hypertensive group without superimposed preeclampsia. Chronic hypertensive women with superimposed severe preeclampsia have a significantly higher incidence of perinatal mortality, abruptio placentae, and growth restriction in infants when compared to severe preeclamptic women without preexisting hypertension (28).

In a study of 44 pregnant women with severe chronic hypertension in the first trimester, in over half severe preeclampsia developed, and those with superimposed preeclampsia experienced higher rates of prematurity (100% versus 38%), small for gestational age infants (78% versus 15%), and perinatal mortality (48% versus 0%) than those in whom superimposed preeclampsia did not develop (29).

Surveillance efforts therefore should be directed toward early detection of superimposed preeclampsia and IUGR in pregnant hypertensive women. The risk of IUGR may be higher among women who take β-blockers, particularly atenolol (30,31).

II. METHODS OF ANTEPARTUM SURVEILLANCE

A. Fetal Movement Assessment

Fetal death is often, but not always, preceded by a reduction in maternal perception of fetal movements (32). Various "kick count" protocols for antenatal fetal assessment have been proposed (32–39). Currently the optimal method for monitoring fetal movements has not been established. The "Count to 10" method (38) is easy and relatively quick to perform, as opposed to counting movements over a 1- or 2-hour period. The patient is instructed to time 10 fetal movements; once 10 movements are perceived, she may discontinue the count. If 10 movements are not perceived in 2 hours, she should contact her care provider immediately for further fetal assessment. As with other forms of antenatal fetal assessment, fetal death secondary to acute events such as umbilical cord compression or placental abruption may not be predictable (39,40).

Thus far, only two randomized trials (Table 4) have assessed the efficacy of fetal movement counts in preventing fetal death (40,41) The Danish study found a significant reduction in stillbirths of normally formed fetuses. The British study found no significant difference in fetal deaths, perhaps as a result of poor compliance in recording and reporting decreased fetal movements. Another unanswered question is whether incorporating fetal movement counts into a regular program of

Table 4 Corrected Stillbirth Rate (per 1000 Pregnancies) in Randomized Clinical Trials of Fetal Movement Count Protocols

Study	Number	Control group (no counting)	Test group (counting)	P
Neldam (1983) (41)	3,111	7.7	1.9	P < 0.05
Grant (1989) (40)	68,000	2.7	2.9	NS[a]

[a]NS = not significant.

antenatal fetal assessment would be of any significant added benefit in reducing antenatal mortality rate.

B. Ultrasound

1. Fetal Biometry

The value of fetal biometric measurements obtained by ultrasound for the purpose of pregnancy dating is dependent upon the gestational age at which the measurements are taken; the earlier the measurements are obtained, the more accurately the pregnancy may be dated (42). Whereas gestational age may be confirmed or determined within ½ to 1 week during the first trimester, the dating error during the third trimester may range by several weeks, with potential for significant error where clinical decision making is concerned. Thus for patients at risk for hypertension-related complications (e.g., chronic hypertension, multifetal gestation, underlying renal disease, antiphospholipid antibody syndrome) early baseline ultrasound is of paramount clinical importance, for decisions regarding timing of delivery and determination of fetal growth by serial ultrasound will be dependent upon precise knowledge of gestational age. For the purpose of evaluating fetal growth, ultrasound biometry should not be performed at less than 3-week intervals.

2. Amniotic Fluid Assessment

Amniotic fluid volume (AFV) may be reduced in cases of chronic uteroplacental insufficiency and thus is an integral part of the monitoring of hypertensive pregnancies during sonographic assessment. Oligohydramnios is associated with adverse pregnancy outcomes (43) and is often associated with nonreassuring intrapartum fetal heart rate (FHR) patterns as a result of umbilical cord compression and/or uteroplacental insufficiency. Sonographic assessment of AFV may be performed by a subjective procedure or by a variety of semiquantitative methods such as the four-quadrant amniotic fluid index (AFI) as described by Rutherford and colleagues (44). There may be a wide margin of error in semiquantitative assessment of amniotic fluid volume using the AFI, especially at the low and high ends of the spectrum (45,46). Normative AFI values have been published for singleton (47,48) and twin gestations (49,50) across the range of gestational ages. Although many clinicians effect delivery when oligohydramnios is diagnosed in terms of a low AFI, there is debate regarding the appropriate threshold of AFI to warrant intervention (e.g., less than 5.0 cm versus 5th centile) (51). Multiple obstetrical variables, including EFM patterns, fetal growth, severity of hypertension, and gestational age, should be considered in the clinical decision making (Fig. 1). At or near term, most clinicians would advocate delivery in those cases in which oligohydramnios complicates hypertension of any cause.

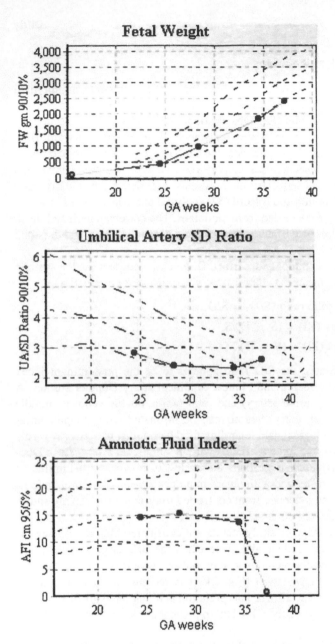

Figure 1 Ultrasonography using estimated fetal weight based on biometry and amniotic fluid volume assessment with the four-quadrant amniotic fluid index (AFI) provides valuable clinical information regarding uteroplacental function and fetal development. Intrauterine growth restriction and oligohydramnios near term should prompt consideration for further fetal assessment and possibly intervention with delivery.

3. Vascular Doppler Ultrasound

There have been numerous reports describing the relationship between umbilical artery Doppler waveforms and perinatal complications since the initial paper published in 1977 from Dublin (52). Observational studies have demonstrated the fetoplacental circulation to be a low-resistance system, with forward flow throughout systolic and diastolic phases of the cardiac cycle under normal circumstances. Some compromised fetuses display reduced diastolic blood flow, and those with absent or reversed diastolic flow may experience particularly poor outcomes (53–56). Thornton and Lilford (57) analyzed published studies in which the Doppler results were concealed from clinicians. The corrected perinatal death rate was 22% in the presence of absent or reversed umbilical artery end diastolic flow ($n = 92$).

There are several commonly described Doppler indices that use the systolic (S), diastolic (D), and mean (M) blood flow velocities in their equations:

Systolic-to-diastolic ratio (S/D) = S/D

Resistance index (RI) = (S − D)/S

Pulsatility index (PI) = (S − D)/M

In the United States, the S/D ratio appears to be the predominant index reported in obstetrical research and clinical umbilical artery Doppler studies. A multitude of maternal (uterine artery) and fetal (aorta, ductus venosus, middle cerebral artery, and renal artery) vessels can be insonated with Doppler ultrasound, providing physiological data regarding fetal blood flow patterns (58). This discussion primarily focuses on experience with the umbilical artery, since Doppler evaluation of this vessel is perhaps the easiest to obtain, most familiar to clinicians, and best characterized with regard to pregnancy-related complications. Moreover, there is yet no evidence from controlled trials that conclusively shows that evaluation of other vessels is of clinical value.

Umbilical artery Doppler study results are considered abnormal when diastolic blood flow is reversed or absent or when the S/D is greater than two standard deviations above the mean for gestational age, which as a rule of thumb is >3 beyond 32 weeks of gestation (Fig. 2). It is recommended that multiple waveforms be assessed to maximize interpretation and that the wall-filter setting be adjusted low enough (typically <150 Hz) to prevent masking of diastolic blood flow (1).

A number of randomized clinical trials of Doppler ultrasound for antepartum management of high-risk pregnancies have been conducted. The updated Cochrane Library review of Doppler for fetal assessment in high-risk pregnancies includes 11 studies involving nearly 7000 women (59). Compared to administration of no Doppler ultrasound, use of Doppler in high-risk pregnancy (especially those complicated by hypertension or presumed impaired fetal growth) was

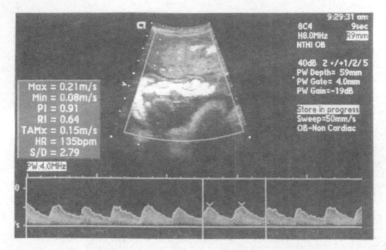

A

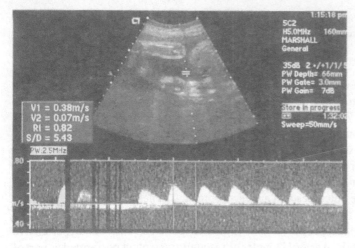

B

Figure 2 Doppler ultrasound of the umbilical artery shows a progressive pathological increase in placental resistance, manifested by decrease in diastolic blood flow. Initially (A), umbilical blood flow and the S/D ratio are normal, but over time (B), the S/D ratio increases. This trend, especially in the absence of end-diastolic blood flow (C) or its reversal, is associated with increased perinatal morbidity and mortality rates.

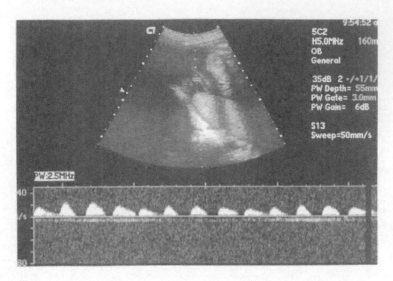

C

Figure 2 Continued

associated with fewer inductions of labor (odds ratio [OR] = 0.83, 95% confidence index [CI] 0.74 to 0.93), fewer antepartum admissions to hospital (OR = 0.56, 95% CI 0.43 to 0.72), and a trend in reduction of perinatal deaths (OR = 0.71, 95% CI 0.50 to 1.01), but no difference in fetal distress during labor (OR = 0.81, 95% CI 0.59 to 1.13) or cesarean delivery (OR = 0.94, 95% CI 0.82 to 1.06). In their review, Neilson and Alfirevic concluded that the addition of Doppler ultrasound to the antenatal fetal surveillance in high-risk pregnancies appears to improve a number of obstetrical care outcomes and appears promising in helping to reduce perinatal deaths (59).

Giles (58) has proposed that high-risk patients, such as hypertensive women, have umbilical artery Doppler ultrasound assessment performed as part of fetal well-being evaluation as often as weekly, with the frequency adjusted depending on concern about fetal well-being. He recommended that in the presence of an abnormal Doppler study finding prior to 32 weeks of gestation, other evidence indicating fetal compromise (e.g., IUGR, abnormal EFM, decreased AFI) be obtained before delivery is effected. He proposed that after 32 weeks of gestation, deteriorating Doppler study results alone would be a reasonable indication for delivery.

A 1999 ACOG Practice Bulletin (1) concluded that "no benefit has been demonstrated for umbilical artery velocimetry for conditions other than suspected intrauterine growth restriction." Given that placental insufficiency and IUGR are more common in hypertensive pregnancies, many clinicians incorporate umbilical artery Doppler into antepartum fetal surveillance programs. The ACOG statement further recommends that if umbilical artery Doppler velocimetry is used, decisions regarding timing of delivery should be made by using a combination of information including other tests of fetal well-being (nonstress test [NST], contraction stress test [CST], AFI, or biophysical profile [BPP]) and maternal condition.

4. Biophysical Profile

The fetal BPP, based on observations of fetal behavior as it relates to hypoxia (61–63), was introduced in 1980 as a method of antenatal fetal assessment (60). The BPP includes five parameters: fetal breathing, fetal movement, fetal tone, amniotic fluid volume, and NST. The first four parameters are assessed by ultrasound (Fig. 3) and the fifth by EFM. Each parameter is designated a value of 0 or 2 (Table 5), and the BPP denominator is totaled as 8 or 10, depending on whether the NST component is included. If the four ultrasound parameters are normal, the NST may be omitted without compromising the validity of the test results (64).

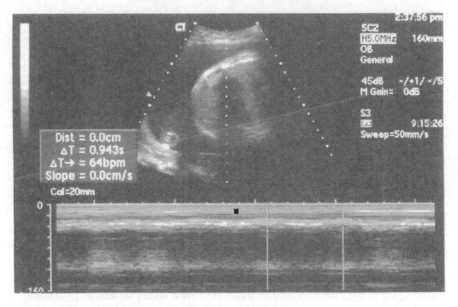

Figure 3 The biophysical profile (BPP) is performed by using real-time sonography and scoring for fetal movement, tone, breathing, and amniotic fluid volume. In this image, adequate amniotic fluid volume is documented by a pocket measuring at least 2 cm and by fetal breathing movements captured by M-mode sonography.

Table 5 The Biophysical Profile Coding Criteria

Biophysical variable	Normal (score = 2)	Abnormal (score = 0)
Fetal breathing movements	One or more episodes of ≥ 20 s duration in 30 min	Absent or no episode of ≥ 20 s duration in 30 min
Gross body movements	Two or more discrete body/limb movements in 30 min (episodes of active continuous movement considered as a single movement)	Less than two episodes of body/limb movements in 30 min
Fetal tone	One or more active episodes of active extension with return to flexion of fetal limb(s) or trunk (opening and closing of hand considered normal tone)	Slow extension with return to partial flexion, movement of limb in full extension, absent fetal movement, or partially open fetal hand
Qualitative amniotic fluid volume	One or more pockets of fluid measuring ≥ 2 cm in vertical axis	Either no pockets or largest pocket < 2 cm in vertical axis
Reactive fetal heart rate	Two or more episodes of acceleration of ≥ 15 bpm and of > 15 s associated with fetal movement in 20 min	One or no episode of acceleration of fetal heart rate or acceleration of < 15 bpm in 20 min

Source: Modified from Ref. 65.

A composite score of 10 or 8 is normal, 6 is equivocal, and 4 or less is abnormal (1). A normal score is managed by repeat testing at the usual interval, except in the case that the score is 8/10, with loss of 2 points for oligohydramnios, in which delivery or additional assessment may be indicated. The management of an equivocal score of 6 is dependent upon gestational age, score composition of individual parameters, and other maternal-fetal factors. An equivocal score requires, at the least, retesting within 24 hours, at which time two-thirds of test results will be found to be normal (65). Generally a score of 4 or less requires delivery. Manning has outlined management recommendations for various clinical scenarios based on BPP score, individual BPP composition, and gestational age (65).

From experience with over 200,000 BPP tests, Manning reports that average testing time was less than 8 minutes, with more than 90% of normal testing completed in the first 4 minutes (65). It is recommended that an abnormal BPP score should not be assigned unless 30 minutes of observation has elapsed.

Observational studies have shown correlation of the BPP with fetal outcome parameters. The BPP score correlates inversely with perinatal mortality rate (66,67) inversely with cerebral palsy (68,69), and directly with umbilical venous pH (70,71). A meta-analysis (72) involving 2839 women from four (73–76) randomized trials on BPP versus NST showed no difference in adverse perinatal outcomes between the BPP and NST; however, significantly larger numbers would be required in order to achieve enough power to demonstrate differences in low-prevalence adverse outcomes such as perinatal death and depressed Apgar score.

The BPP has been proposed by some as a primary method of antenatal fetal surveillance (65). In the United States, where the BPP has been widely incorporated into clinical practice, it is generally used as a backup test for the NST, particularly when the NST is nonreactive, such as in the setting of the premature fetus. The "Modified Biophysical Profile" (77) is a popular primary method of antepartum fetal surveillance (78), which combines the NST (with the option of acoustic stimulation) as an indicator of short-term fetal acid-base condition and the AFI as an indicator of long-term placental function. In a series of 2628 singleton high-risk pregnant women who underwent 5973 tests, there were no unexpected fetal deaths when using this protocol (77).

C. Electronic Fetal Monitoring

Antepartum EFM for the purpose of assessing fetal hypoxia evolved from observations of intrapartum FHR patterns made over the preceding decade (79). The nonstress test (NST) and contraction stress test (CST) are the two EFM methods in current use. The CST and the NST are both performed by recording the FHR via an ultrasound transducer and uterine activity via a tocodynometer placed on the maternal abdomen. The CST preceded the NST in chronological development; however, the popularity of the NST as an antepartum testing method has surpassed that of the CST because of the NST's relative simplicity and reliability (80,81).

The CST is based on the premise that contractions transiently diminish fetal oxygenation, and that the suboptimally oxygenated fetus responds to worsening hypoxemia with late decelerations or, in some cases, with variable decelerations. The CST requires the presence of at least three contractions of 40 seconds' duration in a 10-minute period. If spontaneous contractions of this degree are not present, then contractions are induced by intravenous administration of a dilute oxytocin solution or by nipple stimulation. The CST is relatively contraindicated in conditions associated with the risk of hemorrhage (known placenta previa), uterine rupture (classic cesarean or extensive uterine surgery), or preterm delivery (preterm membrane rupture, preterm labor, or other high-risk factor for preterm delivery). The interpretation of the CST (1) is summarized in Table 6.

The NST is based on the premise that a healthy ·fetus demonstrates FHR accelerations associated with fetal movement. FHR reactivity is generally associated with normal oxygenation and thus normal autonomic nervous system function. Loss of reactivity is often associated with fetal sleep cycles but may be secondary to causes of central nervous system depression, including acidosis. Uncompromised preterm fetuses may have a nonreactive nonstress test result; between 24 and 28 weeks up to 50% may have a nonreactive finding (82), and between 28 and 32 weeks 15% have a nonreactive result (83,84). The interpretation of the NST (1) is summarized in Table 7.

Observational studies (85,86) have demonstrated a correlation between abnormal NST result and measures of poor neonatal outcome. A Cochrane Library meta-analysis (87) of four studies (88–91) involving 1588 pregnancies assessed the effects of antenatal NST on perinatal morbidity and mortality rates. There was a trend to an increase in perinatal deaths in the NST group (OR = 2.85, 95% CI = 0.99 to 7.12). However the reviewers concluded that most of the deaths were not preventable by appropriate intervention. The meta-analysis did not have sufficient power to assess differences in low-prevalence primary outcomes such as perinatal mortality and abnormal neurological outcome, although in one trial there was a reduction in antenatal intervention with fewer hospital admissions and shorter hospital stay duration for women who had antenatal NSTs (89). The reviewers concluded that a study of sufficient size to assess the effect of NST on perinatal mortality rate in a high-risk population is unlikely to be conducted today, because the NST has become an integral component of antenatal care.

Table 6 Interpretation of the Results of the Contraction Stress Test

Result	Definition
Negative	No late or significant variable decelerations
Positive	Late decelerations after 50% or more of contractions (even if the contraction frequency is fewer than three in 10 min)
Equivocal: suspicious	Intermittent late decelerations or significant variable decelerations
Equivocal: hyperstimulatory	Fetal heart decelerations that occur in the presence of contractions more frequent than every 2 min or lasting longer than 90 s
Unsatisfactory	Fewer than three contractions in 10 min or an uninterpretable tracing

Source: Adapted from Ref. 1.

Table 7 Interpretation of the Results of the Nonstress Test

Result	Definition
Reactive (normal)	Two or more FHR accelerations (that peak, but do not necessarily remain, at least 15 bpm above the baseline and last 15 s from baseline to baseline) within a 20-min period, with or without fetal movement discerned by woman
Nonreactive	Lacks sufficient FHR accelerations (as defined) over a 40-min period

Source: Adapted from Ref. 1.

Fetal sleep states may produce falsely nonreactive FHR test results (92–94), potentially leading to unnecessary concern and interventions. A number of methods have been advanced to circumvent this limitation of FHR monitoring. In 1947 Bernard and Sontag (95) first noted FHR acceleration after acoustic stimulation. The fetal scalp stimulation test was reported by Clark and colleagues (96,97) to be beneficial in evaluating nonreassuring intrapartum FHR patterns and a potential alternative to fetal scalp blood sampling. Fetal vibroacoustic stimulation was developed for the purpose of improving the efficiency of antepartum FHR testing. A meta-analysis (98) of seven trials involving 4325 participants showed that vibroacoustic stimulation reduces the incidence of nonreactive antenatal cardiotocography test results (OR = 0.61, 95% CI = 0.49 to 0.75) and reduces overall testing time by 4.55 minutes. However, the data in these trials were insufficient to draw conclusions regarding the effect of vibroacoustic stimulation use on the incidence of fetal distress and perinatal death. Recommendations were made for further studies to assess the optimal testing protocols, as well as the efficacy, safety, predictive reliability, and perinatal outcomes of this test compared with those of other forms of fetal testing. Some perinatal centers incorporate acoustic stimulation in their antepartum testing protocols, primarily for the purpose of reducing NST testing time (77).

Table 8 Corrected Stillbirth Rates for the Methods of Antepartum Fetal Surveillance

Method	Number of tests	Corrected stillbirth rate (per 1000)	Negative predictive value (%)
NST (86)	5,861	1.9	99.8
CST (86)	12,656	0.3	>99.9
BPP (133)	44,828	0.8	>99.9
Modified BPP (78)	54,617	0.8	>99.9
UA Doppler (134)	214	0	100

acoustic stimulation in their antepartum testing protocols, primarily for the purpose of reducing NST testing time (77).

The false-negative rates of the various antepartum fetal testing methods (defined as a stillbirth within 1 week of a normal test result) after correction for lethal congenital anomalies and unpredictable causes of death are very low (Table 8). Maintenance of a low false-negative rate and thus a low stillbirth rate is dependent on an appropriate response to acute changes in maternal or fetal condition and includes either retesting or delivery for worsening condition.

D. Other Modalities to Assess the Fetus at Risk

1. Midtrimester Maternal Serum Screening

Serum screening during the midtrimester was originally devised to detect fetuses with neural tube defects, and later, chromosomal aneuploidy. Fetuses with high maternal serum α-fetoprotein (MS-AFP) level have an increased relative risk for neural tube defects, and those with low MS-AFP and high human chorionic gonadotropin (MS-hCG) levels have an increased relative risk for Down syndrome. It was observed that fetuses with midtrimester "unexplained" elevated MS-AFP or MS-hCG level were at increased risk for adverse third-trimester outcomes such as IUGR, oligohydramnios, fetal death, spontaneous preterm delivery, abruptio placentae, and pregnancy-induced hypertension (99–103). One study of 60,040 patients confirmed previous associations of adverse perinatal outcome with increased MS-AFP (> 2.5 MoM) and increased MS-hCG (> 2.5 MoM), as well as with decreased (< 0.5 MoM) unconjugated estriol levels (104). These complications are thought to be due to placental abnormalities, a defective barrier, or increased placental villous surface, expressed early in pregnancy and detected at the time of midtrimester serum screening (99,105). At present, there are no standardized protocols for monitoring women with "unexplained" elevated MS-AFP and/or MS-hCG level during the third trimester. A small retrospective study in 2001 showed no benefit to increased fetal surveillance (106). Citing a 40% positive predictive value for adverse perinatal outcomes in women with unexplained elevated MS-AFP or MS-hCG level, Dekker and Sibai (107) state that intensified surveillance could be justified. Today it is common practice, but not standard of care, to perform or enhance antenatal fetal surveillance via serial ultrasound and EFM in cases of unexplained elevated midtrimester serum screening.

2. Amniocentesis for Fetal Lung Maturity

Premature delivery for preeclampsia carries a high incidence of neonatal respiratory complications (23,108). Amniocentesis for the purpose of evaluating fetal lung maturation may be of benefit in cases of mild disease near term, when there is no pressing indication for immediate delivery. Although there may be a common perception that hypertension promotes early fetal lung maturation, the presence of preeclampsia does not guarantee lung maturity (109,110). Preeclampsia has not been associated with accelerated fetal development as measured by the Ballard score of neurological and physical development (111).

III. CLINICAL MANAGEMENT STRATEGIES

A. When to Initiate Monitoring

In theory, the optimal time to begin antepartum fetal surveillance during a high-risk pregnancy is dependent on a number of factors, including the false-positive rate of the test for fetal death, the stillbirth rate, and the week-specific neonatal mortality rate (112). There has not been extensive investigation into the question of when to begin testing in hypertensive patients. The clinical recommendations for fetal monitoring of hypertensive pregnancies of the Report of the Working Group on High Blood Pressure in Pregnancy from the National Heart, Lung, and Blood Institute are outlined in Table 9.

Table 9 Recommendations for Fetal Monitoring in Gestational Hypertension and Preeclampsia

---

Gestational hypertension
  Estimation of fetal growth and amniotic fluid volume should be performed at diagnosis.
    If results are normal, repeat testing only if there is significant change in maternal
    condition.
  NST should be performed at diagnosis. If the NST result is nonreactive, perform the BPP.
    If BPP is 8 or if NST result is reactive, repeat testing only if there is significant change
    in maternal condition.
Mild preeclampsia
  Estimation of fetal growth and amniotic fluid volume should be performed at diagnosis.
    If the results are normal, repeat testing every 3 weeks.
  NST, BPP, or both should be performed at diagnosis. If NST is reactive or if BPP is 8,
    repeat weekly. Testing should be repeated immediately if there is abrupt change in
    maternal condition.
  If estimated weight by ultrasound is < 10th percentile for gestational age or if there is
    oligohydramnios (AFI ≤ 5 cm), then testing should be performed at least twice
    weekly.
Severe preeclampsia
  Daily fetal testing (NST and/or BPP)

Source: Modified from Ref. 135.

For patients with chronic hypertension or nonproteinuric pregnancy-induced hypertension, compromise was not detected among 917 women [using the oxytocin challenge test (OCT) as a primary method of surveillance] until after 33 weeks of gestation, in the absence of additional risk factors such as lupus erythematosus, IUGR, diabetes mellitus, or superimposed preeclampsia (113). Theoretical models and clinical studies (112–114) indicate that initiation of testing at 32–34 weeks of gestation is appropriate in most high-risk clinical circumstances. In situations of greater concern, such as chronic hypertension with suspected IUGR, initiation of testing at 26–28 weeks of gestation may be appropriate (1).

A systematic review by the Evidence-Based Practice Center in San Antonio, Texas, did not identify any studies assessing the benefits, harms, or costs of special fetal monitoring techniques for mild chronically hypertensive women during pregnancy (26). Recommendations in a 2001 ACOG Practice Bulletin (115) reflect the Report of the National High Blood Pressure Education Program Working Group on High Blood Pressure in Pregnancy recommendations (9):

> There is no consensus as to the most appropriate fetal surveillance test(s) or the interval and timing of testing in women with chronic hypertension. Thus, such testing should be individualized and based on clinical judgment and on severity of disease. However, other studies have indicated that most of the increased morbidity associated with this condition is secondary to superimposed preeclampsia or IUGR. Thus, these investigators recommend that baseline ultrasonography be obtained at 18–20 weeks of gestation and that ultrasonography should be repeated at 28–32 weeks of gestation and monthly thereafter until delivery to monitor fetal growth. If growth restriction is detected or suspected, fetal status should be monitored frequently with nonstress testing or biophysical profile testing. If growth restriction is not present and superimposed preeclampsia is excluded, these tests are not indicated.

Antepartum fetal surveillance should be implemented when preeclampsia is diagnosed, assuming there is anticipated probability of neonatal survival if delivery is effected.

B. Which Tests to Use

As indicated, at present there is no clear consensus on which test or group of tests is best suited to monitor the fetus of a hypertensive woman (1,9). The NST combined with AFI (modified BPP) is currently a popular method of fetal surveillance employed in the United States. Umbilical artery Doppler is available in many centers, but utilization is not uniform.

C. Frequency of Monitoring

The frequency of monitoring preeclamptic patients is dependent on the severity of the clinical condition as well as on several other factors, including clinical judgment (1). If the CST is the primary method of fetal surveillance, it is usually repeated weekly when the clinical situation is stable and the CST results are normal (116). If the NST is used as the primary method, usually weekly or twice-weekly testing is sufficient (9). Daily fetal movement counts are a useful complement to the NST or BPP. Significant deterioration in maternal condition or acute decrease in fetal activity requires reevaluation, regardless of the time elapsed since the previous test (1).

More frequent antenatal fetal assessment may be appropriate for expectantly managed patients with severe preeclampsia remote from term. Sibai and colleagues reported improved perinatal outcomes, with no increase in the rate of maternal complications, in a select group of women with severe preeclampsia between 24 to 27 weeks of gestation (117) and 28 to 32 weeks of gestation (118) who were managed with intensive fetal and maternal monitoring under strict protocols in a tertiary care center. Chari and colleagues (119) retrospectively assessed whether daily antenatal testing in this subset of preeclamptic women prevented stillbirth or neonatal compromise. They reviewed medical records of 68 women with severe preeclampsia remote from term who underwent expectant management with daily fetal testing until delivery. There were no stillbirths and 31% of patients ultimately had nonreassuring test findings necessitating delivery. Two neonatal deaths occurred, both as a result of prematurity. They recommended that patients with severe preeclampsia managed expectantly undergo daily antepartum testing.

D. Decisions Regarding Delivery

In general, and especially when remote from term, an abnormal NST or Modified BPP finding should usually be further evaluated by either a CST or full BPP (1). Subsequent management is then determined by the cumulative results of the tests of fetal condition (fetal growth, amniotic fluid volume, and fetal testing), gestational age (and fetal lung maturity tests if available), and, specifically in the setting of pregnancy complicated by hypertension, maternal condition. The detection of oligohydramnios requires delivery versus close monitoring, depending on the same multiple maternal-fetal parameters. In the absence of obstetrical contraindications, delivery may be attempted by induction of labor with continuous EFM. If deterioration of fetal condition is noted, for example, by the development of late decelerations, prompt delivery is indicated.

IV. SUMMARY

Pregnancies complicated by maternal hypertension are at increased risk for maternal and fetal-neonatal complications. A number of antepartum fetal surveillance methods, which may help to reduce perinatal morbidity and mortality, exist.

Although a substantial amount of knowledge has been obtained through observational studies about the association of test results with various neonatal complications, there remains a dearth of information regarding optimal management protocols, as a result of the current limited number of prospective clinical trials which would be required to address the issues appropriately. Management recommendations by national entities such as ACOG and the NIH do exist in this regard; however, numerous clinical questions remain. In many clinical cases, a careful, individualized approach to management in general, and fetal surveillance in particular, is warranted.

REFERENCES

1. American College of Obstetricians and Gynecologists. Antepartum fetal surveillance. ACOG Practice Bull Number 9, October 1999.
2. Vintzileos AM. Antenatal assessment for the detection of fetal asphyxia: an evidence-based approach using indication-specific testing. Ann NY Acad Sci 2000; 900:137–150.
3. Ananth CV, Smulian JC, Vintzileos AM. Epidemiology of antepartum fetal testing. Curr Opin Obstet Gynecol 1997; 9:101–106.
4. Boddy K, Dawes GS, Fisher R, Pinter S, Robinson JS. Foetal respiratory movements, electrocortical and cardiovascular responses to hypoxaemia and hypercapnia in sheep. J Physiol 1974; 243:599–618.
5. Natale R, Clewlow F, Dawes GS. Measurement of fetal forelimb movements in the lamb in utero. Am J Obstet Gynecol 1981; 140:545–551.
6. Murata Y, Martin CB Jr, Ikenoue T, et al. Fetal heart rate accelerations and late decelerations during the course of intrauterine death in chronically catheterized rhesus monkeys. Am J Obstet Gynecol 1982; 144:218–223.
7. Manning FA, Platt LD. Maternal hypoxemia and fetal breathing movements. Obstet Gynecol 1979; 53:758–760.
8. Seeds AE. Current concepts of amniotic fluid dynamics. Am J Obstet Gynecol 1980; 138:575–586.
9. Report of the National High Blood Pressure Education Program Working Group on High Blood Pressure in Pregnancy. Am J Obstet Gynecol 2000; 183:S1–S22.
10. Hibbard LT. Maternal mortality due to acute toxemia. Obstet Gynecol 1973; 42:263–270.
11. Kaunitz AM, Hughes JM, Grimes DA, Smith JC, Rochat RW, Kafrissen ME. Causes of maternal mortality in the United States. Obstet Gynecol 1985; 65:605–612.
12. Grimes DA. The morbidity and mortality of pregnancy: still risky business. Am J Obstet Gynecol 1994; 170:1489–1494.
13. Dildy GA, Cotton DB. Hemodynamic changes in pregnancy and pregnancy complicated by hypertension. Acute Care 1988; 15:26–46.
14. Friedman SA. Preeclampsia: a review of the role of prostaglandins. Obstet Gynecol 1988; 71:122–137.
15. Lunell NO, Nylund LE, Lewander R, Sarby B. Uteroplacental blood flow in pre-

eclampsia measurements with indium-113m and a computer-linked gamma camera. Clin Exp Hypertens B 1982; 1:105–117.

16. Lunell NO, Lewander R, Mamoun I, Nylund L, Sarby S, Thornstrom S. Uteroplacental blood flow in pregnancy induced hypertension. Scand J Clin Lab Invest Suppl 1984; 169:28–35.

17. Ferrazzani S, Caruso A, De Carolis S, Martino IV, Mancuso S. Proteinuria and outcome of 444 pregnancies complicated by hypertension. Am J Obstet Gynecol 1990; 162:366–371.

18. Naeye RL, Friedman EA. Causes of perinatal death associated with gestational hypertension and proteinuria. Am J Obstet Gynecol 1979; 133:8–10.

19. Abdella TN, Sibai BM, Hays JM Jr, Anderson GD. Relationship of hypertensive disease to abruptio placentae. Obstet Gynecol 1984;63:365–370.

20. Hurd WW, Miodovnik M, Hertzberg V, Lavin JP. Selective management of abruptio placentae: a prospective study. Obstet Gynecol 1983; 61:467–473.

21. Dildy GA, Cotton DB. Complications of Preeclampsia. In: Clark SL, Cotton DB, Hankins GDV, Phelan JP, eds. Critical Care Obstetrics. Boston: Blackwell Scientific, 1997.

22. Pritchard JA, Weisman R, Ratnoff OD, Vosburgh GJ. Intravascular hemolysis, thrombocytopenia, and other hematologic abnormalities associated with severe toxemia of pregnancy. N Engl J Med 1954; 150:89–98.

23. Weinstein L. Syndrome of hemolysis, elevated liver enzymes, and low platelet count: a severe consequence of hypertension in pregnancy. Am J Obstet Gynecol 1982; 142:159–167.

24. Murphy DJ, Stirrat GM. Mortality and morbidity associated with early-onset preeclampsia. Hypertens Pregnancy 2000; 19:221–231.

25. The sixth report of the Joint National Committee on prevention, detection, evaluation, and treatment of high blood pressure. Arch Intern Med 1997; 157:2413–2446.

26. Ferrer RL, Sibai BM, Mulrow CD, Chiquette E, Stevens KR, Cornell J. Management of mild chronic hypertension during pregnancy: a review. Obstet Gynecol 2000; 96: 849–860.

27. Sibai BM, Abdella TN, Anderson GD. Pregnancy outcome in 211 patients with mild chronic hypertension. Obstet Gynecol 1983; 61:571–576.

28. Sibai BM, Spinnato JA, Watson DL, Hill GA, Anderson GD. Pregnancy outcome in 303 cases with severe preeclampsia. Obstet Gynecol 1984; 64:319–325.

29. Sibai BM, Anderson GD. Pregnancy outcome of intensive therapy in severe hypertension in first trimester. Obstet Gynecol 1986; 67:517–522.

30. Butters L, Kennedy S, Rubin PC. Atenolol in essential hypertension during pregnancy. Br Med J 1990; 301:587–589.

31. Lip GY, Beevers M, Churchill D, Shaffer LM, Beevers DG. Effect of atenolol on birth weight. Am J Cardiol 1997; 79:1436–1438.

32. Pearson JF, Weaver JB. Fetal activity and fetal wellbeing: an evaluation. Br Med J 1976; 1:1305–1307.

33. Sadovsky E, Polishuk WZ. Fetal movements in utero: nature, assessment, prognostic value, timing of delivery. Obstet Gynecol 1977; 50:49–55.

34. Neldam S. Fetal movements as an indicator of fetal wellbeing. Lancet 1980; 1:1222–1224.

35. O'Leary JA, Andrinopoulos GC. Correlation of daily fetal movements and the nonstress test as tools for assessment of fetal welfare. Am J Obstet Gynecol 1981; 139:107–108.
36. Harper RG, Greenberg M, Farahani G, Glassman I, Kierney CM. Fetal movement, biochemical and biophysical parameters, and the outcome of pregnancy. Am J Obstet Gynecol 1981; 141:39–42.
37. Leader LR, Baillie P, Van Schalkwyk DJ. Fetal movements and fetal outcome: a prospective study. Obstet Gynecol 1981; 57:431–436.
38. Moore TR, Piacquadio K. A prospective evaluation of fetal movement screening to reduce the incidence of antepartum fetal death. Am J Obstet Gynecol 1989; 160: 1075–1080.
39. Christensen FC, Rayburn WF. Fetal movement counts. Obstet Gynecol Clin North Am 1999; 26:607–621.
40. Grant A, Elbourne D, Valentin L, Alexander S. Routine formal fetal movement counting and risk of antepartum late death in normally formed singletons. Lancet 1989; 2:345–349.
41. Neldam S. Fetal movements as an indicator of fetal well-being. Dan Med Bull 1983; 30:274–278.
42. Hadlock FP. Sonographic estimation of fetal age and weight. Radiol Clin North Am 1990; 28:39–50.
43. Chamberlain PF, Manning FA, Morrison I, Harman CR, Lange IR. Ultrasound evaluation of amniotic fluid volume. I. The relationship of marginal and decreased amniotic fluid volumes to perinatal outcome. Am J Obstet Gynecol 1984; 150: 245–249.
44. Rutherford SE, Phelan JP, Smith CV, Jacobs N. The four-quadrant assessment of amniotic fluid volume: an adjunct to antepartum fetal heart rate testing. Obstet Gynecol 1987; 70:353–356.
45. Dildy GA III, Lira N, Moise KJ Jr, Riddle GD, Deter RL. Amniotic fluid volume assessment: comparison of ultrasonographic estimates versus direct measurements with a dye-dilution technique in human pregnancy. Am J Obstet Gynecol 1992; 167: 986–994.
46. Croom CS, Banias BB, Ramos-Santos E, Devoe LD, Bezhadian A, Hiett AK. Do semiquantitative amniotic fluid indexes reflect actual volume? Am J Obstet Gynecol 1992; 167:995–999.
47. Brace RA, Wolf EJ. Normal amniotic fluid volume changes throughout pregnancy. Am J Obstet Gynecol 1989; 161:382–388.
48. Moore TR, Cayle JE. The amniotic fluid index in normal human pregnancy. Am J Obstet Gynecol 1990; 162:1168–1173.
49. Porter TF, Dildy GA, Blanchard JR, Kochenour NK, Clark SL. Normal values for amniotic fluid index during uncomplicated twin pregnancy. Obstet Gynecol 1996; 87:699–702.
50. Chau AC, Kjos SL, Kovacs BW. Ultrasonographic measurement of amniotic fluid volume in normal diamniotic twin pregnancies. Am J Obstet Gynecol 1996; 174: 1003–1007.
51. Magann EF, Martin JN Jr. Amniotic fluid volume assessment in singleton and twin pregnancies. Obstet Gynecol Clin North Am 1999; 26:579–593.

52. FitzGerald DE, Drumm JE. Non-invasive measurement of human fetal circulation using ultrasound: a new method. Br Med J 1977; 2:1450–1451.

53. Rochelson B, Schulman H, Farmakides G, et al. The significance of absent end-diastolic velocity in umbilical artery velocity waveforms. Am J Obstet Gynecol 1987; 156:1213–1218.

54. Brar HS, Platt LD. Reverse end-diastolic flow velocity on umbilical artery velocimetry in high-risk pregnancies: an ominous finding with adverse pregnancy outcome. Am J Obstet Gynecol 1988; 159:559–561.

55. Fairlie FM, Moretti M, Walker JJ, Sibai BM. Determinants of perinatal outcome in pregnancy-induced hypertension with absence of umbilical artery end-diastolic frequencies. Am J Obstet Gynecol 1991; 164:1084–1089.

56. Karsdorp VH, van Vugt JM, van Geijn HP, et al. Clinical significance of absent or reversed end diastolic velocity waveforms in umbilical artery. Lancet 1994; 344: 1664–1668.

57. Thornton JG, Lilford RJ. Do we need randomised trials of antenatal tests of fetal wellbeing? Br J Obstet Gynaecol 1993; 100:197–200.

58. Giles WB. Vascular Doppler techniques. Obstet Gynecol Clin North Am 1999; 26: 595–606. vi.

59. Neilson JP, Alfirevic Z. Doppler ultrasound for fetal assessment in high risk pregnancies. Cochrane Database Syst Rev 2000; 2.

60. Manning FA, Platt LD, Sipos L. Antepartum fetal evaluation: development of a fetal biophysical profile. Am J Obstet Gynecol 1980; 136:787–795.

61. Dawes GS, Lewis BV, Milligan JE, Roach MR, Talner NS. Vasomotor responses in the hind limbs of foetal and new-born lambs to asphyxia and aortic chemoreceptor stimulation. J Physiol 1968; 195:55–81.

62. Manning FA. Fetal breathing movements: as a reflection of fetal status. Postgrad Med 1977; 61:116–122.

63. Manning FA, Platt LD. Fetal breathing movements and the abnormal contraction stress test. Am J Obstet Gynecol 1979; 133:590–593.

64. Manning FA, Morrison I, Lange IR, Harman CR, Chamberlain PF. Fetal biophysical profile scoring: selective use of the nonstress test. Am J Obstet Gynecol 1987; 156:709–712.

65. Manning FA. Fetal biophysical profile. Obstet Gynecol Clin North Am 1999; 26: 557–577.

66. Manning FA, Morrison I, Lange IR, Harman CR, Chamberlain PF. Fetal assessment based on fetal biophysical profile scoring: experience in 12,620 referred high-risk pregnancies. I. Perinatal mortality by frequency and etiology. Am J Obstet Gynecol 1985; 151:343–350.

67. Baskett TF, Allen AC, Gray JH, Young DC, Young LM. Fetal biophysical profile and perinatal death. Obstet Gynecol 1987; 70:357–360.

68. Manning FA, Bondagji N, Harman CR, Casiro O, Menticoglou S, Morrison I. Fetal assessment based on the fetal biophysical profile score: relationship of last BPS result to subsequent cerebral palsy. J Gynecol Obstet Biol Reprod 1997; 26:720–729.

69. Manning FA, Bondaji N, Harman CR, et al. Fetal assessment based on fetal biophysical profile scoring. VIII. The incidence of cerebral palsy in tested and untested perinates. Am J Obstet Gynecol 1998; 178:696–706.

70. Vintzileos AM, Fleming AD, Scorza WE, et al. Relationship between fetal biophysical activities and umbilical cord blood gas values. Am J Obstet Gynecol 1991; 165: 707–713.

71. Manning FA, Snijders R, Harman CR, Nicolaides K, Menticoglou S, Morrison I. Fetal biophysical profile score. VI. Correlation with antepartum umbilical venous fetal pH. Am J Obstet Gynecol 1993; 169:755–763.

72. Alfirevic Z, Neilson JP. Biophysical profile for fetal assessment in high risk pregnancies. Cochrane Database Syst Rev 2000; 2.

73. Manning FA, Lange IR, Morrison I, Harman CR. Fetal biophysical profile score and the nonstress test: a comparative trial. Obstet Gynecol 1984; 64:326–331.

74. Platt LD, Walla CA, Paul RH, et al. A prospective trial of the fetal biophysical profile versus the nonstress test in the management of high-risk pregnancies. Am J Obstet Gynecol 1985; 153:624–633.

75. Nageotte MP, Towers CV, Asrat T, Freeman RK. Perinatal outcome with the modified biophysical profile. Am J Obstet Gynecol 1994; 170:1672–1676.

76. Alfirevic Z, Walkinshaw SA. A randomised controlled trial of simple compared with complex antenatal fetal monitoring after 42 weeks of gestation. Br J Obstet Gynaecol 1995; 102:638–643.

77. Clark SL, Sabey P, Jolley K. Nonstress testing with acoustic stimulation and amniotic fluid volume assessment: 5973 tests without unexpected fetal death. Am J Obstet Gynecol 1989; 160:694–697.

78. Miller DA, Rabello YA, Paul RH. The modified biophysical profile: antepartum testing in the 1990s. Am J Obstet Gynecol 1996; 174:812–817.

79. Hon EH, Quilligan EJ. The classification of fetal heart rate. II. A revised working classification. Conn Med 1967; 31:779–784.

80. Evertson LR, Paul RH. Antepartum fetal heart rate testing: the nonstress test. Am J Obstet Gynecol 1978; 132:895–900.

81. Evertson LR, Gauthier RJ, Schifrin BS, Paul RH. Antepartum fetal heart rate testing. I. Evolution of the nonstress test. Am J Obstet Gynecol 1979; 133:29–33.

82. Bishop EH. Fetal acceleration test. Am J Obstet Gynecol 1981; 141:905–909.

83. Lavin JP Jr, Miodovnik M, Barden TP. Relationship of nonstress test reactivity and gestational age. Obstet Gynecol 1984; 63:338–344.

84. Druzin ML, Fox A, Kogut E, Carlson C. The relationship of the nonstress test to gestational age. Am J Obstet Gynecol 1985; 153:386–389.

85. Phelan JP. The nonstress test: a review of 3,000 tests. Am J Obstet Gynecol 1981; 139:7–10.

86. Freeman RK, Anderson G, Dorchester W. A prospective multi-institutional study of antepartum fetal heart rate monitoring. II. Contraction stress test versus nonstress test for primary surveillance. Am J Obstet Gynecol 1982; 143:778–781.

87. Pattison N, McCowan L. Cardiotocography for antepartum fetal assessment. Cochrane Database Syst Rev 2000; 2.

88. Brown VA, Sawers RS, Parsons RJ, Duncan SL, Cooke ID. The value of antenatal cardiotocography in the management of high-risk pregnancy: a randomized controlled trial. Br J Obstet Gynaecol 1982; 89:716–722.

89. Flynn AM, Kelly J, Mansfield H, Needham P, O'Conor M, Viegas O. A randomized

controlled trial of non-stress antepartum cardiotocography. Br J Obstet Gynaecol 1982; 89:427–433.

90. Lumley J, Lester A, Anderson I, Renou P, Wood C. A randomized trial of weekly cardiotocography in high-risk obstetric patients. Br J Obstet Gynaecol 1983; 90: 1018–1026.

91. Kidd LC, Patel NB, Smith R. Non-stress antenatal cardiotocography—a prospective randomized clinical trial. Br J Obstet Gynaecol 1985; 92:1156–1159.

92. Leader LR, Baillie P, Martin B, Molteno C, Wynchank S. Fetal responses to vibrotactile stimulation, a possible predictor of fetal and neonatal outcome. Aust NZ J Obstet Gynaecol 1984; 24:251–256.

93. Smith CV, Phelan JP, Paul RH, Broussard P. Fetal acoustic stimulation testing: a retrospective experience with the fetal acoustic stimulation test. Am J Obstet Gynecol 1985; 153:567–569.

94. Ingemarsson I, Arulkumaran S. Reactive fetal heart rate response to vibroacoustic stimulation in fetuses with low scalp blood pH. Br J Obstet Gynaecol 1989; 96: 562–565.

95. Bernard J, Sontag LW. Fetal reactivity to acoustic stimulation: a preliminary report. J Genet Psychol 1947; 70:205–210.

96. Clark SL, Gimovsky ML, Miller FC. Fetal heart rate response to scalp blood sampling. Am J Obstet Gynecol 1982; 144:706–708.

97. Clark SL, Gimovsky ML, Miller FC. The scalp stimulation test: a clinical alternative to fetal scalp blood sampling. Am J Obstet Gynecol 1984; 148:274–277.

98. Tan KH, Smyth R. Fetal vibroacoustic stimulation for facilitation of tests of fetal wellbeing (Cochrane Review). Cochrane Database Syst Rev 2001; 1.

99. Walters BN, Lao T, Smith V, De Swiet M. alpha-Fetoprotein elevation and proteinuric pre-eclampsia. Br J Obstet Gynaecol 1985; 92:341–344.

100. Waller DK, Lustig LS, Cunningham GC, Golbus MS, Hook EB. Second-trimester maternal serum alpha-fetoprotein levels and the risk of subsequent fetal death. N Engl J Med 1991; 325:6–10.

101. Brazerol WF, Grover S, Donnenfeld AE. Unexplained elevated maternal serum alpha-fetoprotein levels and perinatal outcome in an urban clinic population. Am J Obstet Gynecol 1994; 171:1030–1035.

102. Jauniaux E, Gulbis B, Tunkel S, Ramsay B, Campbell S, Meuris S. Maternal serum testing for alpha-fetoprotein and human chorionic gonadotropin in high-risk pregnancies. Prenat Diagn 1996; 16:1129–1135.

103. Shipp TD, Wilkins-Haug L. The association of early-onset fetal growth restriction, elevated maternal serum alpha-fetoprotein, and the development of severe preeclampsia. Prenat Diagn 1997; 17:305–309.

104. Yaron Y, Cherry M, Kramer RL, et al. Second-trimester maternal serum marker screening: maternal serum alpha-fetoprotein, beta-human chorionic gonadotropin, estriol, and their various combinations as predictors of pregnancy outcome. Am J Obstet Gynecol 1999; 181:968–974.

105. van Rijn M, van der Schouw YT, Hagenaars AM, Visser GH, Christiaens GC. Adverse obstetric outcome in low- and high-risk pregnancies: predictive value of maternal serum screening. Obstet Gynecol 1999; 94:929–934.

106. Huerta-Enochian G, Katz V, Erfurth S. The association of abnormal alpha-fetoprotein and adverse pregnancy outcome: does increased fetal surveillance affect pregnancy outcome? Am J Obstet Gynecol 2001; 184:1549–1553.

107. Dekker G, Sibai B. Primary, secondary, and tertiary prevention of pre-eclampsia. Lancet 2001; 357:209–215.

108. Pritchard JA, Cunningham FG, Pritchard SA. The Parkland Memorial Hospital protocol for treatment of eclampsia: evaluation of 245 cases. Am J Obstet Gynecol 1984; 148:951–963.

109. Piper JM, Langer O. Is lung maturation related to fetal growth in diabetic or hypertensive pregnancies? Eur J Obstet Gynecol Reprod Biol 1993; 51:15–19.

110. Piazze JJ, Maranghi L, Nigro G, Rizzo G, Cosmi EV, Anceschi MM. The effect of glucocorticoid therapy on fetal lung maturity indices in hypertensive pregnancies. Obstet Gynecol 1998; 92:220–225.

111. Chari RS, Friedman SA, Schiff E, Frangieh AT, Sibai BM. Is fetal neurologic and physical development accelerated in preeclampsia? Am J Obstet Gynecol 1996; 174:829–832.

112. Rouse DJ, Owen J, Goldenberg RL, Cliver SP. Determinants of the optimal time in gestation to initiate antenatal fetal testing: a decision-analytic approach. Am J Obstet Gynecol 1995; 173:1357–1363.

113. Pircon RA, Lagrew DC, Towers CV, Dorchester WL, Gocke SE, Freeman RK. Antepartum testing in the hypertensive patient: when to begin. Am J Obstet Gynecol 1991; 164:1563–1569.

114. Lagrew DC, Pircon RA, Towers CV, Dorchester W, Freeman RK. Antepartum fetal surveillance in patients with diabetes: when to start? Am J Obstet Gynecol 1993; 168:1820–1825.

115. ACOG Practice Bulletin. Chronic hypertension in pregnancy. ACOG Committee on Practice Bulletins. Obstet Gynecol 2001; 98 (suppl): 177–185.

116. Freeman RK. The use of the oxytocin challenge test for antepartum clinical evaluation of uteroplacental respiratory function. Am J Obstet Gynecol 1975; 121:481–489.

117. Sibai BM, Akl S, Fairlie F, Moretti M. A protocol for managing severe preeclampsia in the second trimester. Am J Obstet Gynecol 1990; 163:733–738.

118. Sibai BM, Mercer BM, Schiff E, Friedman SA. Aggressive versus expectant management of severe preeclampsia at 28 to 32 weeks' gestation: a randomized controlled trial. Am J Obstet Gynecol 1994; 171:818–822.

119. Chari RS, Friedman SA, O'Brien JM, Sibai BM. Daily antenatal testing in women with severe preeclampsia. Am J Obstet Gynecol 1995; 173:1207–1210.

120. Bryant RD, Fleming JG. Veratrum viride in the treatment of eclampsia: II. JAMA 1940; 115:1333–1339.

121. Bryant RD, Fleming JG. Veratrum viride in the treatment of eclampsia: III. Obstet Gynecol 1962; 19:372–383.

122. Zuspan FP. Treatment of severe preeclampsia and eclampsia. Clin Obstet Gynecol 1966; 9:954–972.

123. Harbert GM, Claiborne HA, McGaughey HS, Wilson LA, Thornton WN. Convulsive toxemia. Am J Obstet Gynecol 1968; 100:336–342.

124. Pritchard JA, Pritchard SA. Standardized treatment of 154 consecutive cases of eclampsia. Am J Obstet Gynecol 1975; 123:543–552.

125. Lopez-Llera M. Complicated eclampsia: fifteen years' experience in a referral medical center. Am J Obstet Gynecol 1982; 142:28–35.

126. Adetoro OO. A sixteen year survey of maternal mortality associated with eclampsia in Ilorin, Nigeria. Int J Gynaecol Obstet 1989; 30:117–121.

127. Sibai BM. Eclampsia. VI. Maternal-perinatal outcome in 254 consecutive cases. Am J Obstet Gynecol 1990; 163:1049–1054.

128. Douglas KA, Redman CW. Eclampsia in the United Kingdom. Br Med J 1994; 309: 1395–1400.

129. MacKenna J, Dover NL, Brame RG. Preeclampsia associated with hemolysis, elevated liver enzymes, and low platelets—an obstetric emergency? Obstet Gynecol 1983; 62:751–754.

130. Weinstein L. Preeclampsia/eclampsia with hemolysis, elevated liver enzymes, and thrombocytopenia. Obstet Gynecol 1985; 66:657–660.

131. Sibai BM, Taslimi MM, el-Nazer A, Amon E, Mabie BC, Ryan GM. Maternal-perinatal outcome associated with the syndrome of hemolysis, elevated liver enzymes, and low platelets in severe preeclampsia-eclampsia. Am J Obstet Gynecol 1986; 155:501–509.

132. Romero R, Vizoso J, Emamian M, et al. Clinical significance of liver dysfunction in pregnancy-induced hypertension. Am J Perinatol 1988; 5:146–151.

133. Manning FA, Morrison I, Harman CR, Lange IR, Menticoglou S. Fetal assessment based on fetal biophysical profile scoring: experience in 19,221 referred high-risk pregnancies. II. An analysis of false-negative fetal deaths. Am J Obstet Gynecol 1987; 157:880–884.

134. Almstrom H, Axelsson O, Cnattingius S, et al. Comparison of umbilical-artery velocimetry and cardiotocography for surveillance of small-for-gestational-age fetuses. Lancet 1992; 340:936–940.

135. Working Group Report on High Blood Pressure in Pregnancy. National Heart, Lung, and Blood Institute. NIH Publication No. 00-3029, July 2000.

11
Hepatic Hemorrhage and Rupture in Pregnancy

Garrett K. Lam and Kenneth J. Moise, Jr.
University of North Carolina, Chapel Hill, North Carolina, U.S.A.

I. INTRODUCTION

During pregnancy, women are vulnerable to a number of unique disease states. The inability of the body to tolerate these stresses leads to sequelae that may result in severe morbidity and, at times, mortality. This unfortunate chain of events is well illustrated by spontaneous subcapsular hepatic hemorrhage and rupture.

This chapter discusses the history and incidence of this uncommon, but potentially lethal phenomenon. The presentation and methods of diagnosis are reviewed. Because of the rarity of occurrence, no etiological explanation has been established. However, theories on the pathophysiological characteristics of this disease are presented. Finally, we suggest management strategies which are based on our previous experience with affected patients.

II. HISTORY

Abercrombie was the first to report hepatic rupture in pregnancy. His case report in 1844 was centered on a 35-year-old patient with a 2-month history of dyspepsia (1). Prior to delivery, the patient complained of intermittent epigastric pain, abdominal distention, and emesis that she had self-treated with tight abdominal binding. The patient proceeded to a vaginal breech delivery without complication, but symptoms of shock quickly developed despite a firm uterus and normal lochia. She was suspected of having intra-abdominal hemorrhage and, despite administration of stimulants, died 3 days later. An autopsy revealed a large hematoma on the superior and anterior surface of the liver, containing approximately "2 pounds of blood." Abercrombie reasoned that hepatic rupture might have resulted from either the external trauma of the patient's abdominal binding or the trauma associated with labor.

Since Abercrombie's original description, approximately 126 additional cases have been reported in the literature. These are reported singly, or in small series (2). Henny and colleagues (3) published an article in 1983 that presented conclusions drawn from case studies of the 75 patients documented in the literature up to that point. However, to date, no comprehensive review has been done to analyze the treatments and outcome of all known affected patients.

III. INCIDENCE

Hepatic hemorrhage with rupture is a rare complication in pregnancy. Estimates of incidence range from 1/45,000 live births to 1/250,000 live births. (4,5) At present, our medical understanding of this disease state is based mainly on case reports.

IV. PATHOPHYSIOLOGY

A review of the literature on hepatic hemorrhage and rupture has identified a number of findings that are common to the disease. Typically, most hematomas involve the right lobe of the liver. In Henny's series, hematomas were found in the right lobe in 75% (3), the left lobe in 11%, and both lobes in 14% of cases. Usually, the anterior and superior areas of the lobes were affected. Microscopic examination of liver biopsy specimens commonly shows areas of acute necrosis, primarily in the portal areas. In many patients disseminated intravascular coagulopathy (DIC), which is associated with widespread fibrin deposition in the hepatic sinusoids and periportal capillaries, develops.

A specific chain of events that explains the development of this disease process has not been delineated. Two models have been proposed to explain the formation and evolution. The first may be described as the "outside-in" theory. In this theory, hepatic rupture is directly caused by an external insult, such as trauma, which results in tissue injury and bleeding. Tissue ischemia results from a steady blood loss, which progresses to local areas of tissue necrosis and subsequently to more hemorrhage. Various case reports have listed the causes for trauma, ranging from significant blunt trauma to simple actions such as transporting the patient to the hospital, moving the patient from the bed to the delivery table, palpating the abdomen, or manually expressing blood clots from the uterus (3).

The second model describes a process that can be characterized as the "inside-out" theory. This model proposes that hemorrhage and rupture stem from an inherent disease process involving the hepatic parenchyma. Specifically, conditions that cause vascular injury or vasospasm (such as the severe hypertension of preeclampsia) or widespread consumption of clotting factors lead to local areas of tissue ischemia. Hemorrhage can result from the sloughing of ischemic, infarcted tissue, or from failure of normal coagulation caused by the excessive consumption of clotting factors. Either way, hepatic rupture ensues as a result of a continuous buildup of pressure from the enlarging hemorrhage under Glisson's capsule.

Pathological analysis of tissue from affected patients has provided evidence to support this second hypothesis. Greenstein and associates (6) found microscopic pseudoaneurysms in a patient with HELLP syndrome (hemolysis, elevated liver enzyme levels, low platelet count) who had recurrent hepatic hemorrhage during pregnancy. His findings support the idea that microscopic angiopathy, in this case from preeclampsia, can lead to hepatic hemorrhage. There is also a clinical report of hepatic hemorrhage and rupture in a patient who used cocaine during pregnancy; that finding suggests that intense vascular spasm can lead to ischemia, organ damage, and subsequent hemorrhage (7).

V. PRESENTATION

Review of the reported cases helps in developing a composite picture of the at-risk patient. Most case reports describe affected women in their late 20s to early 30s (range 21–43 years). Multiparous women are more often affected than primiparous patients; some authors report a 10-fold increase in risk among multiparas (6). However, the most common predisposing condition appears to be preeclampsia: an estimated 80% of the described cases of hepatic hemorrhage and rupture are associated with this disease. Conversely, 1 to 2% of all pre-eclamptic patients are affected (5,8). Those in whom HELLP syndrome develops (4 to 12% of preeclamptic patients) appear to have a worse outcome and are more refractory to treatment for hepatic hemorrhage and rupture (9,10). Other conditions associated with hepatic hemorrhage and rupture include hepatic neoplasms (i.e., hemangiomas, adenomas, and carcinomas), vascular anomalies, biliary tract disease, viral infections, and hepatic abscess. Rare case reports have been published in which malaria, syphilis, amoebic hepatitis, and acute fatty liver have been cited as causes of subcapsular hepatic hemorrhage and rupture during pregnancy.

Unfortunately the clinical presentation of intrahepatic hemorrhage and rupture is nonspecific. Therefore, the key to making the diagnosis is maintaining a high degree of suspicion. Most patients seek medical attention in the third trimester (after 26 weeks), although approximately 20% do so in the initial 48 hours post partum. There have been a few cases diagnosed as early as 18 weeks of gestation, as in a case of hemorrhage caused by a liver hemangioma (11), or as late as 12 days post partum (3).

Patients often present similar lists of symptoms. Henny (3) described a biphasic clinical presentation, with an early, latent phase, followed by a later, acute phase. The initial phase, which can occur up to 1 month before hepatic rupture, consists of vague complaints of right upper quadrant or epigastric pain, at times associated with headache (12). Often the patient has associated nausea and vomiting, leading to a false diagnosis of gastritis, gastric reflux, or cholecystitis. However, the severity of these symptoms progresses as the duration and intensity of the pain increase and relief is not obtained with antacids.

The second, or acute, phase occurs when Glisson's capsule ruptures. At this point, the pain becomes focused in the right upper quadrant and can radiate to the right shoulder and back. On physical examination, peritoneal signs are seen in addition to abdominal tenderness and distention. The patient's condition quickly becomes unstable, with hypotension and shock from acute blood loss and peripheral vascular collapse. Ascites and a right-sided pleural effusion that results in respiratory difficulties may develop, and if delivery is not soon effected, death of the fetus quickly follows (9).

VI. DIAGNOSIS

Early clinical diagnosis is vital for patient outcome. Those who have progressed to hepatic rupture with current or imminent hemodynamic instability require emergency laparotomy. Given the emergent nature of this problem, information that can help identify those patients at special risk would be of immense benefit. Since there are few reliable diagnostic symptoms or signs, it is important to consider the problem when a patient exhibits the clinical findings mentioned. Along with a high level of suspicion, some clinical and laboratory studies may aid diagnosis.

Serial hematocrit and platelet counts are vital for management. Manas and colleagues (2), in their series of seven patients, described an average reduction in hematocrit of 10.8% in the first few hours after the onset of abdominal pain. A peripheral blood smear is helpful since microangiopathic hemolytic anemia, coincident with a platelet count of less than 50,000/mm^3, may be indicative of worsening condition. Interestingly, various studies have shown that liver function test results may exhibit nonspecific changes and are not always significantly elevated. Smith and associates (4) described a series of seven cases, in which three patients had serum aspartate aminotransferase levels between 42 and 99 IU/L.

Imaging techniques such as computed tomography (CT), ultrasonography, and magnetic resonance imaging (MRI) are frequently very useful if there is sufficient time to carry them out. According to recent opinions, CT with contrast may be the most practical because of its almost universal availability in most developed countries and the relative simplicity of the technique (Figure 1). Com-

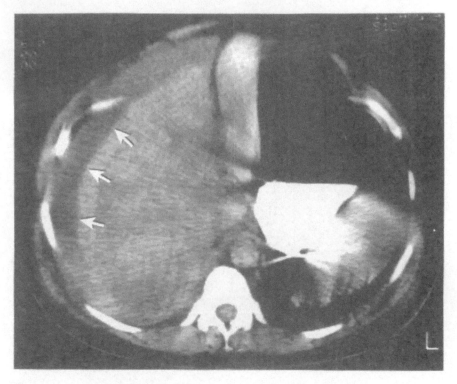

Figure 1 Computed tomography (CT) scan showing hemoperitoneum (arrow) from rupture of the right hepatic lobe.

puted tomography is also extremely sensitive in the detection of acute hemorrhage and allows visualization of the surrounding organs.

MRI has the advantage of not exposing the fetus to radiation. In addition blood collections distinct from nonspecific peritoneal fluid can be clearly identified. However, access, expense, time requirements, and the technical demands of the procedure make it a less common choice.

Ultrasound has also been used for diagnosis. A major advantage is that the machine is portable, allowing bedside diagnosis if the patient's condition is unstable. The major diagnostic sonographic finding of a subcapsular hematoma is an echolucent area near the surface of the liver (see Figure 2). A large fluid collection in the maternal right upper quadrant between the liver and the uterine fundus has also been described as a sign of hepatic rupture (7). Such a finding can, however, be confused with peritoneal bleeding from other intra-abdominal

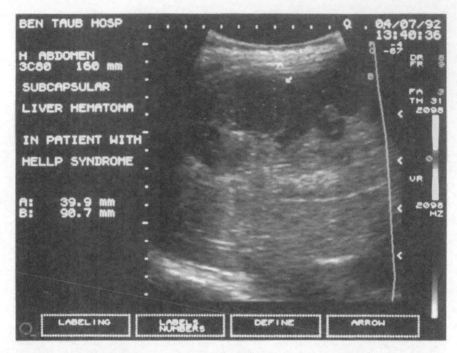

Figure 2 Ultrasound demonstrating hemoperitoneum from hepatic rupture (see arrow).

sources such as a ruptured uterus. This may be circumvented by CT, which enables most of the abdomen to be imaged simultaneously, allowing an overall survey of the abdomen and pelvis.

Other diagnostic tests that have proved useful include peritoneal lavage and selective angiography. Herbert and Brenner (13) noted that the diagnostic accuracy of lavage is greater than 95% with less than a 0.5% complication rate. These authors suggest that culdocentesis is equally reliable and that positive findings should result in laparotomy.

Angiography has been used to identify specific sites of hemorrhage in the hepatic vasculature (see Figure 3). The advantage is that bleeding sites can be directly identified and accessed for embolization. Loevinger (14) was one of the earliest to report the use of angiography to confirm hepatic rupture, which was then treated by transcatheter embolization of the hepatic artery. Graham and coworkers (11) also reported the use of angiography to diagnose hepatic hemorrhage in a patient with a cavernous hemangioma at 18 weeks gestation. Embolization of the bleeding point was successfully undertaken, and the patient survived without complication.

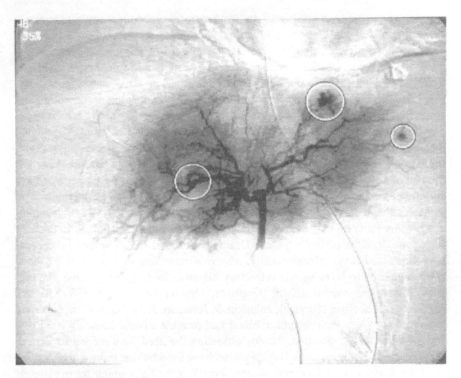

Figure 3 Angiogram showing areas of focal hemorrhage from the vascular branches of the left and right hepatic arteries (see circled areas).

VII. MANAGEMENT

The general approach to treating acute hepatic hemorrhage and rupture in pregnancy has changed over time as more cases have been documented in the literature. A review of the early case reports reveals that such events were regarded as highly refractory to treatment, and most cases had a poor outcome. Some of the inherent characteristics of the hepatic vasculature may contribute to the high complication rates. Specifically, hepatic blood vessels do not contain valves and are thin-walled. After interruption of their integrity they do not efficiently retract into the surrounding parenchyma nor contract to improve hemostasis. Thus, a hepatic hematoma may result in major blood loss. Given the liver's inability to self-regulate hemostasis, surgical ligation of the arteries supplying the bleeding area was initially thought to be the optimal treatment.

Dodson and O'Leary (15) published one of the first case reports with a successful outcome. They recommended laparotomy though a large midline incision to expose the liver adequately to ligate specific bleeding points and oversew raw areas of rupture. They also suggested abdominal delivery of the fetus since most of these patients also had preeclampsia, a major etiological factor in the pathophysiological features of the rupture. The risk of rapid maternal hemodynamic decompensation with consequent fetal loss also mandates delivery.

Subsequent authors have reinforced the need for surgical intervention and emphasized the importance of packing laparotomy sponges around the liver to put pressure on the bleeding surface and to further tamponade bleeding. Continued bleeding may increase tension on Glisson's capsule, eventually causing rupture; the latter significantly worsens the prognosis (3). The earlier literature describes the use of a number of tissues, including omentum, fat, and muscle; and of oxycellulose and laparotomy sponges to affect hemostasis (13). The literature also supports liberal drainage of the hepatic bed with Penrose drains (rather than cholecystostomy tubes and T-tubes) to prevent the reaccumulation of blood in the area of rupture or in the pericolic gutters. Drainage of blood should reduce postoperative sepsis and fever. More recently, new materials and surgical methods have been suggested to be helpful in refractory hepatic bleeding. Hemostatic material such as purified animal gelatin (Gelfoam, Upjohn Co., Kalamazoo, MI) and regenerated cellulose (Surgicel, Johnson & Johnson, New Brunswick, NJ) may absorb many times their weight in blood and provide a basic framework for clot formation. Both are resorbed, thereby obviating the need for a second surgery to remove the packing material. Other authors have used bovine thrombin or bovine microfibrillar collagen (Avitene, Alcon, Fort Worth, TX), which traps platelets within a molecular meshwork, allowing clot formation and hemostasis (13).

Many of the operative techniques described are based on methods used for traumatic liver rupture. The Pringle maneuver may improve visualization in cases complicated by heavy bleeding. In this maneuver, the surgeon grasps the hepatic artery and portal vein as they course under the liver, thus occluding blood flow to the organ. Compression for 15–20 minutes allows a reduction in blood loss without significant ischemic damage to the hepatic parenchyma (4).

Hepatic lobectomy or partial resection has been proposed for the treatment of hepatic hemorrhage and rupture. Though each is effective, there is a high risk of ischemic necrosis of the gallbladder and the remaining hepatic parenchyma. These can occur because control of bleeding in the commonly affected right lobe of the liver necessitates ligation of the right hepatic artery. Some surgeons who use this method routinely include cholecystectomy in an attempt to prevent postoperative complications that result from ischemia (16). Because of the continued advances in surgical technique and the excellent reparative properties of the liver, partial or lobular resection is no longer regarded as an appropriate first line therapy. Of 1000 patients with traumatic liver injury treated at Ben Taub General Hospital in Houston, those who underwent lobectomy, with selective vascular ligation, had a mortality rate of 33.6%, compared to 7.6% in those who had conservative surgical therapy (hepatic packing/drainage and hemostatic agents) (17). Hepatic rupture in pregnancy is less common, but Smith and colleagues (4) have reported 7 cases, and 23 others have been reported since 1976. A significantly improved survival rate is reported from packing and drainage compared with lobectomy (82% vs. 25%).

The review by Smith and colleagues (4) illustrates the advances that allow effective treatment of hepatic hemorrhage and rupture with more conservative methods. Recent literature supports this assertion. Manas and associates (2) reported on seven patients with preeclampsia in whom subcapsular hematomas developed. Two were diagnosed post partum. All were monitored with computerized tomography and were treated with fluid and blood product resuscitation in addition to abdominal delivery. All seven survived without hepatic rupture, and five of the seven infants survived. In a 1989 review by Neerhof and coworkers (18) two patients survived without surgical treatment, two had leaking subcapsular hematomas, and another had a ruptured liver. All survived with intensive medical treatment. Nevertheless, this approach should only be considered in the appropriate circumstances.

Loevinger and colleagues (14) reported the first case of hepatic rupture in pregnancy (confirmed by CT) that was successfully treated with transcatheter embolization of the hepatic artery. The patient had a decreasing platelet and hematocrit count associated with elevated liver enzymes. Hemoperitoneum was confirmed by peritoneal lavage. A CT scan and celiac angiogram showed bleeding from the right lobar intrahepatic arteries. The patient had pledgets (Gelfoam) directly injected into the common hepatic artery through a vascular catheter, resulting in rapid stabilization. A second case (11) was reported in 1993. The patient was found to have a hemangioma in the left lobe of the liver, which bled at 18 weeks gestation. She had selective embolization of the left hepatic artery with a good result and was delivered at term by cesarean section without any complications.

Clearly there is evidence, though limited, that less invasive therapy can be effective in the management of patients with hepatic hemorrhage. On the basis of our literature review and cumulative experience, we recommend the following approach to hepatic hemorrhage and rupture in pregnancy (see Figure 4). The diagnosis must be considered particularly in older multiparous women with preeclampsia and right upper quadrant pain. If her condition is hemodynamically stable, the patient should have a CT or MRI scan. Appropriate arrangements should be made with radiology, surgical, and anesthetic services to manage any emergency during or after the investigation. If such imaging is not available, ultrasound or peritoneal lavage may be useful to determine whether there is a hemoperitoneum or an unruptured hepatic hematoma. A negative ultrasound examination finding does not exclude hepatic hematoma or hemorrhage, since small bleeds may not be seen, and rupture without subcapsular hemorrhage may be difficult to diagnose.

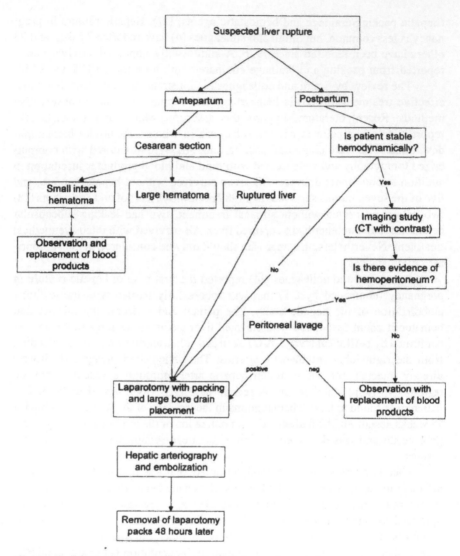

Figure 4   Management algorithm of hepatic hemorrhage and rupture in pregnancy.

In those antepartum patients in whom a diagnosis of liver hematoma is made, cesarean section using a midline incision should be undertaken. The liver should be visualized (usually by elevation of the anterior abdominal wall) and evidence of active bleeding sought. If a small hematoma is found with Glisson's capsule intact, the patient may be observed and treated medically. If an extensive (or obviously enlarging) hematoma, or overt rupture, is found, visualization needs to be optimized, usually by extension of the incision. The liver capsule should be opened and the hematoma gently evacuated. The liver should be packed with multiple laparotomy sponges placed above and below the involved lobe. Large-diameter closed drains should be placed in the right paracolic gutter and above the right lobe of the liver. Drains such as the Duvall system (Bard, Cranston, RI) can be used and connected to continuous low-pressure suction. We have also used standard chest tubes (oversewn with a latex drain to prevent adhesion to omentum or bowel) (see Figure 5). Smaller-caliber drains such as the Hemovac (Snyder Labs, Dover, OH) or Jackson-Pratt (Bard, Cranston, RI) systems are not appropriate as they readily become obstructed. Additional hemostasis can be achieved with topical hemostatic agents, such as Avitene or Gelfoam, placed under the lapatotomy packs on the raw hepatic surface. The abdominal wall is closed with towel clips if the abdomen requires reopening within 48 hours to remove packs. As the most common cause of death is uncontrollable hemorrhage, we recommend that

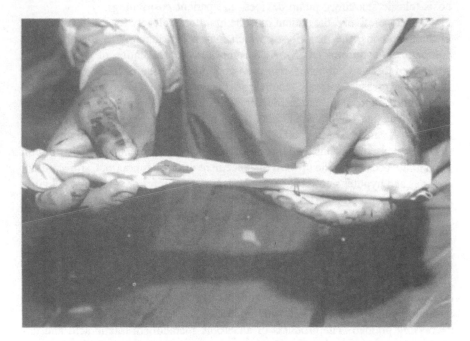

Figure 5 Example of a system to provide continuous drainage of the abdomen. A large-caliber chest tube is covered by a Penrose drain, in which large holes have been cut. The drain is sutured to the chest tube. The latex drain prevents aspiration of omentum into the tube. This system allows continuous drainage of large amounts of blood that can accumulate in the abdomen, without obstruction by large clots.

the patient be taken from the operating suite to interventional radiology for hepatic arteriography and selective embolization of the involved hepatic artery. The laparotomy packs are removed approximately 48 hours later via a second laparotomy procedure.

The intraoperative anesthetic management of such cases is extremely important and is vital to the success of the surgical procedure. Adequate large-bore intravenous (IV) lines and invasive monitoring catheters are essential where there has been massive blood loss. Appropriate and preemptive replacement of blood and coagulation products significantly improves the outcome. An established coagulopathy is very difficult to reverse, and all efforts should be directed to prevent dilutional and/or disseminated intravascular coagulation. To this end the patient's body temperature should be kept within normal limits and hypothermia prevented. This may require warming devices for the patient and for fluid delivery systems, use of warmed rinse fluids, and maintenance of the operating room temperature at a higher level than usual. Other anesthetic issues are the administration of intraoperative antibiotics and measures to prevent deep venous thrombosis (elastic stockings, pump devices, and patient positioning).

Postoperatively, the patient must be monitored closely for the development of complications, the majority of which may be attributable to the abdominal compartment syndrome (ACS). ACS comprises a constellation of problems that are related to a sudden increase in intra-abdominal pressure. In the case of liver rupture, the pressure increase results from the presence of a large amount of blood in the abdomen from the damaged liver (see Figure 6). As more and more pressure is placed on the abdominal organs, their perfusion is reduced, and ischemia develops. A variety of signs and symptoms are noted as a result of the involvement of different organ systems. Patients become hypercarbic and increasingly difficult to ventilate because of the upward displacement of the diaphragm. Cardiac output declines and hypotension results from collapse of the inferior vena cava. Oliguria results as renal artery perfusion is compromised, and ureteral and renal venous outflow are obstructed. An increase in intracranial pressure may also occur. Thus, for a patient with a concomitant head injury (i.e., hemorrhagic stroke from eclamptic seizure or HELLP), there is a profound risk of permanent central nervous system (CNS) damage (19,20).

Treatment of ACS consists primarily of abdominal decompression via celiotomy. However, surgical intervention carries a considerable risk. When the intra-abdominal pressure is suddenly released, the abdominopelvic veins expand, decreasing preload. The products of anaerobic metabolism (lactic acid and potassium from cell destruction) are released into the circulation. Reduced pressure on the diaphragm causes a precipitous increase in the patient's tidal volume, which results in respiratory alkalosis. Together, these sequelae, dubbed the "reperfusion syndrome," can be fatal. Eddy and colleagues (19) reported that in 12% of 34 patients in their series, asystole developed after surgical treatment. Clearly, pre-

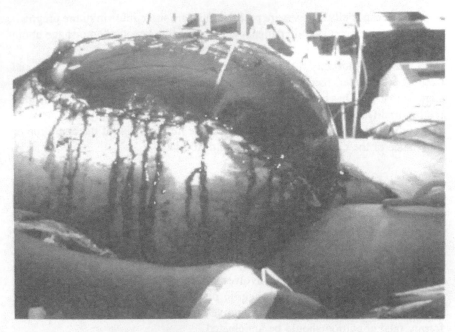

Figure 6 Abdominal compartment syndrome caused by the accumulation of a large amount of blood in the abdomen. The plastic sutured to the fascial edges is a Bogota bag made from a sterile urology irrigation bag.

vention of the increase in intra-abdominal pressure is vital to the management of patients with hepatic rupture. This necessity further underscores the importance of ensuring good drainage of the abdomen.

VIII. RECURRENCE

There has only been one published case of a patient who experienced recurrent intrahepatic hemorrhage. Greenstein and colleagues (6) described a preeclamptic patient in whom a hepatic hematoma developed at term during her second pregnancy. She was treated conservatively without further surgical therapy. In the postpartum period of her next pregnancy, the patient was noted to have active hemorrhage from numerous pseudoaneurysms of the left hepatic lobe. Her condition did not stabilize with replacement of blood products and embolization of the left hepatic artery. Surgical treatment was effective and she made a full recovery. Given that this is the only reported case, the risk of recurrence cannot be estimated. However, this case suggests that patients previously affected by hepatic hematoma, especially if they were preeclamptic, are susceptible in future pregnancies. We advise preeclamptic patients who have had a hepatic hemorrhage about the risk and observe them carefully during any future pregnancy.

Maternal mortality rate was previously estimated to be between 59% and 62% (21); however, recent estimates incorporating data from the last 20 years suggest that there has been a decrease to 33 to 49% (9). It is interesting to note that fetal mortality rate has remained relatively constant at 60% despite the improvement in maternal outcome. This may reflect the inherent risk of the condition or reluctance of the clinician to intervene until too late.

IX. CONCLUSIONS

Overall, although the literature on hepatic hemorrhage and rupture consists mainly of case reports, there is a clear trend toward improved survival rate with less invasive, conservative therapy. The algorithm described in this chapter is based on a multidisciplinary approach that involves a variety of exploratory techniques and imaging modalities, all of which help to preclude the need for radical surgical therapy. With careful management improved outcomes of what was once a uniformly fatal condition should be anticipated.

REFERENCES

1. Abercrombie J. Hemorrhage of the liver. London Med Gazette 1844; 34:792–794.
2. Manas KJ, Welsh JD, Rankin RA, Miller DD. Hepatic hemorrhage without rupture in preeclampsia. N Engl J Med 1985; 312:424–426.
3. Henny CP, Lim AE, Brummelkamp WH, Buller HR, Ten Cate JW. A review of the importance of acute multidisciplinary treatment following spontaneous rupture of the liver capsule during pregnancy. Surg Gynecol Obstet 1983; 156:593–598.
4. Smith LG Jr, Moise KJ Jr, Dildy GAD, Carpenter RJ Jr. Spontaneous rupture of liver during pregnancy: current therapy. Obstet Gynecol 1991; 77:171–175.
5. Westergaard L. Spontaneous rupture of the liver in pregnancy. Acta Obstet Gynaecol Scand 1980; 59:559–561.
6. Greenstein D, Henderson JM, Boyer TD. Liver hemorrhage: recurrent episodes during pregnancy complicated by preeclampsia. Gastroenterology 1994; 106:1668–1671.
7. Moen MD, Caliendo MJ, Marshall W, Uhler ML. Hepatic rupture in pregnancy associated with cocaine use. Obstet Gynecol 1993; 82:687–689.
8. Rolfes DB, Ishak KG. Liver disease in pregnancy. Histopathology 1986; 10:555–570.
9. Sheikh RA, Yasmeen S, Pauly MP, Riegler JL. Spontaneous intrahepatic hemorrhage and hepatic rupture in the HELLP syndrome: four cases and a review. J Clin Gastroenterol 1999; 28:323–328.

10. Wilson RH, Marshall BM. Postpartum rupture of a subcapsular hematoma of the liver. Acta Obstet Gynaecol Scand 1992;71:394-397.

11. Graham E, Cohen AW, Soulen M, Faye R. Symptomatic liver hemangioma with intratumor hemorrhage treated by angiography and embolization during pregnancy. Obstet Gynecol 1993; 81:813–816.

12. Stevenson JT, Graham DJ. Hepatic hemorrhage and the HELLP syndrome: a surgeon's perspective. Am Surg 1995; 61:756–760.

13. Herbert WN, Brenner WE. Improving survival with liver rupture complicating pregnancy. Am J Obstet Gynecol 1982; 142:530–534.

14. Loevinger EH, Vujic I, Lee WM, Anderson MC. Hepatic rupture associated with pregnancy: treatment with transcatheter embolotherapy. Obstet Gynecol 1985; 65: 281–284.

15. Dodson MG, O'Leary JA. Hepatic rupture during pregnancy. Obstet Gynecol 1969; 33:827–829.

16. Lucas CE, Ledgerwood AM. Prospective evaluation of hemostatic techniques for liver injuries. J Trauma 1976; 16:442–451.

17. Feliciano DV, Mattox KL, Jordan GL Jr, Burch JM, Bitondo CG, Cruse PA. Management of 1000 consecutive cases of hepatic trauma (1979–1984). Ann Surg 1986; 204: 438–445.

18. Neerhof MG, Zelman W, Sullivan T. Hepatic rupture in pregnancy. Obstet Gynecol Surv 1989; 44:407–409.

19. Eddy V, Nunn C, Morris JA Jr. Abdominal compartment syndrome: the Nashville experience. Surg Clin North Am 1997; 77:801–812.

20. Sugerman HJ, Bloomfield GL, Saggi BW. Multisystem organ failure secondary to increased intraabdominal pressure. Infection 1999; 27:61–66.

21. Bis KA, Waxman B. Rupture of the liver associated with pregnancy: a review of the literature and report of 2 cases. Obstet Gynecol Surv 1976; 31:763–773.

12

Intensive Care of the Patient with Complicated Preeclampsia

John Anthony and Rosie Burton
University of Cape Town, Cape Town, South Africa

Preeclampsia affects 2 to 6% of pregnant women. It is amongst the leading causes of maternal mortality in industrialized nations, whereas in developing countries it is the single most common obstetrical cause of death (1–5). Confidential inquiries have shown that substandard care contributed to 80% of deaths in both industrialized and developing parts of the world, and expert opinion holds that many deaths were potentially preventable (6–8). This is justification enough to make knowledge and training in obstetrical critical care prerequisites of any health service or training program.

I. THE CLINICAL SYNDROME

Preeclampsia is a reversible clinical syndrome characterized by sustained hypertension (diastolic pressure in excess of 90 mmHg) and proteinuria (more than 300 mg excreted per 24 hours) during the latter half of pregnancy. Delivery of the fetus always results in remission of the clinical syndrome (9).

The features that define preeclampsia may be the only manifestations of the disease. In some women, however, the disease may develop into a syndrome of multiorgan failure (including neurological, renal, hepatic, hematological, cardiorespiratory, and fetoplacental abnormalities). Seizure activity and renal failure may be the predominant clinical features, although the cardinal signs of preeclampsia (hypertension and proteinuria) are invariably also present.

Maternal mortality reports attribute preeclamptic deaths to all forms of organ failure. Eclampsia (with or without intracranial hemorrhage) remains the single most lethal complication.

II. PATHOPHYSIOLOGY OF SEVERE PREECLAMPSIA

This chapter does not provide an exhaustive review of the pathogenesis of preeclampsia. Certain concepts are highlighted because they may be important in understanding, managing, and counseling the critically ill woman and her family.

Preeclampsia is a condition of genetic predisposition; it is more common among women whose mother or siblings had eclampsia (10–13). Paternal antigen exposure is also relevant, and immunological mechanisms are implicated to the extent that preeclampsia may be construed as a disease of primipaternity rather than primigravidity (14) (see Chapter 3). Those in whom preeclampsia develops follow a hierarchical pathophysiological pattern. The earliest anatomical changes occur in the blood vessels of the placental bed. These vessels normally dilate after the sixteenth week of pregnancy in association with the second wave of trophoblast invasion. In preeclamptic women, these changes are partially or completely absent. In addition, other forms of vascular abnormality, typically the lesion of acute atherosis, develop (15,16). Acute atherosis is analogous to atherosclerosis and gives rise to partial luminal obstruction of the artery by lipid-laden myointimal cells. This abnormality defines the vascular basis of placental insufficiency characteristic of preeclampsia.

The hypertension that subsequently develops probably reflects a hyperdynamic circulation, evolving into the typical pattern of severe preeclampsia characterized by increasing vasospasm, intravascular dehydration, and a low cardiac output. There is abundant evidence that endothelial perturbation and altered vascular reactivity precede and accompany these clinical events (17–21). Immunological changes may play a pivotal role in severe disease. Markers of granulocyte activation are common in preeclampsia and may contribute to the endothelial damage in fulminant preeclampsia. Endothelial perturbation may contribute to impaired prostacylin production with augmented release of a host of vasoconstrictors (including platelet-derived thromboxane, endothelin, and serotonin) (17–21). Endothelial expression of cell adhesion molecules provides for interaction between activated leukocytes and platelets (22–25). Consequently, platelet turnover increases and may result in overt thrombocytopenia. Both the endothelium and activated platelets release a range of cytokines that mediate intravascular coagulation, manifested as increasing levels of circulating thrombin-antithrombin III complexes, falling antithrombin III levels, and increased levels of fibrin degradation products (26,27).

Initially there may be no apparent clinical disease in women with preeclampsia. The clinical syndrome usually evolves from uncomplicated proteinuric hypertension progressing slowly or rapidly to a syndrome of fulminant disease characterized by multiorgan failure. The most consistent anatomical pathological condition in women who die of severe preeclampsia is widespread ischemia. Postmortem studies reveal evidence of vascular injury (commonly fibrinoid necrosis), hemorrhage, and ischemic necrosis in the liver, brain, kidney, and placenta (28–33).

Widespread vascular injury is associated with the development of interstitial edema leading to intravascular dehydration, intensified peripheral vasospasm, and diminished cardiac output. Global hemodynamic changes associated with a low cardiac output result in a critically low rate of oxygen delivery to the peripheral tissues that further aggravates diminished perfusion through the damaged vasculature (34–37).

III. ORGAN FAILURE IN SEVERE PREECLAMPSIA

Maternal mortality reports highlight eclampsia, pulmonary complications, hemolysis, elevated liver enzyme levels, low platelet count (HELLP) syndrome, and renal failure as the leading causes of death (7,8).

A. Eclampsia

1. Pathophysiology

Because eclampsia is the event most likely to result in the death of the women with complicated preeclampsia, it is important to review the pathophysiologic characteristics, clinical presentation, and management in detail.

The anatomical pathological features of eclampsia include a swollen, pale brain with evidence of petechial hemorrhage into the cortex, meninges, and white matter (29,30). Histological evaluation confirms ring hemorrhage around small vessels, fibrinoid necrosis of arteriolar vessel walls, as well as microhemorrhages and infarcts. These findings are consistent with ischemic damage to neuronal tissue and vessel walls (29).

Further information regarding pathogenesis may be gained from radiological investigation: computed tomography and magnetic resonance imaging (MRI) reveal a range of abnormalities that commonly include cerebral edema and occasionally show development of large hematomata or intraventricular hemorrhage (38–42). Cerebral edema typically affects the occipital lobes and the white matter but may occur in a "watershed" pattern. The latter picture represents the development of edema between the distribution territories of the major vessels supplying blood to the brain.

It is debated whether eclamptic abnormality is different from hypertensive encephalopathy in nonpregnant patients (29). In the latter condition, the development of severe systemic hypertension exceeds the capacity of the cerebral vasculature to autoregulate flow. This results in high flow rates and barotrauma to the vessel walls. The alternative view is that preeclamptic vasospasm alone may give rise to ischemic change.

The evidence favoring flow-related or vasogenic edema is based on several observations. The most commonly observed changes occur in the posterior vertebro-basilar circulation, which has less sympathetic innervation and a lower autoregulatory blood pressure threshold (29,43). Single-photon emission computed tomography (SPECT) and other studies have shown increased cerebral blood flow in eclamptic compared to preeclamptic patients (41,44,45). One publication establishes a positive correlation between cerebral blood flow and mean arterial pressure although the majority of these patients have systemic mean arterial blood pressure of less than 150 mmHg (45). The authors conclude that the increased flow results from loss of normal endothelial homeostatic function rather than severe systemic hypertension that exceeds the normal upper limit of cerebral autoregulation.

By contrast, Morriss and colleagues could find no evidence of either vasospasm or increased flow in a group of patients subject to phase-contrast MRI examination although all eight of the eclamptic patients in this group had abnormal T2-weighted brain imaging findings (46). Although these authors questioned the role of vasospasm, they also acknowledged that all patients investigated had been treated with magnesium sulfate. Sibai and others point out that as many as 20% of women have seizure activity when their diastolic blood pressure is below 90 mmHg (47). Blood pressure as low as this would render failure of the cerebral vascular autoregulatory function unlikely. Older angiographic studies as well as the newer techniques of magnetic resonance imaging angiography demonstrate vasospasm of the large and medium-sized cerebral arteries (41,48–50). However, more recent Doppler ultrasound studies document increased flow rather than vasospasm (51). The only exception are reports showing that the ophthalmic vessels and central retinal vessels exhibit increased pulsatility indices that decrease after the administration of vasodilators (52,53). Combined transcranial ultrasonography and MRI angiography has documented resolving postpartum vasospasm after eclampsia in an individual case report (54). There are now data available that suggest that cerebral perfusion pressure (CPP) is increased in severe preeclampsia and that abnormal cerebral autoregulation may lead to an overperfusion state. It appears that in most preeclamptic women, the increased CPP does not result in an overperfusion state since it is controlled by cerebral autoregulation. In some cases, however, overperfusion may result from a failure of autoregulation and an uncontrolled increase in cerebral blood flow. In these rare cases it is assumed that overperfusion leads to vessel barotrauma, vasogenic edema, and possibly recalcitrant vasospasm (125,126).

Certain caveats apply to all the published studies. These include the notion that vasospasm may only affect the cerebral microcirculation and may not be susceptible to investigation by transcranial imaging (45). The influence of drugs such as magnesium sulfate and dihydralazine may also confound the results of many studies. The use of dihydralazine is of particular concern because of evidence that it may diminish cerebral autoregulation and has been associated with increasing intracranial pressure when administered to nonpregnant neurosurgical patients with elevated intracranial pressure (55,56).

In summary, the evidence of endothelial dysfunction in preeclampsia/eclampsia is compelling and both microcirculatory vasospasm as well as diminished autoregulation of cerebral blood flow are probably implicated in eclamptic seizures. In the future, it may be possible to delineate different groups of patients with predominant vasogenic or cytotoxic edema; this distinction may influence management significantly (43).

2. Clinical Presentation

Eclampsia is the occurrence of generalized tonic-clonic epileptiform seizures in a pregnant patient with proteinuric hypertension. Most seizures occur antenatally, although 40% of those who experience convulsions do so within 24 hours of delivery. *Late postpartum eclampsia* which has also been described, is defined as the occurrence of seizure activity between 48 hours and 4 weeks after delivery (57–59). Eclampsia may be preceded by prodromal symptoms ("imminent" eclampsia), which consist of headaches and visual disturbances (blurred vision, photopsia, scotomata, and diplopia) (29,49,60,61).

The blood pressure at the time of seizure activity varies. Pregnant women may have convulsions with a blood pressure that is mildly elevated (or even normal), although they more commonly have moderate to severe hypertension (53). The seizure itself is associated with a surge in blood pressure and a fall in peripheral oxygen saturation during the tonic-clonic phase. This is of concern because the occurrence of severe hypertension has been clearly linked to the risk of cerebrovascular hemorrhage (24, 62).

The differential diagnosis of seizure activity in pregnancy is extensive and ranges from the obvious (epilepsy) to rare but important conditions that include systemic lupus erythematosus, thrombotic thrombocytopenic purpura, fatty liver of pregnancy, amniotic fluid embolism, cerebral venous thrombosis, malaria, and cocaine intoxication (63–66).

3. Investigation

Investigations should document the presence or absence of multiorgan disease and may be necessary to document neuropathological conditions and complications arising from the eclamptic seizures. Hence renal and liver function tests, changes in coagulation, respiratory function (chest radiograph, peripheral arterial oxygen saturation, arterial blood gas) and fetal well-being are all routinely required.

Specific neuroradiological investigation should be restricted to those women who have atypical presentations, persistent neurological signs, seizures that develop at the time of therapeutic magnesium sulfate blood concentration, convulsions that continue after magnesium sulfate is started, or development of late postpartum eclampsia. Abnormal neuroradiological investigation results are found in upward of 45% of such cases; however, several papers show a lack of correlation between the degree of hypertension and the number of seizures compared to neuroradiological abnormality. The most consistently seen changes are those affecting the posterior cerebral circulation giving rise to parieto-occipital edema (40,41). This picture may be associated with symptoms of visual disturbance (61,62). Other changes, which vary considerably, include white matter and basal ganglia lesions (41,50,67). Petechial hemorrhage is also reported in MRI studies. Major hemorrhage, not always evident at the time of first investigation, is associated with persistent clinical neurological abnormality (69).

The investigation of late postpartum "eclampsia" may show changes typically associated with eclampsia even in the absence of those clinical features (hypertension and proteinuria) considered essential to the diagnosis of eclampsia. Raps and associates reported a series of four postpartum patients with MRI findings of subcortical and occipitoparietal high signal foci; of these patients three had no proteinuria yet exhibited radiological features consistent with a diagnosis of eclampsia (38).

4. Management

There are three pillars of management: prevention of seizures, acute management, and supportive measures (68).

a. Prevention

In the broader context, prevention of eclampsia is clearly related to the prevention of preeclampsia. This chapter does not address this issue other than by allusion to the putative utility of low-dose aspirin, calcium supplementation, eicosopentanoic acid derivatives, and antioxidants (70).

Management aimed at the prevention of eclamptic seizures is empirical. In the United States of America up to 5% of women may be treated with magnesium sulfate prior to delivery (71). The efficacy and risks of magnesium sulfate use for this indication are currently being tested in a randomized trial (the MAGPIE trial). Smaller studies seem to show the efficacy of magnesium sulfate use for this indication. The largest published randomized study demonstrated that even patients with severe disease had a low incidence of seizures despite treatment with placebo (3.2%) (72). Despite this, the addition of magnesium sulfate to the regimen resulted in an 11-fold reduction in the relative risk of seizure activity.

The prevention of recurrent eclamptic seizures is less controversial. The Collaborative Eclampsia Trial has shown that magnesium sulfate should now be the accepted drug of choice for preventing recurrent seizures. This study compared magnesium sulfate to diazepam and phenytoin for the prevention of recurrent seizures in eclamptic patients (73). Rate of recurrent seizures was reduced by more than 50% when magnesium sulfate was compared to either of the control drugs; this reduction in seizure rate did not affect the maternal or fetal mortality rate, although there was a significant reduction in neonatal morbidity rate in the magnesium sulfate arm.

The action of magnesium sulfate (discussed later) is unclear, and it was proposed that seizures could perhaps be prevented by vasodilatation alone. One drug that could have such benefits is nimodipine. This dihydropyridine calcium channel blocker acts as a systemic vasodilator with unique effects on the cerebral vasculature and neurons. Given the theory that vasospasm is responsible for the majority of eclamptic seizures, nimodipine was compared with magnesium sulfate as a seizure prophylaxis agent in a large international multicenter randomized study. The study was stopped because of an increased rate of eclampsia in the nimodipine group. This was unexpected and suggests that vasospasm may not be as important as hypertensive encephalopathy in the pathophysiological features of eclampsia (73a). It is possible that the increased vascular resistance noted in the cerebral circulation of most preeclamptic women is actually protective vasoconstriction rather than pathological vasospasm. Furthermore, interfering with this vasoconstriction may put the patient at increased risk of seizure activity. Clearly there are women with status eclampticus who have vasospasm that is responsible for cerebral ischemia. These eclamptic patients may benefit from drugs that induce cerebral vasodilatation. In general, however, specific cerebral vasodilator drugs are best not used by most preeclamptic women, especially if they have elevated blood pressure that is difficult to control.

b. Acute Management

The objectives of management are self-evident: terminate the seizure, protect the patient from injury, and secure the airway.

Seizure activity (although likely to terminate spontaneously within 3 to 4 minutes) may be arrested by parenteral benzodiazepines (74). The dose required to terminate the seizure will vary and repeated doses may be necessary. These drugs sedate the mother and the fetus and can induce neonatal respiratory depression (75). In the United States it is common to avoid the use of such drugs in favor of securing an airway, protecting the mother from injury, and awaiting spontaneous resolution of the seizure.

The prevention of aspiration pneumonia is extremely important and revolves around positioning the patient on her side and suctioning the oropharynx once the seizure has been arrested. Patients who remain neurologically obtunded after the convulsion or who have recurrent seizures may be better managed by endotracheal intubation and elective ventilation in order to prevent aspiration pneumonia (76).

c. Supportive Measures

Besides the prevention of recurrent seizures, supportive therapy includes managing severe hypertension, deciding on the mode and timing of delivery, together with managing associated complications.

Hemodynamic management.   Antihypertensive therapy is imperative when severe hypertension threatens the development of hypertensive encephalopathy and cerebrovascular hemorrhage. By contrast, an excessive reduction in blood pressure may also be harmful because cerebral edema may cause raised intracranial pressure, requiring elevated systemic pressure to ensure cerebral perfusion (77,78). A mean arterial pressure of at least 100 mmHg is necessary to maintain cerebral perfusion in the face of cerebral edema (79). Mild hypertension may also be necessary in order to preserve perfusion in the face of preeclamptic microvascular disease, especially acute atherosis in the placental vascular bed. This condition may lead to partial luminal obstruction of the vessel resulting in diminished perfusion, partially compensated by a higher systemic perfusing pressure (15,77).

Antihypertensive therapy should be considered in all patients with mean arterial pressure greater than 126 mmHg. It is essential in all eclamptic and preeclamptic women with a mean arterial pressure equal to or greater than 140 mmHg. The goal of antihypertensive therapy should be to maintain systemic pressure between 100 and 126 mmHg. Patients admitted to intensive care units and managed with the benefit of invasive hemodynamic monitoring should have vasodilator therapy titrated against both systemic blood pressure and derived parameters such as systemic vascular resistance (SVR). The SVR should be restored to normal levels (1000 and 1200 dyne $\cdot$ sec/cm^{-5}), providing the MAP remains above 100 mmHg (76).

Plasma volume expansion is an essential adjunct to antihypertensive therapy. Diminishing peripheral perfusion may result from vasodilator therapy because of an excessive reduction in blood pressure but more commonly occurs because the necessary rise in cardiac output and stroke volume fails to occur (77). Many severe preeclamptic/eclamptic patients have a contracted intravascular blood volume, incompatible with a dilated vasculature. In these women, vasodilatation leads to falling venous return together with low preload and stroke volume. Clinically this is often evident when the pulse rate rises soon after commencing of vasodilatation and typically leads to fetal distress and development of oliguria (77). These adverse effects can be prevented by prior plasma volume expansion to increase ventricular preload. Plasma volume expansion may have beneficial effects because it reduces vascular resistance and increases cardiac output and oxygen delivery to the peripheral tissues (35,77,78). It remains an essential adjunct to safe vasodilatation and is probably a more important determinant of the efficacy and safety of vasodilators than the specific characteristics of individual drugs themselves.

Plasma volume expansion, however, increases the risk of iatrogenic pulmonary edema. Patients with preeclampsia/eclampsia are susceptible to the development of pulmonary edema because left-sided ventricular filling pressures rise sharply in response to plasma volume expansion even when small volumes of fluid are infused (as little as 400–500 mL of intravenous fluid). The reasons for this are unclear but presumably reflect changes in left ventricular compliance in severe preeclampsia. Right-sided filling pressures (central venous pressure) are not similarly affected and do not change rapidly in response to volume expansion. These disparate effects are evident when monitoring central venous pressure and pulmonary artery pressure measurements. Hemodynamic monitoring based on the use of central venous pressure lines only may be misleading and is likely to increase the risk of iatrogenic pulmonary edema (35,77).

In practice, volume expansion should precede vasodilatation and may be considered against a background rate of fluid administration (urinary output plus insensible loss) in addition to which small aliquots of fluid (300 mL) may be given for rapid volume expansion. This may take place without invasive monitoring on one or two occasions. In those who require greater volumes of fluid intravenously or have positive fluid balance pulmonary edema is less likely to develop if the clinician has knowledge of the pulmonary capillary wedge pressure.

Ventilatory support.   Sustained ventilatory care may be necessary in patients with a depressed level of consciousness, laryngeal edema (discussed later), or respiratory distress. Patients who suffer multiple seizures are often restless, semiconscious, and unable to protect their airway. Mechanical ventilation of these patients not only protects the airway against aspiration but also allows the introduction of heavy sedation. Patients who experience recurrent seizures in spite of magnesium sulfate administration are best ventilated while sedated by a continuous high-dose benzodiazepine or pentothal infusion. These patients may have cerebral edema and care should be taken to maintain a mean arterial pressure in excess of 100 mmHg in order to preserve cerebral blood flow in the face of raised intracranial pressure (79). Ventilatory care should be maintained until at least 24 hours postpartum.

Timing and mode of delivery.   Although some argue in favor of conservative management of severe preeclampsia, eclampsia is strongly correlated with maternal mortality, and resolution of the disease depends on termination of the pregnancy (80).

The timing and mode of delivery are empirical obstetrical decisions. There are no randomized trials that bias management in any particular direction. It would not be unreasonable to attempt vaginal delivery in favorable circumstances; the patient who has had one seizure without other complications or fetal distress may undergo induction of labor providing the cervix is favorable and delivery foreseeable. An attempt at induction of labor should not be protracted, and, although arbitrary, a time limit should be set beyond which lack of progress should lead to the diagnosis of failed induction of labor.

The risk of anesthetic complications attends cesarean delivery in eclamptic women. Upper airway edema may render endotracheal intubation difficult and can lead to failed intubation. Laryngeal edema, identified at the time of intubation or developing during cesarean section, is an indication for postoperative mechanical ventilation. Extubation of these women should be delayed until the airway is sufficiently patent to allow the patient to breathe past the endotracheal tube with the cuff deflated (68). The second problem associated with general anesthesia is the pressor response related to endotracheal intubation. This response can be obtunded in a number of ways, including the combined use of a bolus dose of intravenous magnesium sulfate and alfentanil given immediately prior to intubation (81). Regional anesthesia is not commonly advocated for eclamptic patients because of the risk of recurrent seizures and hemodynamic abnormality. The development of coagulopathy and severe thrombocytopenia (platelet count $< 50 \times 10^6$/mL) may also be a contraindication to regional procedures.

Because of the anesthetic risks inherent in managing these patients, cesarean delivery should never be precipitate, it should be carried out after the patient's condition has been stabilized in the labor ward. Stability includes arresting seizure activity, controlling hypertension, and investigating the patient for respiratory complications, renal failure, and coagulopathy.

B. Respiratory Complications

Respiratory complications frequently lead to critical care admission. They include upper airway edema, pulmonary edema, and aspiration pneumonia.

1. Pathophysiology

Patients with severe preeclampsia may have low oncotic pressure and altered capillary permeability with or without left ventricular dysfunction (systolic or diastolic) (34,35). Consequently, these women are predisposed to the development of pulmonary edema. Clinically unrecognized left ventricular diastolic dysfunction is particularly common and frequently documented in hemodynamic studies. As a result, rapid plasma volume expansion may increase the risk of pulmonary edema. This may occur after the administration of intravenous fluids; even small aliquots have been repeatedly shown to cause a sharp rise in left-sided filling pressures, usually without any changes in central venous pressure (34,35).

This may occur despite evidence of normal systolic ventricular function and reflects changes in left ventricular compliance during diastole. Iatrogenic fluid overload is consequently a frequent cause of pulmonary edema among these patients.

Some patients show evidence of cardiomyopathy; however, this condition is not typical of preeclampsia. The condition is likely to be undiagnosed without echocardiography or invasive monitoring. Occult valvular disease may also precipitate pulmonary edema in pregnancies complicated by hypertension.

Atelectasis giving rise to respiratory distress may occur in the critically ill preeclamptic patient. This can be a postoperative complication but is occasionally seen among patients with HELLP syndrome, who often splint the right hemidiaphragm because of pain associated with hepatic ischemia. Aspiration pneumonia is another obvious differential diagnosis in any eclamptic patient in whom respiratory distress develops. In the latter case, initial radiological signs may be unimpressive.

Adult respiratory distress syndrome (ARDS) is often cited as a complication of preeclampsia. This is unlikely to be a primary complication of the disease but may follow aspiration pneumonia or prolonged ventilation. Mabie and associates reported the occurrence of ARDS in an obstetrical intensive care unit (82). Over a 6-year period, 16 cases of respiratory distress attributable to ARDS were diagnosed (after exclusion of fluid overload and left ventricular dysfunction). Only 4 of these 16 cases were linked to preeclampsia/eclampsia. Three of the four patients had additional complications that may have contributed to the development of ARDS (including aspiration pneumonia, lupus nephritis, sepsis, and a ruptured liver hematoma with massive blood transfusion). The fourth patient had pulmonary edema that developed into ARDS after the patient had a respiratory arrest. These observations are important because most cases of respiratory distress have a cardiogenic component amenable to intervention. ARDS should never be used as a primary diagnosis in preeclampsia/eclampsia.

Laryngeal edema may be present in severe preeclampsia at the time of first presentation or may develop during the course of the disease. It is of particular importance in relation to anesthesia for delivery as well as the need for postoperative ventilation.

2. Presentation, Investigation, and Management

Patients who have respiratory distress frequently present a clinical diagnostic challenge; when the diagnosis remains in doubt after clinical examination and initial investigation (chest radiograph and electrocardiogram), echocardiography or pulmonary artery catheterization is required (68).

Women with pulmonary edema should be managed according to the specific hemodynamic findings (83). Hence, those who have high SVR may require vasodilation as primary therapy. Elevated SVR combined with impaired left ventricular function may be treated similarly. By contrast, elevated preload resulting from fluid overload requires diuretic therapy. These different hemodynamic subsets cannot be identified by studying blood pressure and pulse rate variables alone.

In all circumstances the differential diagnosis must be considered carefully. The development of localized signs and purulent sputum should alert the clinician to the possibility of aspiration pneumonia, especially in eclamptic women. Radiological findings in these circumstances may vary from normal lung fields to unilateral shadowing, atelectasis, and collapse. Investigation of women with suspected aspiration pneumonia may necessitate bronchoscopy if aspiration of particulate matter is suspected. Respiratory physicians should participate in the management of this complication; the principles of treatment include the use of broad-spectrum antibiotics (including anerobic cover).

C. Renal Complications

Oliguric renal failure frequently complicates severe preeclampsia.

1. Pathophysiology

Renal abnormality is the result of anatomical change in the glomerulus combined with changes in perfusion. The renal lesion held to be pathognomonic of preeclampsia is glomerular capillary endotheliosis (32). This lesion gives rise to glomeruli that are partially obstructed by lipid-laden mesangial cells. Intrinsic ischemia is aggravated by prerenal events, notably vasospasm and a low cardiac output. These changes create a cycle of ischemia that may end in acute tubular necrosis. The patients most susceptible to acute tubular necrosis are those with underlying preeclamptic changes who then suffer a superimposed hypovolemic insult (such as abruptio placentae or ruptured subcapsular liver hematoma). Hemoglobinuria in patients with the HELLP syndrome may also give rise to renal impairment.

2. Clinical Presentation, Investigation, and Management

Renal impairment commonly is associated with oliguria that is sometimes associated with marked hematuria (among patients with severe HELLP syndrome). Prerenal ischemia is usually the initiating event; if the patient is not already in positive fluid balance, plasma volume expansion should be attempted. If two fluid challenges (300 mL fluid, 30 minutes apart) do not improve the urinary output, low-dose dopamine may be commenced at an infusion rate of 1–5 µg/kg/min. Although dopamine is now regarded as a drug of questionable benefit in general critical care, at least two studies have demonstrated efficacy without adverse effects in the oliguric preeclamptic patient (84,85). Patients who do not respond to either of these measures require hemodynamic monitoring. The use of pulmonary artery catheter monitoring allows optimal fluid and vasodilator therapy aimed at normalizing ventricular preload and afterload (86).

The volume-replete vasodilated patient who does not pass urine has an intrinsic renal abnormality, usually acute tubular necrosis. A single large dose of frusemide (0.5 to 1 g intravenously) may lead to high-output renal failure. Should this measure also fail, care must be taken to prevent fluid overload and the patient should be prepared for dialysis.

D. Hepatic Complications

Weinstein first appended the acronym *HELLP* to the hepatic complications of preeclampsia in 1982 (31). This describes the subset of preeclamptic women who typically have symptoms of epigastric pain in association with evidence of microangiopathic hemolytic anemia, thrombocytopenia, and elevated liver enzyme level. It is by far the dominant hepatic pathological condition. Ruptured liver hematoma is a rare and devastating complication of preeclampsia/eclampsia.

1. Pathophysiology

HELLP syndrome results from the development of hepatic ischemia in a periportal distribution. Examination of the liver surface also shows multiple areas of subcapsular petechial hemorrhage. Large subcapsular hematomas presumably develop from enlarging hemorrhages that become confluent. The histological findings are periportal hemorrhage and necrosis (31). The vasculature in the areas of ischemic change shows evidence of fibrinoid necrosis. Microangiopathic changes result in platelet consumption and low-grade intravascular coagulation with consequent hemolysis.

Hemolysis and hemoglobinuria contribute to the development of renal failure and the characteristic passage of dark-colored urine.

2. Clinical Presentation, Investigation, and Management

The diagnosis is easy when patients with severe HELLP syndrome are obviously ill: the occurrence of epigastric pain in the setting of severe proteinuric hypertension with typical laboratory features raises little doubt about the diagnosis. However, the original description of these patients noted that the syndrome might be associated with relatively mild hypertension, leading to mistaken diagnoses such as peptic ulcer disease.

Severe derangement of liver enzymes can lead to persistent hypoglycemia.

Coagulopathy is less likely and partial thromboplastin and prothrombin times are usually normal. Excessive operative ooziness may nevertheless occur as a result of thrombocytopenia. The platelet count in women with HELLP syndrome should be interpreted with the recognition that preeclamptic platelets are qualitatively abnormal and cannot be equated with similar low counts in conditions such as idiopathic thrombocytopenia.

Respiratory distress may also develop in the patient with HELLP syndrome. This may be cardiogenic but can also result from right basal atelectasis because subdiaphragmatic pain causes rapid shallow respiration with consequent splinting of the right hemidiaphragm. Women with HELLP also have an increased risk of development of all the other complications of preeclampsia, including renal failure and eclampsia. The renal failure (characterized by rising urea and creatinine levels and passage of small quantities of blood-stained or cola-colored urine) may result in hyperkalemia that may require treatment with ion exchange resins. Fluid restriction (and abolition of all potassium-bearing intravenous fluids) is usually sufficient to preclude dialysis unless the patient has established acute tubular necrosis (ATN). Eclampsia associated with HELLP should be managed according to standard protocols (discussed earlier). Thrombocytopenia may provoke concern in the patient at risk of seizure activity; in the setting of severe hypertension, the criteria for administering platelet support should be relaxed because of the association between severe hypertension and cerebrovascular hemorrhage.

Ruptured liver hematoma is a devastating but rare complication. This may become evident as a result of the development of severe epigastric pain and sudden hypovolemia; alternatively, hemoperitoneum detected at the time of operative delivery may indicate the diagnosis.

The management of HELLP syndrome is primarily obstetrical because delivery is always curative. The thrombocytopenia should attain its nadir within 72 hours of delivery, and persistently low counts should provoke consideration of alternative diagnoses (87). Supportive therapy is necessary while effecting delivery. This includes attention to the hemodynamic principles of volume expansion and vasodilatation, especially in patients with renal failure. Each individual affected organ system requires supportive therapy according to the pattern of clinical disease. Seizure prophylaxis should be provided to all women with HELLP syndrome.

The issue of differential diagnosis is of particular concern because unrelated diseases requiring specific therapy can mimic HELLP syndrome. Hence, persistent postpartum thrombocytopenia should lead to a search for sepsis or folate deficiency. Thrombotic thrombocytopenic purpura, systemic lupus erythematosus, and acute fatty liver of pregnancy are also part of the differential diagnosis (88,89). Obstetrical cholestasis and viral hepatitis may enter the differential diagnosis in milder cases.

E. The Hypovolemic Preeclamptic Patient

Women with severe untreated preeclampsia tolerate hypovolemia poorly because of the contracted intravascular volume and low cardiac output. Peripheral oxygenation is critically impaired, and hypovolemia is often the trigger for multiorgan ischemia, especially renal ischemia. In developing countries, the hypovolemic preeclamptic patient has a significant mortality risk. Resuscitation of these women is complicated by ventricular dysfunction, necessitating some form of hemodynamic monitoring.

Women with severe preeclampsia complicated by obstetrical hemorrhage (usually abruptio placentae, postpartum hemorrhage, excessive operative blood loss, or, more rarely, ruptured subcapsular liver hematoma) should be recognized as critically ill and require access to intensive care.

IV. DRUG THERAPY IN SEVERE PREECLAMPSIA

A. Magnesium Sulfate

Parenteral magnesium results in systemic vasodilatation, cerebral vasodilatation, neuronal cell calcium channel blockade, and antiplatelet effects. Individually or collectively, these properties account for the anticonvulsant properties of magnesium sulfate (90).

Magnesium is a weak calcium channel blocker that increases cyclic guanosine monophosphate (GMP) levels, indicating a possible nitric oxide–mediated mechanism of vasodilatation (91,92). Magnesium sulfate infusions have also been shown to cause transient changes in both the renin-angiotensin system and endothelin 1 levels, both of which decrease after magnesium sulfate infusion (93–95). Magnesium sulfate–induced vasodilatation results in improved cardiac output. Cerebral vasodilatation distal to the middle cerebral artery has been demonstrated and retinal artery vasospasm has been reversed by magnesium sulfate infusion (96–98). The myocardial effects of parenteral magnesium include slowing of the cardiac conduction times, prolongation of the atrioventricular nodal refractory period and increase in sinoatrial conduction times (99). In high doses magnesium is significantly negatively inotropic (100).

Neuronal ischemia leads to a loss of intracellular potassium, magnesium, glucose, and adenosine triphosphate (ATP). Rising intracellular levels of sodium and calcium may be important determinants of ischemic neuronal injury (101). Calcium channel blockers, including magnesium sulfate, may prevent neuronal injury by regulating the intracellular calcium flux through N-methyl-D-aspartate receptor blockade (102,103).

Magnesium sulfate reduces serum calcium levels, leading to rising parathyroid hormone and vitamin D levels (104,105). These changes may be the result of increased renal magnesium and calcium excretion. Falling serum calcium levels inhibit acetylcholine release at the motor endplate, the extent of which is directly related to the level of the serum magnesium and inversely proportional to the calcium concentration (106,107).

Dosing regimens and therapeutic levels of magnesium sulfate are controversial. Higher serum levels may be associated with greater anticonvulsant efficacy as well as greater toxicity. There are several regimens commonly advocated. The Pritchard regimen requires the combined intramuscular (IM) and intravenous (IV) use of magnesium sulfate (4 g IV and 10 IM followed by 5 g IM four hourly thereafter) (108). Pritchard described the therapeutic serum magnesium level as between 2 and 3.5 mmol/L. Intramuscular administration of magnesium is unusually painful, and many other regimens advocate intravenous use only. These regimens usually combine a 4-g loading dose with a constant intravenous infusion of magnesium sulfate in doses ranging from 1 to 3 g per hour (108). The Pritchard regimen generally results in higher serum levels than intravenous regimens unless a 3-g/h maintenance dose is utilized (109). The Collaborative Eclampsia Trial used an intravenous regimen consisting of a 4-g loading dose followed by a constant infusion of 1 g/h. This treatment regimen was significantly more effective than either phenytoin or diazepam administration without adverse effects. Arguably, patients who continued to have convulsions on this treatment might have been better managed with a higher dose of magnesium sulfate, but the risks of adverse effects would also have increased. The balance of epidemiological data therefore favors the regimen used in the Collaborative Eclampsia Trial, although individual circumstances may dictate a different approach.

Toxicity of magnesium sulfate depends on the serum level of magnesium. This is determined by the dose, the distribution of the drug, and excretion. Parenterally administered magnesium is widely distributed in all body fluids, including the cerebrospinal fluid (110). The kidney excretes magnesium; glomerular filtration is followed by tubular reabsorption. The fractional reabsorbtion of magnesium depends on the serum magnesium level, renal perfusion, and tubular function (100,106). Toxic levels of magnesium may lead to respiratory arrest by blocking neuromuscular transmission (106,111,112). Even therapeutic levels of magnesium can affect neuromuscular function, leading to measurable changes in respiratory function as well as neuro-ophthalmological muscle weakness (113–115). Therapeutic doses of magnesium sulfate may unmask myasthenia gravis in women with no other clinical manifestations of the disease (116).

There are few direct adverse effects of parenteral magnesium on the cardiovascular system. The combined use of magnesium and dihydropyridine calcium channel blockers has led to several case reports detailing both neuromuscular blockade and iatrogenic hypotension; this may be an idiosyncratic reaction, and some units continue to use the two drugs in combination (117–119). Magnesium sulfate used together with neuromuscular blocking agents prolongs the action of succinylcholine. This effect is confined to preeclamptic patients and may be related to a reduced level of plasma cholinesterase activity (120–123).

Magnesium sulfate may vasodilate the uterine circulation and may have direct fetal effects as a result of transplacental passage. These effects are more typically seen after prolonged tocolytic therapy using magnesium sulfate than in treatment for preeclampsia/eclampsia. Hence, prolonged therapy results in higher amniotic fluid and cord blood levels than those found in maternal serum (124). Fetal hypermagnesemia leads to elevated levels of fetal parathyroid hormone with neonatal bone demineralization and metaphyseal changes (125). Neurobehavioral changes (changes in the biophysical profile associated with loss of short-term variability patterns in the fetal heart rate) are also described (126–128).

B. Phenytoin

Although phenytoin is an accepted anticonvulsant drug, it may lack efficacy in managing eclampsia because of the unique pathophysiological characteristics of the disease as well as pharmacodynamic factors (129).

The therapeutic range of phenytoin (the dose required to stop seizure activity, usually defined as 10–20 mg/L) shows wide variation, depending on the nature and severity of seizure activity (130). Pregnancy results in an increased volume of drug distribution as well as accelerated clearance by hepatic hydroxylation and increased urinary excretion. Protein binding decreases, resulting in a greater amount of free drug (131). A loading dose of 17.5 mg/kg results in levels above the therapeutic range 30 minutes after drug administration in 31% of cases, where lower doses (15 mg/kg) lead to subtherapeutic levels in 22% of patients 12 hours after initiation of therapy (132).

Phenytoin has adverse effects, including lower folate levels and interference with vitamin K–dependent clotting factors in the neonate, leading to an increased risk of neonatal hemorrhage (131).

The Collaborative Eclampsia Trial used a fixed regimen of phenytoin, which may not have attained therapeutic levels in many patients (73). Considering the difficulty inherent in securing a therapeutic level, there would seem to be little place for phenytoin as a first-line treatment in patients with severe preeclampsia/eclampsia.

C. Benzodiazepines

Benzodiazepines have been used to arrest seizure activity and prevent recurrent seizures (90). Both efficacy and adverse effects of benzodiazepines are dose related; the most important disadvantage of high-dose benzodiazepine infusion is heavy maternal and neonatal sedation, which increases the risk of aspiration pneumonia and neonatal respiratory depression.

The Collaborative Eclampsia Trial showed the magnesium sulfate regimen to be more effective than a fixed dosage regimen of diazepam (73). Diazepam therefore should not be used as the drug of first choice in managing the eclamptic patient.

Benzodiazepines, however, still have a role to play in women who experience recurrent seizures despite treatment with magnesium sulfate. These patients (often semiconscious and restless between seizures) require endotracheal intubation and mechanical ventilation. High doses of benzodiazepines given under these circumstances sedate the patient for the purposes of ventilation and also prevent recurrent seizures. Shorter-acting drugs such as midazolam may prove a better choice than longer-acting agents like diazepam.

D. Dihydralazine

Dihydralazine is an effective direct acting vasodilator. It is infused in normal saline solution at a rate of 2.5 to 7.5 mg per hour after an initial loading dose of 5 to 10 mg. The dose can be titrated against blood pressure, although care should be exercised once the total infused dose reaches 10 to 12 mg, beyond which there may be a sharp fall in blood pressure (77).

The tachycardia that commonly follows the administration of dihydralazine is usually the result of an inadequate blood volume and low preload, although there are reports of increased levels of noradrenaline associated with the administration of the drug (133). One disadvantage of dihydralazine is that it may diminish the capacity of the cerebral circulation to autoregulate blood flow (55). Although an old drug, dihydralazine remains effective and free of adverse drug interactions (77).

E. Calcium Channel Blockers

Orally administered dihydropyridine calcium channel blockers such as nifedipine are effective vasodilators and have a rapid onset of action. Hypotensive episodes can follow the administration of nifedipine in patients with a contracted intravascular blood volume who are inadequately preloaded prior to vasodilation. Hypotensive episodes have also been attributed to the interaction between nifedipine and magnesium sulfate in several anecdotal reports (118,134). These episodes may reflect the negative inotropic properties of both drugs combined with the individual susceptibility of the occasional patient who has severe preeclampsia and impaired left ventricular function. Despite these reports some obstetrical units routinely use the two drugs in combination.

Nimodipine, a second-generation dihydropyridine, has been investigated as a combined antihypertensive/anticonvulsant drug in the management of preeclampsia/eclampsia. This drug has been used to prevent ischemic neurological deficit after subarachnoid hemorrhage and successfully used in the management of small groups of eclamptic patients (135–138). Nimodipine, like magnesium sulfate, is both a vasodilator and an inhibitor of calcium transport in neuronal tissue (134). Despite the initial enthusiasm, nimodipine did not prevent postpartum convulsions in preeclamptic women, and it is not recommended as a first-line treatment.

F. Labetalol

Intravenous labetalol has combined α- and β-blocking action. The mechanism of action (in doses required to reduce blood pressure) is that of negative chronotropism rather than any negative inotropic effect. The use of labetalol is typically confined to the treatment of patients who have hypertension on the basis of a high cardiac output (78). This is an unusual circumstance, usually recognized after pulmonary artery catheterization. It is nevertheless conceivable that such patients with hypertensive encephalopathy may be better managed with β-blockade than with vasodilator drugs

β-blockers may also reduce the incidence of ventricular arrhythmias in patients with preeclampsia. A small randomized study has shown a significant reduction in the incidence of arrhythmias when labetalol was compared to dihydralazine in the management of eclampsia (140). Ventricular arrhythmias, however, are rarely observed clinically and do not in themselves justify the selection of β-blockers ahead of other vasodilators because of the adverse influence of β-blockers on the preterm fetus (141).

G. Other Drugs

Potent antihypertensive drugs such as sodium nitroprusside are rarely required in the management of severe preeclampsia. Intravenous nitroglycerin may have a small role to play in those patients who have pulmonary edema, high pulmonary capillary wedge pressure (PCWP), and normal left ventricular function (142). Nitroglycerin acts as a vasodilator and venodilator; this action diminishes venous return, leading to a fall in left ventricular preload.

V. ANESTHETIC CONSIDERATIONS

Many critically ill preeclamptic patients require operative delivery (143). General anesthesia is complicated by the hypertensive surge associated with endotracheal intubation and is clearly undesirable in women already severely hypertensive. There is also a possibility of failed intubation in those patients with upper airway edema.

Regional anesthesia is widely held to be the method of choice in managing these patients; however, it is more difficult because of the preload sensitivity of women with severe disease; in the absence of hemodynamic monitoring inadequate preloading may further aggravate peripheral ischemia. Additional concerns arise from coagulopathy and thrombocytopenia. General anesthesia is reserved for patients with eclampsia and those who have platelet counts of less than 100,000/L. The pressor response to intubation has been controlled in a number of ways, including the combined use of bolus dose magnesium sulfate and alfetanil during the induction of anesthesia, immediately prior to intubation.

VI. MONITORING OF THE WOMAN WITH SEVERE PREECLAMPSIA

The intensive care management of severe preeclampsia poses questions regarding routine monitoring. Some of these issues have been debated (CVP versus PCWP monitoring), others largely ignored (automated blood pressure monitoring).

A. Role of Blood Pressure Monitoring

It is critically important to be able to measure blood pressure accurately in women whose risk of complications, especially cerebrovascular hemorrhage, is directly related to their degree of hypertension. At Groote Schuur Hospital, blood pressure determined by two automated blood pressure monitors (the auscultatory Welch-Allyn QuietTrak and the oscillometric SpaceLabs 90207) was compared to blood pressure measured by means of both sphygmomanometry and direct intra-arterial pressure readings in women with preeclampsia (144). Compared to mercury, the auscultatory Quiet Trak consistently underread systolic and diastolic blood pressure by 13 (±15) mmHg. The oscillometric 90207 also underread systolic by 10 (±10) mmHg and diastolic pressure by 8 (±7) mmHg. Compared to intra-arterial readings, both monitors significantly underread systolic and mean arterial pressure. These data have important implications for those involved in the care of women with severe preeclampsia. Automated blood pressure monitoring devices are generally inaccurate and blood pressure determination in the critically ill preeclamptic should take place by mercury sphygmomanometry or intra-arterial recording.

B. Invasive Monitoring

Left ventricular systolic and diastolic dysfunction complicates severe preeclampsia. Even small volumes of intravenous fluids result in a sharp rise in left-sided ventricular filling pressures. In critically ill patients it is important to measure cardiac output and pulmonary artery wedge pressure as a guide to fluid management. In women with severe pre-eclampsia and pulmonary edema, knowledge of cardiac function and filling pressures is an essential adjunct to rational therapy.

Pulmonary artery catheterization is regarded as the gold standard in hemodynamic monitoring. Recent evidence has, however, suggested that morbidity and mortality directly attributable to the use of the catheter require assessment of the risk-benefit ratio. The Pulmonary Artery Catheter Consensus Meeting subsequently evaluated the evidence for or against the use of pulmonary artery catheters in selected circumstances (145). The use of the catheter in the management of preeclampsia was curiously described in relation to "perioperative management," and the participants concluded that there was no evidence favoring the *routine* use of the catheter. The caveat was allowed that expert opinion deemed the catheter useful in certain circumstances, notably persistent oliguria, pulmonary edema, and resistant hypertension.

A 3-year review of catheters used for invasive monitoring at Groote Schuur Hospital showed that 19.5% of intensive care unit (ICU) patients had invasive monitoring (146). The most common indications for invasive monitoring were renal failure (56%) and pulmonary edema (32%). After catheterization over half the patients monitored were considered to have some form of ventricular dysfunction, and the information obtained by catheterization was deemed clinically relevant in 93% of cases. Among the patients studied there was no catheter-related mortality, and only three minor complications (two cases of thrombophlebitis from long-line insertions through the antecubital fossa and one case of cellulitis) occurred.

Alternative forms of monitoring may be relevant. Rapid echocardiographic assessment of left ventricular function is a useful although less accessible tool for monitoring ventricular function in preeclampsia. More recently, transoesophageal Doppler assessment of the aortic waveform has been proposed to allow estimation of cardiac output and derived estimates of vascular resistance. This form of monitoring, which is less invasive, has been compared to pulmonary artery catheterization. One study showed that the Doppler readings consistently underestimated cardiac output by 20% although the trends in hemodynamic changes were consistently similar (147).

In summary, the pulmonary artery catheter remains the most immediately available and accurate tool for monitoring women with severe preeclampsia. The indications include persistent oliguria, pulmonary edema, and resistant hypertension. Central venous pressure monitoring on its own is less important in the management of severe preeclampsia because of the disparate findings between central venous and pulmonary artery wedge pressures after acute volume expansion.

VII. SCORING SYSTEMS IN PREECLAMPSIA/ECLAMPSIA

Scoring systems are commonly employed by critical care units to categorize severity of illness and assess outcome, most commonly mortality rates, in relation to treatment. Several scoring systems have been used, including the Acute Physiology and Chronic Health Evaluation (APACHE), the Simplified Acute Physiology Scores (SAPS), and the Logistic Organ Dysfunction Score (LODS) (148–150). None of these scoring systems has been specifically validated in obstetrical intensive care. Unpublished data from Groote Schuur Hospital evaluated the SAPS in the prediction of maternal mortality rate in an obstetrical ICU; 661 women, admitted to the obstetrical ICU over a 3-year period, were scored by the SAPS acute health score. Of this cohort, 387 women had severe preeclampsia. Although the mortality rate was low (1.96% for the whole group), the overall data showed that the area under the receiver operator characteristic curve was 0.87, a finding that suggests that SAPS is able to discriminate well between survivors and nonsurvivors. However, using a cutoff SAPS score of 7, the positive predictive value was only 0.09 because of the low maternal mortality rate. SAPS overestimated maternal mortality rate when compared with the original SAP database. The prediction of morbidity was more consistent (see Table 1): using a cutoff of 7 there was a relative risk of central hemodynamic monitoring, inotropic support, ventilation, and dialysis of 1.96, 4.48, 3.63, and 3.49, respectively.

Further research is required to establish whether scoring systems can more reliably identify women who need critical care.

Another study, from Durban, South Africa, studied the utility of scoring systems among eclamptic patients. This study utilized APACHE scoring systems and found that only the Glasgow Coma Scale (GCS) reliably identified the risk of mortality in this specific group of women. Notably, there were no fatalities in women who had a GCS score greater than 10 (151).

Table 1 Relative Risk of the Need for Hemodynamic Monitoring, Inotropic Support, Ventilation, and Dialysis in Women who Survived with a SAPS Score ≥ 7 Compared to Women with a SAPS Score < 7[a]

	SAPS score < 7 $n = 544$ (%)	SAPS score ≥ 7 $n = 104$ (%)	Relative risk (95% confidence intervals)
Hemodynamic monitoring	96 (17.6)	36 (34.6)	1.96 (1.42–2.70)
Inotropic support	7 (1.2)	6 (5.8)	4.48 (1.54–13.07)
Ventilation	30 (5.5)	21 (20.1)	3.63 (2.16–6.08)
Dialysis	6 (1.1)	4 (3.8)	3.49 (1.00–12.14)

[a]SAPS = Simplified Acute Physiology Scores.

VIII. DIFFERENTIAL DIAGNOSIS OF SEVERE
PREECLAMPSIA/ECLAMPSIA

There are a number of conditions that may closely resemble preeclampsia. These conditions are outlined briefly in the following sections.

A. Thrombotic Thrombocytopenic Purpura

Thrombotic thrombocytopenic purpura (TTP) is part of a spectrum of microangiopathic conditions that include hemolytic uremic syndrome (HUS) (89). TTP presents a clinical pentad of features: microangiopathic hemolytic anemia, fever, transitory neurological disturbance, renal impairment, and thrombocytopenia. Mild hypertension and proteinuria may make the condition clinically indistinguishable from HELLP syndrome. The presence of pronounced hemolysis and unusually large multimers of von Willebrand factor is a pointer to the diagnosis of TTP. Unlike preeclampsia patients, patients who have TTP do not improve after delivery, and this is an important diagnosis to consider in the thrombocytopenic patient whose platelet count does not begin to rise 3 days after delivery. Without appropriate management TTP has a high mortality rate. Treatment consists of plasmaphoresis, infusion of fresh frozen plasma, and high-dose steroids.

B. Acute Fatty Liver of Pregnancy

Acute fatty liver of pregnancy (AFLP) is a condition that occurs in the latter half of pregnancy and is characterized by microvesicular fatty infiltration of the liver (88). The typical presentation is that of mild right upper quadrant discomfort associated with prodromal nausea and vomiting. More than 50% of affected patients have symptoms and signs suggestive of preeclampsia (hypertension and proteinuria), which may make the distinction from HELLP syndrome difficult. Jaundice is commonly present at the time of first presentation, whereas it is an uncommon feature of HELLP syndrome. Hypoglycemia and coagulopathy due to rapidly developing fulminant liver failure may give rise to a clinical bleeding diathesis and prolonged clotting times (APTT and INR). Other hematological markers include microangiopathic hemolytic anemia, neutrophil leukocytosis, and elevated levels of fibrin degradation products that result from disseminated intravascular coagulation. Liver enzymes levels are raised; transaminase levels may be elevated several-fold; values above 1000 IU/L may occur in severe cases. Renal failure and pancreatitis may further complicate the clinical picture.

The management principles do not differ from those of severe preeclampsia because they revolve around delivery and supportive therapy. In some circumstances making the clinical distinction between HELLP and AFLP may be difficult; if deemed to be clinically relevant, liver biopsy may contribute to establishment of the diagnosis. Acute fatty liver is characterized by microvesicular fatty infiltration, whereas HELLP results in periportal necrosis and hemorrhage.

C. Amniotic Fluid Embolus

Amniotic fluid embolus (AFE) is a rare but potentially lethal condition in which an anaphylactoid response develops in the mother in the presence of amniotic fluid in the circulation.

The clinical syndrome is diagnosed in every 1 in 8000 to 1 in 80,000 pregnancies. Because of the rarity of the condition a national registry of cases was opened in the United States of America; this remains the most authoritative single source of information about this condition (66). The condition usually appears during labor but may occur during cesarean delivery. Rarely, it can manifest itself immediately after childbirth. In approximately half the patients seizure activity develops; it is the single most common presenting symptom in patients in whom AFE develops before delivery of the fetus.

Despite the abrupt onset of this syndrome, the distinction from eclampsia is aided by the presence of hypotension, which is universally present. In almost all patients pulmonary edema with cyanosis develops, and the other cardinal clinical feature is the development of profound coagulopathy, which should immediately alert the attending obstetrician to the diagnosis.

D. Other Conditions

Systemic lupus erythematous, malaria, and sickle cell disease are all conditions that may to some extent mimic preeclampsia/eclampsia. These differential diagnoses should be considered in all cases of atypical preeclampsia and in women whose disease does not remit after delivery.

IX. CONCLUSIONS

Severe preeclampsia is a dangerous, complex multiorgan disorder best managed by experienced clinicians. Obstetrical intensive care units fulfill this requirement but are rarities in many parts of the world. In the absence of dedicated units, women with preeclampsia are most likely to benefit from a team approach involving obstetricians, physicians, intensivists, and anesthesiologists.

This chapter reflects the clinical practice of one center and much of the therapy advocated may be regarded as empirical. Despite the high prevalence of preeclampsia, too few critically ill patients are treated in any single center (or even several centers) to make randomized studies easily feasible. In the absence of such evidence, much of clinical practice depends on expert opinion and smaller studies.

There are also many opinions about every aspect of management described in this chapter, and the practice advocated here is likely to change with improving knowledge derived from both randomized clinical trials and basic science studies. This chapter is therefore dedicated to all the critically ill women whose lives are entrusted to our care and for whom we must strive to practice to the limits of our knowledge and ability at all times.

REFERENCES

1. MacGillivray I. Some observations on the incidence of preeclampsia. J Obstet Gynaecol Br Commonwealth 1958; 65:536–539.
2. MacGillivray I. Preeclampsia: The Hypertensive Disease of Pregnancy. London: W.B. Saunders, 1983.
3. Duley L. Maternal mortality associated with hypertensive disorders of pregnancy in Africa, Latin America and the Caribbean. Br J Obstet Gynaecol 1992; 99: 547–553.
4. World Health Organization. Geographic variation in the incidence of hypertension in pregnancy: International Collaborative Study of Hypertensive Disorders of pregnancy. Am J Obstet Gynecol 1988; 158:80–83.
5. Hogberg U, Innala E, Sandstrom A. Maternal mortality in Sweden, 1980–1988. Obstet Gynecol 1994; 84(2):240–244.
6. Bashir A, Aleem M, Mustansar M. A 5-year study of maternal mortality in Faisalabad City, Pakistan. Int J Gynaecol Obstet 1995; 50(suppl 2):S93–S96.
7. Department of Health. Report on Confidential Enquiries into Maternal Deaths 1991–1993. London: HMSO, 1996.
8. Pattinson B, ed. Saving Mothers: Report on Confidential Enquiries into Maternal Deaths in South Africa 1998. Department of Health, South Africa, 1999.
9. Davey DA, MacGillivray I. The classification and definition of the hypertensive disorders of pregnancy. Am J Obstet Gynecol 1988; 158(4):892–898.
10. Chesley LC, Cooper DW. Genetics of hypertension in pregnancy: possible single gene control of pre-eclampsia and eclampsia in descendants of eclamptic women. Br J Obstet Gynaecol 1986; 93:898–908.
11. Cooper DW, Liston WA. Genetic control of severe pre-eclampsia. J Med Genet 1979; 16:409–416.
12. Humphrey KE, Harrison GA, Cooper DW, Wilton AN, Brennecke SP, Trudinger BJ. HLA-G deletion polymorphism and pre-eclampsia/eclampsia. Br J Obstet Gynaecol 1995; 102(8):707–710.
13. Harrison GA, Humphrey KE, Jones N, Badenhop R, Guo G, Elakis G, Kaye JA, Tuner RJ, Grehan M, Wilton AN, Brennecke SP, Cooper DW. A genomewide linkage study of pre-eclampsia/eclampsia reveals evidence for a candidate region on 4q. Am J Hum Genet 1997; 60(5):1158–1167.
14. Robillard PY, Dekker GA, Hulsey TC. Revisiting the epidemiological standard of preeclampsia: primigravidity or primipaternity? Eur J Obstet Gynecol Reprod Biol 1999; 84:37–41.

15. Pijnenborg R, Anthony J, Davey DA, Rees A, Tiltman A, Vercruysse L, van Assche A. Placental bed spiral arteries in the hypertensive disorders of pregnancy. Br J Obstet Gynaecol 1991; 98:648–655.

16. Robertson WB, Brosens, I, Dixon G. Uteroplacental vascular pathology. Eur J Obstet Gynecol Reprod Biol 1975; 5:47–65.

17. Nova A, Sibai BM, Barton JR, Mercer BM, Mitchell MD. Maternal plasma level of endothelin is increased in preeclampsia. Am J Obstet Gynecol 1991; 165(3): 724–727.

18. Clark BA, Halvarson L, Sachs B, Epstein FH. Plasma endothelin levels in pre-eclampsia: elevation and correlation with uric acid levels and renal impairment. Am J Obstet Gynecol 1992; 166(3):962–968.

19. Walsh SW. Preeclampsia: an imbalance in placental prostacyclin and thromboxane production. Am J Obstet Gynecol 1985; 152:335–340.

20. Gujrati VR, Shanker K, Vrat S, Chandravati, Parmar SS. Novel appearance of placental nuclear monamine oxidase: biochemical and histochemical evidence for hyperserotonomic state in pre-eclampsia–eclampsia. Am J Obstet Gynecol 1996; 175(6):1543–1550.

21. Nasiell J, Nisell H, Blanck A, Lunell NO, Faxen M. Placental expression of endo-thelial constitutive nitric oxide synthase mRNA in pregnancy complicated by pre-eclampsia. Acta Obstet Gynaecol Scand 1998; 77:492–496.

22. Redman CWG. Platelets and the beginnings of preeclampsia (editorial). N Engl J Med 1990; 323:478–480.

23. Lyall F, Greer IA, Boswell F, Macara LM, Walker JJ, Kingdom JCP. The cell adhesion molecule VCAM-1 is selectively elevated in serum in pre-eclampsia: does this indicate the mechanism of leucocyte activation. Br J Obstet Gynaecol 1994; 101:485–487.

24. Halim A, Kanayama N, el Maradny E, Nakashima A, Bhuiyan AB, Khatun S, Terao T. Plasma P selectin (GMP-140) and glycocalicin are elevated in pre-eclampsia and eclampsia: their significances. Am J Obstet Gynecol 1996; 174(1 pt 1):272–277.

25. Halim A, Kanayama N, el Maradyn E, Maehara K, Bhuiyan AB, Terao T. Correlated plasma elastase and sera cytotoxicity in eclampsia: a possible role of endothelin-1 induced neutrophil activation in pre-eclampsia–eclampsia. Am J Hypertens 1996; 9(1):33–38.

26. Halligan A, Bonnar J, Sheppard B, Darling M, Walshe J. Haemostatic, fibrinolytic and endothelial variables in normal pregnancies and pre-eclampsia. Br J Obstet Gynaecol 1994; 101(6):488–492.

27. Taylor RN, Casal DC, Jones LA, Varma M, Martin JN Jr, Roberts JM. Selective effects of preeclamptic sera on human endothelial cell procoagulant protein expres-sion. Am J Obstet Gynecol 1991; 165(6 pt 1):1705–1710.

28. Sheehan H, Lynch J. Cerebral lesions. In: Sheehan H, Lynch J, eds. Pathology of Toxemia of Pregnancy. Baltimore: Williams & Wilkins; 1973: 524–553.

29. Donaldson JO. The brain in eclampsia. Hypertens Pregn 1994; 13(2):115–133.

30. Richards AM, Graham DI, Bullock MRR. Clinicopathological study of neurological complications due to hypertensive disorders in pregnancy. J Neurosurg Psychol 1988; 51:416.

31. Weinstein L. Syndrome of hemolysis, elevated liver enzymes and low platelet count:

a severe consequence of hypertension in pregnancy. Am J Obstet Gynecol 1982; 142: 159–167.

32. Spargo BH, McCartney C, Winemiller R. Glomerular capillary endotheliosus in toxemia of pregnancy. Arch Pathol 1959; 13:593–599.

33. Barton JR, Sibai BM. Cerebral pathology in eclampsia. Clin Perinatol 1991; 18: 891–910.

34. Visser W, Wallenburg HCS. Central hemodynamic observations in untreated preeclamptic patients. Hypertension 1991; 17:1072–1077.

35. Belfort MA, Anthony J, Kirshon B. Respiratory function in severe gestational proteinuric hypertension: the effects of rapid volume expansion and subsequent vasodilatation with verapamil. Br J Obstet Gynaecol 1991; 98:964–972.

36. Belfort MA, Saade GR, Wasserstrum N, Johanson R, Anthony J. Acute volume expansion with colloid increases oxygen delivery and consumption but does not improve the oxygen extraction in severe pre-eclampsia. J Matern Fetal Med 1995; 4: 57–64.

37. Belfort MA, Anthony J, Saade GR, Wasserstrum N, Johanson R, Clark S, Moise KJ. The oxygen consumption/oxygen delivery curve in severe pre-eclampsia: evidence for a fixed oxygen extraction state. Am J Obstet Gynecol 1993; 169:1448–1455.

38. Raps EC, Galetta SL, Broderick M, Atlas SW. Delayed peripatum vasculopathy: cerebral eclampsia revisited. Ann Neurol 1993; 33(2):222–225.

39. Milliez J, Dahoun A, Boudraa M. Computed tomography of the brain in eclampsia. Obstet Gynecol 1990; 75:975–980.

40. Crawford S, Varner MW, Digre KB, Servais G, Corbett JJ. Cranial magnetic resonance imaging in eclampsia. Obstet Gynecol 1987; 70:474–477.

41. Schwartz RB, Jones KM, Kalina P, Bajakian RL, Mantello MT, Garada B, Holman BL. Hypertensive encephalopathy: findings on CT, MR imaging and SPECT imaging in 14 cases. Am J Radiol 1992; 159:379–383.

42. Akan H, Kucuk M, Bolat O, Selcuk MB, Tunali G. The diagnostic value of cranial computed tomography in complicated eclampsia. J Belge Radiol 1993; 76(5):304–306.

43. Schaefer PW, Buonanno FS, Gonzales RG, Schwamm LH. Diffusion-weighted imaging discriminates between cytotoxic and vasogenic edema in a patient with eclampsia. Stroke 1997; 28:1082–1085.

44. Williams KP, Wilson S. Maternal cerebral blood flow changes associated with eclampsia. Am J Perinatol 1995; 12(3):189–191.

45. Zunker P, Ley-Pozo J. Louwen F, Schuierer G, Holzgreve W, Ringelstein EB. Cerebral hemodynamics in pre-eclampsia/eclampsia syndrome. Ultrasound Obstet Gynecol 1995; 6(6):411–415.

46. Morriss MC, Twickler DM, Hatab MR, Clarke GD, Peshock RM, Cunningham FG. Cerebral blood flow and cranial magnetic resonance imaging in eclampsia and severe pre-eclampsia. Obstet Gynecol 1997 89(4):561–568.

47. Sibai BM. Eclampsia VI. Maternal and perinatal outcome in 254 consecutive cases. Am J Obstet Gynecol 1990; 163:1049–1054.

48. Kanayama N, Nakajima A, Maehara K, Halim A, Kajiwara Y, Isoda H, Masui T, Terao T. Magnetic resonance imaging angiography in a case of eclampsia. Gynecol Obstet Invest 1993; 36(1):56–58.

49. Duncan R, Hadley D, Bone I, Symonds EM, Worthington BS, Rubin PC. Blindness

in eclampsia: CT and MRI imaging. J Neurol Neurosurg Psychiatry 1989; 52: 899–902.

50. Lewis L, Hinshaw D, Will A, Hasso A, Thompson J. CT and angiographic correlation of severe neurological disease in toxemia of pregnancy. Neuroradiology 1988; 30:59–64.

51. Belfort MA, Saade GR. Retinal vasospasm associated with visual disturbance in preeclampsia: color flow doppler findings. Am J Obstet Gynecol 1993; 169(3):523–525.

52. Belfort MA, Saade GR, Moise KJ, Arcadia Cruz RVT, Adam K, Kramer W, Kirshon B. Nimodipine in the management of pre-eclampsia: maternal and fetal effects. Am J Obstet Gynecol 1994; 171:417–424.

53. Belfort MA, Saade GR, Moise KJ. The effect of magnesium sulfate on maternal retinal blood flow in pre-eclampsia: a randomized placebo-controlled study. Am J Obstet Gynecol 1992; 167:1548–1553.

54. Hashimoto H, Kuriyama Y, Naritoma H, Sawada T. Serial assessments of middle cerebral artery flow velocity with transcranial doppler ultrasonography in the recovery stage of eclampsia: a case report. Angiology 1997; 48(4):355–358.

55. Rowe GG, Maxwell GM, Crumpton CW. The cerebral haemodynamic response to administration of hydralazine. Circulation 1963; 25:970–972.

56. Overgaard J, Skinhoj E. A paradoxical cerebral hemodynamic effect of hydralazine. Stroke 1975; 6:402–404.

57. Douglas KA, Redman CW. Eclampsia in the United Kingdom. Br Med J 1994; 309 (6966):1395–1400.

58. Lubarsky SL, Barton JR, Friedman SA, Nasreddine S, Ramadan MK, Sibai BM. Late postpartum eclampsia revisited. Obstet Gynecol 1994; 83(4):502–505.

59. Tetzschner T, Felding C. Postpartum eclampsia: impossible to eradicate? Clin Exp Obstet Gynecol 1994; 21(2):74–76.

60. Dieckmann WJ. The Toxemias of Pregnancy, 2nd ed. St. Louis: C. V. Mosby, 1952.

61. Chang WN, Lui CC, Chang JM. CT and MRI findings of eclampsia and their correlation with neurologic symptoms. Chung Hua I Hsueh Tsa Chih 1996; 57(3): 191–197.

62. Unal M, Senakayli OC, Serce K. Brain MRI findings in two cases with eclampsia. Australas Radiol 1996; 40(3):348–350.

63. Hauser WAS, Kurland LT. The epidemiology of epilepsy in Rochester, Minnesota 1935 through 1967. Epilepsia 1975; 16:1–66.

64. Towers CV, Pircon RA, Nageotte MP, Porto M, Garite TJ. Cocaine intoxication presenting as pre-eclampsia and eclampsia. Obstet Gynecol 1993; 81(4):545–547.

65. Gamba G. Acute thrombocytopaenias and thrombotic thrombocytopenic purpura: differential diagnosis. Transfus Sci 1992; 13:13–16.

66. Clark SL, Hankins GDV, Dudley DA, Dildy GA, Flint Porter T. Amniotic fluid embolism: analysis of the national registry. Am J Obstet Gynecol 1995; 172:1158–1169.

67. Thomas SV, Somanathan N, Rao VR, Radhakurmari K. Reversible nonenhancing lesions without focal neurological deficits in eclampsia. Indian J Med Res 1996; 103:94–97.

68. Linton DM, Anthony J. Critical care management of severe pre-eclampsia. Intensive Care Med 1997; 23:248–255.

69. Drislane FW, Wang AM. Multifocal cerebral hemorrhage in eclampsia and severe pre-eclampsia. J Neurol 1997; 244(3):194–198.

70. Lindheimer MD. Pre-eclampsia–eclampsia 1996: preventable? Have disputes on its treatment been resolved? Curr Opin Nephrol Hypertens 1996; 5:452–458.

71. Lucas MJ, Leveno KI, Cunningham FG. A comparison of magnesium sulphate with phenytoin for the prevention of eclampsia. N Engl J Med 1995; 333:205–210.

72. Coetzee EJ, Dommisse J, Anthony J. A randomised controlled trial of intravenous magnesium sulphate versus placebo in the management of patients with severe pre-eclampsia. Br J Obstet Gynaecol 1998; 105(3):300–303.

73. Eclampsia Trial Collaborative Group. Which anticonvulsant for women with eclampsia? Evidence from the Collaborative Eclampsia Trial 1995. Lancet 1995; 345 (8969):1455–1463.

73a. Belfort M, Anthony J, Allen J and the Nimodipine Study Group. Magnesium sulfate is more effective at preventing eclampsia than the selective cerebral vasodilator nimodipine. J Soc Gynecol Invest 2001; 8:73A.

74. Browne TR, Penry JK. Benzodiazepines in the treatment of epilepsy: a review. Epilepsia 1973; 14:277–310.

75. Cree JE, Meyer J, Hailey DM. Diazepam in labor: its metabolism and effect on the clinical condition and thermogenesis of the newborn. Br Med J 1973; 4:251–255.

76. Anthony J, Johanson R, Domisse J. Critical care management of severe pre-eclampsia. Fetal Matern Med Rev 1994; 6:219–229.

77. Wallenburg HCS. Hemodynamics in hypertensive pregnancy. In: Rubin PC ed, Handbook of Hypertension. Vol. 21. Hypertension in Pregnancy. Amsterdam: Elsevier Science; 2000.

78. Wasserstrum N, Cotton DB. Hemodynamic monitoring in severe pregnancy-induced hypertension. Clin Perinatol 1986;13(4):781–799.

79. Richards AM, Moodley J, Graham DI, Bullock MRR. Active management of the unconscious eclamptic patient. Br J Obstet Gynaecol 1986; 93:554–562.

80. Visser W, Wallenburg HC. Temporizing management of severe preeclampsia with and without HELLP syndrome. Br J Obstet Gynaecol 1995; 102:111–117.

81. Allen RW, James MFM, Uys PC. Attenuation of the pressor response to intubation in hypertensive proteinuric pregnant patients by lignocaine, alfentanyl and magnesium sulphate. Br J Anaest 1991; 66:216–223.

82. Mabie WC, Barton JR, Sibai BM. Adult respiratory distress syndrome in pregnancy. Am J Obstet Gynecol 1992; 167:950–957.

83. Clark SL, Cotton DB. Clinical indications for pulmonary artery catheterisation in the patient with severe pre-eclampsia. Am J Obstet Gynecol 1988; 158:453–458.

84. Kirshon B, Lee W, Mauer MB, Cotton DB. Effects of low dose dopamine therapy in the oliguric patient with preeclampsia. Am J Obstet Gynecol 1988; 159:604–607.

85. Mantel G, Makin J. A double blind randomised controlled trial of the use of low dose dopamine in post partum pre-eclamptic or eclamptic women with oliguria. Presented at the 10th World Congress of the International Society for the Study of Hypertension in Pregnancy, Seattle, 1996.

86. Clark SL, Greenspoon JS, Aldahl D, Phelan JP. Severe preeclampsia with persistent oliguria: management of hemodynamic subsets. Am J Obstet Gynecol 1986; 154: 490–494.

87. Chandron R, Serra-Serra V, Redman CWG. Spontaneous resolution of pre-eclampsia related thrombocytopaenia. Br J Obstet Gynaecol 1992; 99:887–890

88. Kaplan MM. Acute fatty liver of pregnancy. N Engl J Med 1985; 313:367–370.

89. Atlas M, Barkai G, Menczer J, Houlu N, Lieberman P. Thrombotic thrombocytopaenic purpura in pregnancy. Br J Obstet Gynaecol 1982; 89:476–479.

90. Anthony J, Johanson RB, Duley L. Role of magnesium sulphate in seizure prevention in patients with eclampsia and pre-eclampsia. Drug Saf 1996; 15(3):188–199.

91. Reinhart RA. Clinical correlates of the molecular and cellular actions of magnesium on the cardiovascular system. Am Heart J 1991; 121:1513–1521.

92. Barton JR, Sibai BM, Ahokas RA, Whybrew WD, Mercer BM. Magnesium sulfate therapy in preeclampsia is associated with increased urinary cyclic guanosine monophosphate excretion. Am J Obstet Gynecol 1992; 167(4 Pt 1):931–934.

93. Fuentes A, Goldkrand JW. Angiotensin-converting enzyme activity in hypertensive subjects after magnesium sulfate therapy. Am J Obstet Gynecol 1987; 156(6):1375–1379.

94. Sipes SL, Weiner CP, Gellhaus TM, Goodspeed JD. The plasma renin-angiotensin system in preeclampsia: effects of magnesium sulfate. Obstet Gynecol 1989; 73(6):934–937.

95. Mastrogiamnis DS, Kalter CS, O'Brien WF, Carlan SJ, Reece EA. Effect of magnesium sulfate on plasma endothelin-1 levels in normal and preeclamptic pregnancies. Am J Obstet Gynecol 1992; 167(6):1554–1559.

96. Naidu S, Payne AJ, Moodley J, Hoffmann M, Gouws E. Randomised study assessing the effect of phenytoin and magnesium sulphate on the maternal cerebral circulation in eclampsia using transcranial doppler ultrasound. Br J Obstet Gynaecol 1996; 103(2):111–116.

97. Belfort MA, Moise KJ Jr. Effect of magnesium sulfate on maternal brain blood flow in preeclampsia: a randomized, placebo-controlled study. Am J Obstet Gynecol 1992; 67(3):661–666.

98. Belfort MA, Saade GR, Moise KJ Jr. The effect of magnesium sulfate on maternal retinal blood flow in preeclampsia: a randomized placebo-controlled study. Am J Obstet Gynecol 1992; 167(6):1548–1553.

99. Kulick DL, Hong R, Ryzen E, et al. Electrophysiologic effects of intravenous magnesium in patients with normal conduction systems and no clinical evidence of significant cardiac disease. Am Heart J 1988; 115(2):367–373.

100. Arsenian MA. Magnesium and cardiovascular disease. Prog Cardiovasc Dis 1993; 35(4):271–310.

101. Altura BT, Altura BM. Interactions of Mg and K on cerebral vessels—aspects in view of stroke. Review of present statutus and new findings. Magnesium 1984; 3(4–6):195–211.

102. de Jonge MC, Traber J. Nimodipine: cognition, aging, and degeneration. Clin Neuropharmacol 1999; 16(suppl 1):S25–S30.

103. Lipton SA, Rosenberg PA. Excitatory amino acids as a final common pathway for neurologic disorders. N Engl J Med 1994; 330:613–622.

104. Smith LG Jr, Burns PA, Schanler RJ. Calcium homeostasis in pregnant women receiving long-term magnesium sulfate therapy for preterm labor. Am J Obstet Gynecol 1992; 167(1):45–51.

105. Cruikshank DP, Chan GM, Doerrfeld D. Alterations in vitamin D and calcium metabolism with magnesium sulfate treatment of preeclampsia. Am J Obstet Gynecol 1993; 168(4):1170–1176.

106. Mordes JP, Wacker WC. Excess magnesium. Pharmacol Rev 1978; 29:273–300.

107. Ramanathan J, Sibai BM, Pillai R, Angel JJ. Neuromuscular transmission studies in preeclamptic women receiving magnesium sulfate. Am J Obstet Gynecol 1988; 158(1):40–46.

108. Pritchard JA. The use of magnesium sulfate in pre-eclampsia/eclampsia. J Reprod Med 1979; 23:107–111.

109. Sibai BM, Lipshitz J, Anderson GD, Dilts PV. Reassessment of intravenous MgSo4 therapy in preeclampsia–eclampsia. Obstet Gynecol 1981; 57:199–202.

110. Thurnau GR, Kemp DB, Jarvis A. Cerebrospinal fluid levels of magnesium in patients with preeclampsia after treatment with intravenous magnesium sulfate: a preliminary report. Am J Obstet Gynecol 1987; 157(6):1435–1438.

111. Richards A, Stather-Dunn L, Moodley J. Cardiopulmonary arrest after the administration of magnesium sulfate. a case report. S Afr Med J 1985; 67(4):145.

112. Swartjes JM, Schutte MF, Bleker OP. Management of eclampsia: cardiopulmonary arrest resulting from magnesium sulfate overdose. Eur J Obstet Gynecol Reprod Biol 1992; 47(1):73–75.

113. Ramanthan J, Sibai BM, Duggirala V, Maduska AL. Pulmonary function in preeclamptic women receiving MgSO4. J Reprod Med 1988; 33(5):432–435.

114. Herpolsheimer A, Brady K, Yancey MK, Pandian M, Duff P. Pulmonary function of preeclamptic women receiving intravenous magnesium sulfate prophylaxis. Obstet Gynecol 1991; 78(2):241–244.

115. Digre KB, Varner MW, Schiffman JS. Neuroophthalmologic effects of intravenous magnesium sulfate. Am J Obstet Gynecol 1990; 163(1):1848–1852.

116. Bashuk RG, Krendel DA. Myasthenia gravis presenting as weakness after magnesium administration. Muscle Nerve 1990; 13(8):708–712.

117. Ben-Ami M, Giladi Y, Shalev E. The combination of magnesium sulphate and nifedipine: a cause of neuromuscular blockade. Br J Obstet Gynaecol 1994; 101(3): 262–263.

118. Waisman GD, Mayorga LM, Camera MI, Vignola CA. Magnesium plus nifedipine: potentiation of hypotensive effect in preeclampsia? Am J Obstet Gynecol 1988; 159 (2):308–309.

119. Bhalla AK, Dhall GI, Dhall K. A safer and more effective treatment regimen for eclampsia. Aust NZ J Obstet Gynaecol 1994; 34(2):144–148.

120. Kabam JR, Perry SM, Entman S, Smith BE. Effect of magnesium on plasma cholinesterase activity. Am J Obstet Gynecol 1988; 159 (2):309–311.

121. James MF, Schenk PA, van der Veen BW. Priming of pancuronium with magnesium. Br J Anaest 1991; 66(2):247–249.

122. Fuchs-Buder T, Wilder-Smith OH, Borgeat A, Tassonyi E. Interaction of magnesium sulfate with vecuronium-induced neuromuscular block. Br J Anaest 1995; 74(4): 405–409.

123. James MF, Cork RC, Dennet JE. Succinylcholine pretreatment with magnesium sulfate. Anesth Analg 1986; 65(4):373–376.

124. Hankins GD, Hammond TL, Yeomans ER. Amniotic cavity accumulation of magne-

sium with prolonged magnesium sulfate tocolysis. J Reprod Med 1991; 36(6): 446–449.

125. Santi MD, Henry GW, Douglas GL. Magnesium sulfate treatment of preterm labor as a cause of abnormal neonatal bone mineralization. J Pediat Orthop 1994; 14(2): 249–253.

126. Sherer DM. Blunted fetal response to vibroacoustic stimulation associated with maternal intravenous magnesium sulfate therapy. Am J Perinatol 1994; 11(6): 401–403.

127. Peaceman AM, Meyer BA, Thorp JA, Parisi VM, Creasy RK. The effect of magnesium sulfate tocolysis on the fetal biophysical profile. Am J Obstet Gynecol 1989; 161(3):771–774.

128. Lin CC, Pielet BW, Poon E, Sun G. Effect of magnesium sulfate on fetal heart rate variability in preeclamptic patients during labor. Am J Perinatol 1988; 5(3):208–213.

129. Rall TW, Schleifer LS. Drugs effective in the therapy of the epilepsies. In: Goodman AG, Rall TW, Nies AS, Taylor P, eds. Goodman and Gilman's The Pharmacological Basis of Therapeutics, 8th ed. New York: Pergamon Press; 1990: 426–444.

130. Hayes G, Kootsikas ME. Reassessing the lower end of the phenytoin therapeutic range: a review of the literature. Ann Pharmacother 1993; 27(11):1389–1392.

131. Hopkins A. Neurological disorders. In: de Swiet M, ed. Medical Disorders in Obstetric Practice, 2nd ed. Oxford, London, Edinburgh, Boston, Melbourne: Blackwell Scientific; 1989: 737–746.

132. Robson SC, Redfern N, Seviour J, Campbell M, Walkinshaw S, Rodeck C, de Swiet M. Phenytoin prophylaxis in severe pre-eclampsia and eclampsia. Br J Obstet Gynaecol 1993; 10(7):623–628.

133. Lin MS, McNay JL, Shepherd AM, Musgrave GE, Keeton TK. Increased plasma norepinephrine accompanies persistent tachycardia after hydralazine. Hypertension 1983; 5:257–263.

134. Snyder SW, Cardwell MS. Neuromuscular blockade with magnesium sulfate and nifedipine. Am J Obstet Gynecol 1989; 161(1):35–46.

135. Belfort MA, Carpenter RJ Jr, Kirshon B, Saade GR, Moise KJ Jr. The use of nimodipine in a patient with eclampsia: color flow Doppler demonstration of retinal artery relaxation. Am J Obstet Gynecol 1993; 169(1):204–206.

136. Anthony J, Mantel G, Johanson R, Dommisse J. The haemodynamic and respiratory effects of intravenous nimodipine used in the treatment of eclampsia. Br J Obstet Gynaecol 1996; 103(6):518–522.

137. Hongo K, Kobayashi S. Calcium antagonists for the treatment of vasospasm following subarachnoid haemorrhage. Neurol Res 1993; 15(4):218–224.

138. Horn EH, Filshie M, Kerslake RW, Jaspan T, Worthington BS, Rubin PC. Widespread cerebral ischemia treated with nimodipine in a patient with eclampsia. Br Med J 1990; 301(6755):794.

139. Disterhoft JF, Moyer JR Jr, Thompson LT, Kowalska M. Functional aspects of calcium-channel modulation. Clin Neuropharmacol 1993; 16(suppl 1):S12–S24.

140. Bhorat IE, Naidoo DP, Rout CC, Moodley J. Malignant ventricular arrhythmias in eclampsia: a comparison of labetolol with dihydralazine. Am J Obstet Gynecol 1993; 168(4):1292–1296.

141. Stevens TP, Guillet R. Use of glucagon to treat neonatal low-output congestive heart failure after maternal labetalol therapy. J Pediatr 1995; 127(1):151–153.

142. Cotton DB, Johnes MM, Longmire S, Dorman KF, Tessem J, Joyce TH. Role of intravenous nitroglycerin in the treatment of severe pregnancy-induced hypertension complicated by pulmonary edema. Am J Obstet Gynecol 1986; 154:91–93.
143. Neumark J. Anaesthesia for caesarean section. Curr Opin Anaest 1996; 9:202–206.
144. Natarajan P, Shennan AH, Penny JA, Halligan AW, De Swiet M, Anthony J. Comparison of an auscultatory and oscillometric automated blood pressure monitor in the setting of pre-eclampsia. Am J Obstet Gynecol 1999; 181(5):1203–1210.
145. Pulmonary Artery Catheter Consensus Conference: Consensus Statement. Crit Care Med 1997; 24:910–925.
146. Gilbert WM, Towner DR, Field NT, Anthony J. The safety and utility of pulmonary artery catheterization in severe pre-eclampsia/eclampsia. Am J Obstet Gynecol 2000; 182:1397–1403.
147. Penny JA, Anthony J, Shennan AH, De Swiet M, Singer M. A comparison of hemodynamic data derived by pulmonary flotation catheter and the esophageal Doppler monitor. Am J Obstet Gynecol 2000; 183:658–661.
148. Le Gall J, Loirat P, Alperovitch A, et al. A simplified acute physiology score for ICU patients. Crit Care Med 1984; 12:975–977.
149. Wagner D, Draper E, Knaus W. APACHE III study design: analytic plan for evaluation of severity and outcome in intensive care unit patients. Development of APACHE III. Crit Care Med 1989; 17:s199–s203.
150. Le Gall JR, Klar J, Lemeshow S, et al. The Logistic Organ Dysfunction system: a new way to assess organ dysfunction in the intensive care unit: ICU Scoring Group. JAMA 1996; 276:802–810.
151. Bhagwanjee S. ICU Considerations in pre-eclampsia/eclampsia. In: Care of the Critically Ill Pregnant Patient: 1999 Refresher Course. Department of Anaesthesia, University of Natal.

13

Echocardiography and Pregnancy: A Simple, Rational Approach to Assessing Central Hemodynamics

Roxann Rokey
University of Wisconsin, Madison, and Marshfield Clinic, Marshfield, Wisconsin, U.S.A.

Michael A. Belfort
University of Utah Health Sciences Center, Salt Lake City, and Utah Valley Regional Medical Center, Provo, Utah, U.S.A.

Echocardiography is a powerful noninvasive tool that can be used in the evaluation and management of pregnant women with known or suspected cardiac disease. In this chapter we show that in addition, this modality can be used to evaluate the central hemodynamics of pregnant women with preeclampsia, oliguria, and/or cardiac failure. In this context, we demonstrate that with a little training and experience, the practicing obstetrician can master the rudiments of echocardiography to the extent that the state of filling of the vasculature, the cardiac output, the ejection fraction, and the peripheral vascular resistance can be assessed. This information can be invaluable in an obstetrical setting when it is important to know the state of filling of the vasculature or the status of cardiac function in order to make a decision regarding fluid therapy. Since most pregnant women have a healthy myocardium, it is often unnecessarily invasive to place a pulmonary artery catheter simply to determine whether the patient can tolerate a further fluid bolus infusion to treat oliguria. Under most circumstances a single evaluation of the state of vascular filling and of the cardiac function is sufficient to allow therapeutic adjustments and to eliminate the need for invasive hemodynamic monitoring. Thus, a knowledge of evaluation of the maternal heart and inferior vena cava is of significant value to the clinician. Since most recently trained obstetricians, and many who trained prior to the general availability of ultrasound, have now acquired fetal imaging skills, the learning curve for maternal functional echocardiography is relatively steep.

Two-dimensional, M-mode, and Doppler echocardiography are used in concert to produce clinically relevant information. The terminology and imaging information have been defined by the American Society of Echocardiography and are not reviewed here. Instead, the basic information that is needed for acquisition and interpretation of data is presented. The fundamental intention of this chapter is to explain the utility of this methodology for the rapid assessment of basic cardiac function and selected central hemodynamic parameters, and to indicate how it may be introduced into the clinical practice of those involved in the care of preeclamptic women.

I. TWO-DIMENSIONAL ECHOCARDIOGRAPHY

Two-dimensional echocardiography is the mainstay of cardiac imaging of the pregnant patient. The imaging positions used are similar to those used for other studies such as M-mode and Doppler echocardiography, with minor modifications for preventing the supine hypotension syndrome (aortocaval compression). In general, the patient is placed in the left lateral decubitus position at about a 30-degree angle in order to move the heart closer to the chest wall. This position varies, depending on the individual. It is sometimes useful to raise the patient's left arm above her head to allow better access to her chest wall. Since in most cases obstetrical suites are not equipped with cardiac imaging tables (which have a cut-out that allows easier access to the chest wall), it may be necessary to move the patient close to the edge of the bed so that her left side projects over the edge. In this way access to the lateral chest wall is improved.

In the adult patient, higher-frequency transducers generally produce the best images (3–5 MHz). The images are optimally obtained when the ultrasound beam is oriented perpendicularly to the cardiac structures. The two basic transducer positions are the parasternal and apical windows (Figures 1–5) (1,2).

In the parasternal view, the images acquired include the parasternal long axis (Figure 1) and parasternal short axis (Figure 2) views. The parasternal long axis is parallel to, and the parasternal short axis is perpendicular to, the long axis of the heart. In these views, the aortic valve can be best visualized, as can the left and right ventricular outflow tract, and the tricuspid and pulmonic valves. The left ventricular and atrial sizes are well defined through these windows as well. The posterior and septal wall motion is also easily visualized.

In order to obtain the parasternal images, the transducer is placed between the third and fourth intercostal spaces just along the left parasternal border. The transducer is rotated and tipped until the image in Figure 1 is obtained. Ideally the apex of the left ventricle is horizontally aligned at a 0-degree angulation. Further

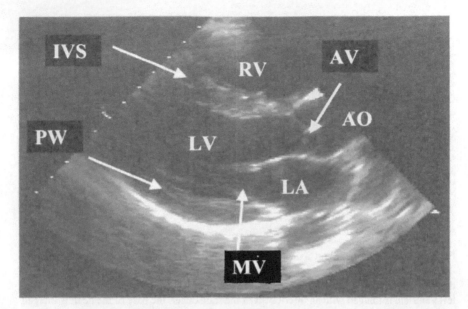

Figure 1 Parasternal long-axis echocardiographic image. Images are acquired as described in the text. In this view, the aortic/mitral valves, size of three cardiac chambers, and interventricular/posterior walls can be seen. RV = right ventricle; IVS = interventricular septum; LV = left ventricle; PW = posterior wall; AO = aorta, AV = aortic valve; MV = mitral valve.

adjustments are made to obtain this alignment by moving the transducer either toward or away from the sternum and up or down an interspace. Additionally, a slight clockwise or counterclockwise rotation of the transducer results in a more modified four-chamber "off-axis" view, depending on the initial placement of the transducer. A common error in obtaining the parasternal long axis image is made by placing the transducer at a position that is too low and lateral, yielding an "off-axis" four-chamber view. The apex of the heart is shown in a vertical position. However, because there are multiple anatomical variants, even one's best attempts to obtain the true alignment of the heart in the parasternal long axis view may not allow acquisition of an ideal image.

Once the parasternal long axis view is obtained, rotation of the transducer in a clockwise manner allows the parasternal short axis to become visible. In this view the left ventricle can be identified usually as a circular structure in the center of the image (Figure 2, left panel). With inferior angulation of the transducer, a more apical view of the left ventricle is seen. Superior angulation yields images of the heart base with the aorta and aortic valves shown as a central circle (Figure 2, right panel).

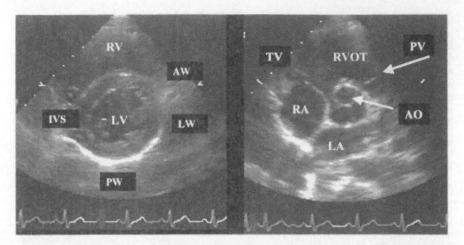

Figure 2 Parasternal short-axis echocardiographic images. After the parasternal long
-axis image is optimized, rotation of the transducer through 90 degrees allows imaging of
the heart in the short-axis plane at the level of the left ventricle. The more distal aspect of the
left ventricle is imaged with an inferior tilt of the transducer; the base of the heart is imaged
with superior tilt of the transducer. The left ventricle at the level of the papillary muscles is
depicted in the left panel, and the base of the heart in the right panel. RV = right ventricle;
LV = left ventricle; AW = anterior wall; LW = lateral wall; PW = posterior wall; IVS =
interventricular septum; AO = aorta; RVOT = right ventricular outflow tract; PV = pulmonic valve; TV = tricuspid valve; LA = left atrium.

Echocardiographic images showing all four chambers of the heart can be
visualized through the apical window. Via the apical window, four-chamber, five-
chamber, and two-chamber views can be acquired for evaluation of cardiac valve
morphological characteristics, chamber sizes, and wall motion. Both the right and
left ventricles and atria are seen in the apical four-chamber view. The mitral and
tricuspid valves as well as the septal, lateral, and apical walls of the ventricles are
also assessed in this view (Figure 3). To obtain the apical four-chamber view, the
transducer is placed at the apex of the heart with a slight upward tilt. The standard
view of the heart in adults is presented with the apex pointing toward the top of the
screen and the atria toward the bottom. The left ventricle is generally to the right.
The left ventricle has more myocardial mass and in normal patients is easily
recognized as such. If this left-right orientation is not seen, then the transducer is
rotated 180 degrees. In the apical four-chamber view, both ventricles, atria,
ventricular septum, left ventricular lateral wall, and apex are well visualized.

From the four-chamber view, with sight anterior angulation of the transducer, the apical five-chamber view can be acquired, and the left ventricular
outflow and aortic valve can be better observed (Figure 4). Moving the transducer

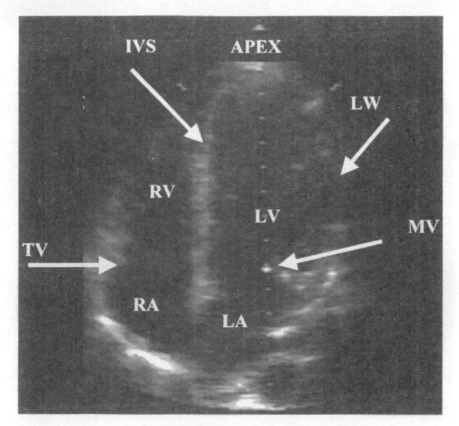

Figure 3   Apical four-chamber echocardiographic image. To obtain the apical four-chamber view, the transducer is placed at the apex of the heart with a slight upward tilt. In the standard view of the heart in adults the apex points toward the top and the atria towards the bottom of the screen. Suggestions for adjustments necessary to acquire an optimal image are described in the text. RV = right ventricle; LV = left ventricle; IVS = interventricular septum; LW = lateral wall; TV = tricuspid valve; MV = mitral valve.

back to the optimal plane for four-chamber imaging and then rotating 90 degrees puts the left ventricle, left atrium, apical anterior, and inferior walls in view (Figure 5).

For complete echocardiographic imaging, additional transducer positions and views are necessary. However, the two basic imaging positions described provide sufficient information to allow most management decisions required in the treatment of the preeclamptic patient.

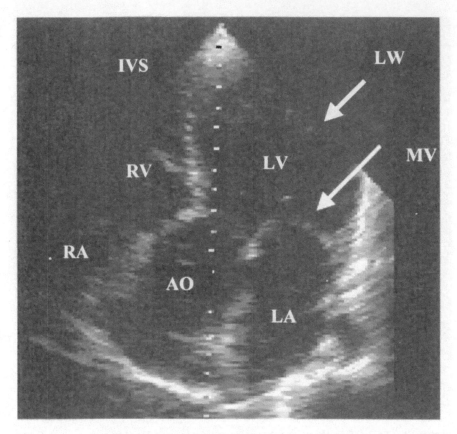

Figure 4 Apical five-chamber echocardiographic image. From the apical four-chamber image, slight superior angulation of the transducer draws the aorta and left ventricular outflow tract into view. The more anterior aspects of the interventricular septum and lateral wall are also seen in this view. RV = right ventricle; LV = left ventricle; IVS = interventricular septum; LW = lateral wall; AO = aorta; MV = mitral valve; LA = left atrium; RA = right atrium.

II. M-MODE ECHOCARDIOGRAPHY

The M-mode echocardiographic imaging technique is ancillary to the two-dimensional imaging procedure and involves using the two-dimensional image as a reference. The M-mode images are obtained primarily in the parasternal views. The technique is superior in its temporal resolution and subsequent ability to visualize movement of the cardiac valves and wall motion. In pregnancy we have found it useful for evaluation of the chamber sizes and wall motion and for

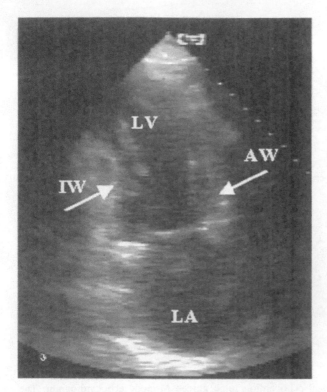

Figure 5 Apical two-chamber view. Once the apical four-chamber view is optimized, a 90-degree rotation of the transducer yields this view. The inferior and anterior and apical walls are observed. The left ventricle and atrium are also seen. IW = inferior wall; AW = anterior wall; LV = left ventricle; LA = left atrium.

estimation of ejection fraction when the apical views are technically difficult to analyze (Figure 6). A thorough review of M-mode echocardiography is, however, beyond the scope of this chapter.

III. DOPPLER ECHOCARDIOGRAPHY

The Doppler echocardiographic technique provides qualitative and quantitative information about intracardiac blood velocity. From this, intracardiac pressures, valve dynamics, and other additional information can be obtained. With Doppler echocardiographic evaluation, the best results are obtained with a lower-frequency transducer than is used when structural detail is important. In order to evaluate

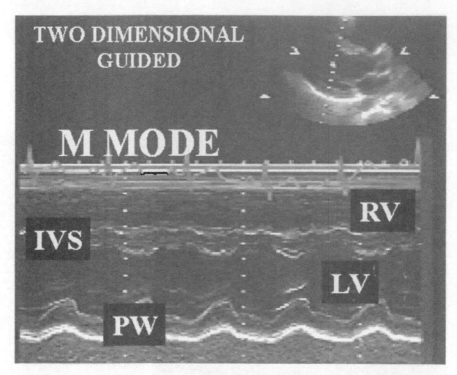

Figure 6 Two-dimensional echocardiographic guided M-mode echocardiogram. The parasternal long-axis view (upper right) is used to guide the M-mode. The structures on the M-mode follow the anterior-posterior structures seen on the parasternal two-dimensional image. RV = right ventricle; LV = left ventricle; IVS = interventricular septum; PW = posterior wall.

and quantitate flow best, the ultrasound beam is oriented parallel to the column of blood being evaluated. This avoids the error introduced by the angle of insonation and subsequent division by the Cos θ (which is contained in the denominator of the Doppler shift equation).

Continuous wave Doppler produces an ultrasound beam that is much better suited to the measurement of high-velocity signals than pulsed Doppler ultrasound. It cannot localize a signal from a specific location as can pulsed Doppler ultrasound, but allows the highest velocity signal within the entire ultrasound beam to be detected (Figure 7). Pulsed Doppler provides short bursts of ultrasound and allows localization of the signal as well as quantitation of flow. This allows discrimination among multiple signals since the operator is able to place the cursor within the area of interest and exclude interference from others in the near

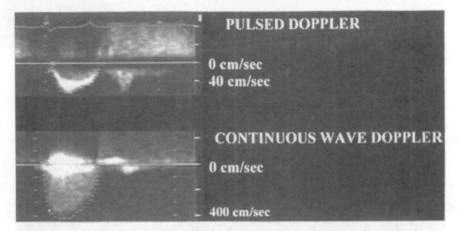

PULSED DOPPLER

0 cm/sec
40 cm/sec

CONTINUOUS WAVE DOPPLER

0 cm/sec

400 cm/sec

Figure 7 Difference between pulsed and continuous wave Doppler. By using pulsed wave Doppler, flow and volume may often be obtained since the velocities are low enough and the signal is acquired in a specific location. However, if velocities are too high, as can often be seen with aortic stenosis, mitral/ tricuspid regurgitation, or other disease states, the technique is unable to discriminate velocities accurately and pressure calculations are inaccurate. Continuous wave Doppler provides an alternative method for calculation of velocities since it is ideal in detection of high velocities that cannot be detected with the pulsed Doppler technique. However, the continuous method of velocity detection prevents accurate localization of the Doppler signal. Shown here is a pulsed Doppler sample from the left ventricular outflow tract with maximal velocities of about 70 cm/s. The continuous wave Doppler detects higher velocities (which are not seen with pulsed Doppler).

proximity. However, if the velocity of the flow is too high with pulsed Doppler, turbulence is observed and accurate quantitation of intracardiac pressures is not feasible (Figure 7). Thus the choice of the type of Doppler ultrasound most suitable in any particular situation depends on the anticipated velocity of the blood and the need for accurate range discrimination.

Color Doppler is a variant of pulsed Doppler ultrasound. Multiple pulsed scan lines are superimposed on a two-dimensional image with a color assigned to identify the direction of blood flow. Commonly, flow toward a transducer is coded red, and that away from the transducer is blue. When flow is turbulent, or the velocity is too high to discriminate velocities, then the flow appears as a mosaic of colors (Figure 8).

In the Doppler examination, color Doppler imaging is helpful in identifying turbulent blood flow and direction of flow. In the pregnant woman, pulsed and continuous wave Doppler are commonly used to evaluate intracardiac hemo-dynamics, stroke volume. and valve area.

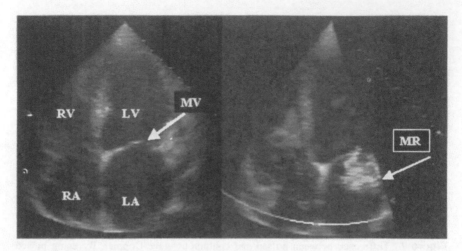

Figure 8 Color Doppler image of mitral regurgitation. An apical four-chamber view of ventricular systole is seen on the left (mitral valve leaflets are closed). Color Doppler is superimposed on the two-dimensional image. When flow is turbulent or the velocity is too high to allow discrimination of velocities, then the flow appears as a mosaic of colors. In this example, the mitral regurgitation that occurs during systole causes a mosaic of colors. RV = right ventricle; LV = left ventricle; LA = left atrium; RA = right atrium; MV = mitral valve; MR = mitral regurgitation.

A. Hemodynamic Measurements

1. Stroke Volume

Stroke volume through a valve can be estimated as the product of the orifice cross-sectional area and the integral of the pulsed Doppler inflow signal or time velocity integral (TVI). The stroke volume calculation is easily obtained by using software packages on most echocardiographic machines. Stroke volume can be measured at any annular orifice but is most accurate in the left ventricular outflow site and aortic annulus. The aortic diameter is measured in the parasternal long-axis view (Figure 9) at the level of the aortic valve annulus. The cursors should be placed at the insertion of the aortic valve leaflets during maximal systole in order to ensure the most accurate reading. Most normal pregnant women have an aortic annulus diameter in the range of 1.8 to 2.2 cm. The aortic annulus area is subsequently calculated by using the formula for area of a circle (πr^2). Most normal pregnant women have an aortic annulus area of 2.54 to 3.80 cm^2. If significant chronic aortic valvular regurgitation, dilatation of the aortic root, or congenital stenotic lesions is present, the annulus size and area may be larger.

The stroke volume is calculated by multiplying the annulus area by the TVI

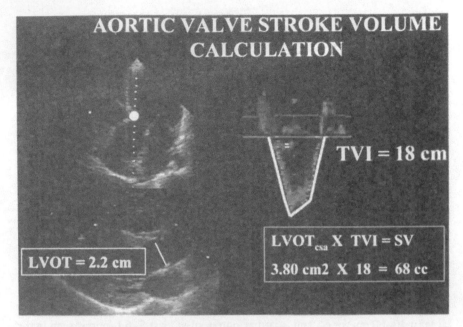

AORTIC VALVE STROKE VOLUME CALCULATION

TVI = 18 cm

LVOT = 2.2 cm

LVOT$_{csa}$ X TVI = SV

3.80 cm2 X 18 = 68 cc

Figure 9 Left ventricular outflow tract stroke volume calculation (aortic valve stroke volume). In the absence of significant valvular insufficiency, stroke volume through any particular valve can be calculated by the formula SV = CSA × TVI, where SV = stroke volume; CSA = cross-sectional area; TVI = time velocity integral. For estimates of left ventricular stroke volume, the CSA of the left ventricular outflow tract (LVOT) and TVI in the LVOT are obtained. The diameter of the aortic annulus is measured in the parasternal long-axis view at the aortic leaflet insertion (lower left panel). This diameter is used to calculate LVOT CSA. The LVOT TVI is obtained by using pulsed-wave Doppler in the left ventricular outflow tract at a level just below the aortic leaflets (upper left panel). The resulting signal is outlined with commercially available software to obtain the TVI. The stroke volume is the product of the cross-sectional area and the TVI.

of the Doppler waveform generated by blood leaving the heart in systole. The Doppler waveform is acquired by placing the cursor within the left ventricular outflow tract (LVOT) as seen in the apical five-chamber view (Figure 9). The signal generated by the movement of blood out of the heart has a characteristic waveform shape that can be easily distinguished from other systolic signals. It is triangular in shape, peaks relatively early in the cycle, and occupies only the period of systolic ejection (Figure 9). It is important to obtain the optimal outflow tract waveform signal, and this can be done by ensuring that the Doppler sample volume is aligned parallel to the direction of blood flow and placed within 1 cm of the aortic valve leaflet insertion in the five-chamber view. Error in subsequent quantitative measurements using an incorrect signal can be introduced when the signal obtained is not parallel to the direction of flow, when the sample volume is too low in the left ventricle, or when in the presence of aortic stenosis, the sample volume is placed too close to the aortic valve leaflets. The latter error results in detection of accelerating velocities and a suboptimal waveform. Other systolic events that may be detected with pulsed wave Doppler such as mitral/tricuspid regurgitation, ventricular septal defects, or abnormal flow from hypertrophic cardiomyopathy are usually quite turbulent with very high velocities. Pulsed Doppler of these abnormalities does not yield the characteristic waveform from the left ventricular outflow tract as described. Once the correct LVOT waveform is identified, different methods can be used to calculate the TVI. By far the easiest of these methods is to use the software supplied in most cardiac calculation packages. By simply outlining the waveform and pushing a button, the TVI is displayed on the ultrasound screen. The stroke volume (SV) is defined by the formula SV (cm^3 or cc) = VTI (cm) × annulus area (cm^2). In the absence of significant regurgitation, the stroke volume multiplied by the heart rate is equivalent to the cardiac output (Figure 9). Although there is variation of stroke volume and cardiac output during pregnancy, typically a VTI of at least 16–18 cm, a stroke volume of at least 40–60 cm^3 or cc, and a cardiac output of at least 5–6 L/min is seen in the normal pregnant patient early in the first trimester of pregnancy

2.   Calculating Stroke Volume of Other Valves

Occasionally, calculation of stroke volume from other cardiac valves is necessary. The technique of determining stroke volume at the pulmonic, tricuspid, or mitral valves is similar to that employed at the aortic valve. Several studies have shown that the measurement of stroke volume from these locations is similar but most accurate in descending order for the aortic, pulmonic, mitral, and tricuspid locations. For measurement of stroke volume from the pulmonic, mitral, and tricuspid valves, the basic concept of measuring annulus diameter and acquiring the pulsed sample volume at the annulus is similar. However, there are some differences. For these valves, annulus measurement and pulsed Doppler acquisition are in the same location. In the pulmonic location, the two-dimensional image and Doppler acquisition are in the short-axis view at the base of the heart, where the pulmonary artery appears as a vertical structure. The annulus measurement is obtained at or just proximal to the pulmonic valve leaflet insertion in maximal systole. The pulsed Doppler signal is attained by placing the sample volume at the same location centrally and parallel to the direction of flow (Figure 10). For the mitral and tricuspid valves, the measurement of annulus diameter is made during maximal diastole with the leaflets widely open. The pulsed Doppler sample is placed centrally within the annulus and parallel to the direction of blood flow (Figure 11).

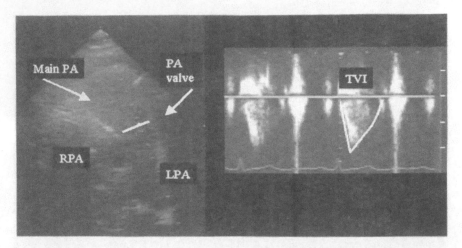

Figure 10 Pulmonary artery stroke volume. In the absence of significant valvular insufficiency or shunt, stroke volume should be similar through each cardiac valve and the calculation of this value is as described in Figure 9. The diameter of the pulmonary artery annulus (solid line) is measured during systole, and from this value, the cross-sectional area is determined (left panel). The pulsed wave Doppler sample volume is placed at the annulus parallel to flow and in the center of the lumen (right panel). The resultant signal is processed to determine TVI. The product of the CSA and TVI yields stroke volume, as described in Figure 9. PA = pulmonary artery; LPA = left pulmonary artery; RPA = right pulmonary artery; TVI = time velocity integral.

3. Valve Regurgitation

Mitral or aortic regurgitation severity can be calculated from knowing the stroke volume of a normal valve and the stroke volume of the regurgitant valve. This requires assessment of SV at two sites. For example, if the patient has a regurgitant mitral valve and a normal aortic valve, these two valves can be used. The difference yields regurgitant volume: regurgitant volume = SV (normal valve) − SV (regurgitant valve).

Regurgitant orifice area is calculated when regurgitant volume is divided by the time velocity integral of the regurgitant jet: regurgitant orifice area = SV (normal valve) − SV (regurgitant valve)/TVI (regurgitant valve).

The regurgitant fraction of the regurgitant valve is the quotient of regurgitant volume divided by the regurgitant valvular stroke volume multiplied by 100:

regurgitant fraction = regurgitant volume/SV (regurgitant valve) × 100.

Regurgitant orifice area and regurgitant volume are also assessed by using color and continuous wave Doppler.

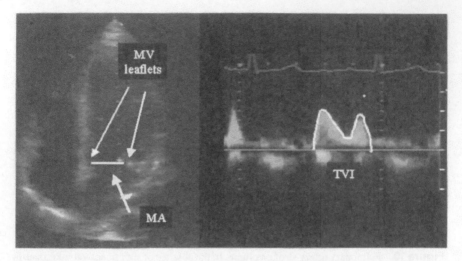

Figure 11 Mitral valve stroke volume. Stroke volume through the mitral and tricuspid valves requires annulus measurement during diastole. A two-dimensional image is acquired during diastole and the diameter is measured at the leaflet insertion site (solid line) (left panel). The pulsed Doppler sample volume is placed at this location, ideally centrally and parallel to inflow. The TVI of the Doppler signal (right panel) is obtained and, when multiplied by the cross-sectional area, gives the mitral valve stroke volume. MA = mitral annulus; TVI = time velocity integral; MV = mitral valve.

4. Pressure Measurements

a. Right Atrial Pressure

Estimates of right atrial pressure (RAP) in nonpregnant patients are obtained by measuring the maximal and minimal sizes of the inferior vena cava during inspiration and expiration. Because the gravid uterus can affect the size of the inferior vena cava (IVC), estimation of right atrial pressure may not be accurate unless the patient is tilted to one or the other side to prevent the aortocaval compression syndrome. Estimates specifically designed for pregnant women have been published (1).

The technique of imaging the IVC is as follows: The transducer should be placed above the fundus of the uterus and angled toward the heart. The IVC can be identified beneath the liver coursing toward the right atrium (RA). The correct region in which to measure the diameter is the first 2 to 3 cm of the IVC below the right atrial confluence (Figure 12). If the measurement is too close to the RA, the diameter is overestimated and the RAP is artificially high. If the measurement is too far from the RA, the diameter of the IVC is too small and the RAP is underestimated. Once the correct region of the IVC is identified, the patient should

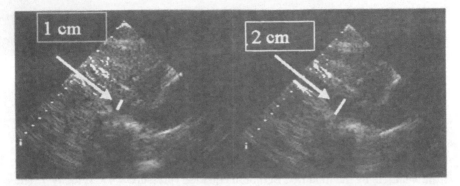

Figure 12 Estimation of right atrial pressure for pulmonary artery systolic pressure measurement for pregnant women has been previously reported and is reflected by the size of the inferior vena cava during inspiration and expiration. If the inferior vena cava size is normal in expiration (≤2.5 cm) and reduced by 50% during inspiration, right atrial pressure is considered to be normal (0–5 mmHg.) If the inferior vena cava size is ≤2.5 cm and not reduced by 50% during inspiration, right atrial pressure is considered to be 6–10 mmHg. When the inferior vena cava size is >2.5 cm and reduced by ≥50% during inspiration, right atrial pressure is assigned a value of 11–15 mmHg. A right atrial pressure of 20 mmHg is assumed if the inferior vena cava diameter is more than 2.5 cm throughout the respiratory cycle.

be asked to inhale sharply through the nose. This allows measurement of the IVC diameter during expiration and inspiration.

 If the inferior vena caval diameter is normal in expiration (≤ 2.5 cm) and is reduced by 50% during inspiration, right atrial pressure is considered to be 0 to 5 mmHg. If the inferior vena cava size is ≤ 2.5 cm but not reduced by 50% during inspiration, right atrial pressure is considered to be 6 to 10 mmHg. When the inferior vena cava size is > 2.5 cm and is reduced by ≥ 50% during inspiration, right atrial pressure is assigned a value of 11 to 15 mmHg. A right atrial pressure of 20 mmHg is assumed if the inferior vena caval diameter is more than 2.5 cm throughout the respiratory cycle (see Table 1 and Figure 12).

b. Pulmonary Artery Pressure

The pressure difference between two regions is obtained by using the modified Bernoulli equation, where $P = 4(V^2)$. This information is vital in the determination of the pulmonary artery systolic pressure and is also used to estimate valve area and chamber pressures (discussed later).

 Both Doppler and two-dimensional measurements are usually obtained to estimate pulmonary artery systolic pressure. In this estimation the peak velocity of the tricuspid regurgitant jet can be converted to reflect the peak pressure within the

Table 1 Central Venous Pressure

Starting diameter	Inspiration decrease in diameters	Estimated CVP
< 2.5 cm	> 50%	0–5 mmHg
	≤ 50%	6–10 mmHg
> 2.5 cm	> 50%	11–15 mmHg
	≤ 50%	12–20 mmHg
> 2.5 cm	No change	> 20 mmHg

right ventricle by the modified Bernoulli equation (pressure $= 4 \times$ velocity^2). The tricuspid regurgitant jet is identified as a jet of turbulent flow seen escaping between the closed valve leaflets during systole. With color Doppler, this is shown as a burst of mosaic color indicating high velocity (Figure 13). The continuous wave Doppler cursor is placed in alignment as parallel as possible to the regurgitant flow, and the peak velocity of the resultant waveform is measured (Figure 14). Common errors in this technique include acquisition of a suboptimal signal so that the true peak velocity is not measured and acquisition of the signal at an angle greater than 20 degrees parallel to the direction of flow. Another common error is

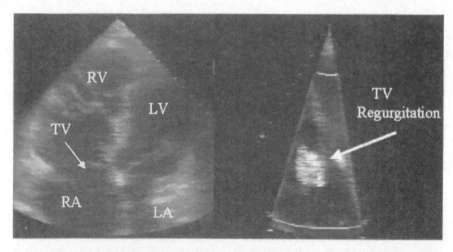

Figure 13 Estimation of pulmonary artery systolic pressure. Several methods are used to measure pulmonary artery systolic pressure. The easiest is that employing the tricuspid regurgitant jet. The two-dimensional echocardiographic image is acquired (left panel) and then color Doppler is applied to determine when regurgitation is present in that field (right panel). RV = right ventricle; LV = left ventricle; LA = left atrium; RA = right atrium; TV = tricuspid valve.

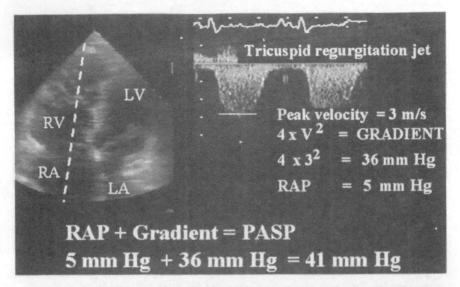

Figure 14 Estimation of pulmonary artery systolic pressure. With this method, both Doppler and two-dimensional measurements are required to estimate pulmonary artery systolic pressure. In this estimation, the peak velocity of the tricuspid regurgitant jet is converted to reflect the peak pressure within the right ventricle by using the modified Bernoulli equation (pressure = 4 × peak velocity^2). The continuous wave Doppler is used to examine the tricuspid valve/right atrial area for peak regurgitant velocities (left panel). From the signal obtained, an estimate of right ventricular systolic pressure is made by the modified Bernoulli equation. Pulmonary artery systolic pressure is determined as the sum of right atrial pressure (Figure 12) and right ventricular pressure. RV = right ventricle; LV = left ventricle; LA = left atrium; RA = right atrium; RAP = right atrial pressure; PASP = pulmonary artery systolic pressure; V = velocity.

sole reliance on color flow to place the continuous wave Doppler. The color should be used as a guide, but the continuous wave Doppler should be moved about slightly to ensure that the optimal signal is acquired.

The regurgitant jet must initially overcome the right atrial pressure before it can penetrate the right atrium. Therefore, in order to estimate the pulmonary artery pressure, the calculated pressure from the regurgitant jet $[P = 4(V^2)]$ must be added to the right atrial pressure (PA pressure = $4V^2 + RAP$)

5. Valve Area

Valve area can be calculated in a number of ways. The most common left-sided stenotic lesion in pregnant women in the United States is in the aortic position. Knowledge of valve area and gradient across the valve is extremely important

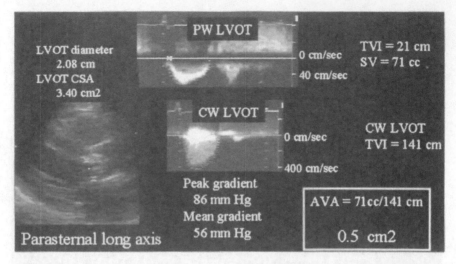

Figure 15 Aortic valve area calculation using two-dimensional and pulsed/continuous wave Doppler. Stroke volume is first calculated by using left ventricular outflow tract dimension and pulsed wave Doppler. Continuous wave Doppler of the aortic outflow velocity is also acquired. Using these data, aortic valve area is mathematically derived. In this example, the aortic valve area is 0.5 cm². $CSA_{LVOT} \times TVI_{LVOT}/TVI_{AV} = CSA_{AV}$, where SV = stroke volume; LVOT = left ventricular outflow tract; AV = aortic valve; TVI = time velocity integral; CSA = cross-sectional area; PW = pulsed wave; CW = continuous wave; other abbreviations as previously.

information in management decisions of the pregnant woman. Doppler echocardiography allows estimation of both parameters (Figure 15). Unfortunately, the simple formula $CSA_{AV} \times TVI_{AV}$ is inaccurate because the flow detected after passing the aortic valve is quite turbulent. As the flow through the stenotic valve emerges, the velocities substantially increase and peak and mean velocities can usually only be detected by continuous wave Doppler. Because these velocities represent turbulence, the simple formula $CSA_{AV} \times TVI_{AV}$ is not accurate for calculating aortic valve area. With transthoracic echocardiography, CSA of the aortic valve is calculated by using the Doppler-continuity equation. In simplest terms, stroke volume is equivalent immediately before and after a stenotic valve. Doppler echocardiography takes advantage of this condition since the formula for the estimation of stroke volume is known (CSA × TVI) both before and after the stenotic lesion and Doppler/two-dimensional echocardiography provides three of the four values (CSA_{LVOT}, TVI_{LVOT}, and TVI_{AV}) (Figure 15). Calculation of stroke volume in the left ventricular outflow tract has been discussed earlier (Figure 9). The TVI_{AV} is obtained with continuous wave Doppler through the aortic valve, usually in the five-chamber view. The one remaining variable, CSA_{AV}, is a mathematically derived value.

$$SV_{LVOT} = SV_{AV}$$

$$CSA_{LVOT} \times TVI_{LVOT} = CSA_{AV} \times TVI_{AV}$$

$$(CSA_{LVOT} \times TVI_{LVOT})/TVI_{AV} = CSA_{AV}$$

Where SV = stroke volume; LVOT = left ventricular outflow tract; AV = aortic valve; TVI = time velocity integral; and CSA = cross-sectional area.

Aortic valve area may also be calculated by using the peak velocities of the pulsed wave and continuous wave Doppler as well.

Peak and mean pressure gradients across the aortic valve are obtained from continuous wave Doppler of the aorta. As previously discussed, the pressure difference between two regions is calculated by using the modified Bernoulli equation, where $P = 4(V^2)$. By using commercially available packages, the peak and mean aortic valve gradient estimates based on the Doppler signal are easily acquired (Figure 15). In the pregnant state, in which stroke volume and cardiac output are expected to be increased, these gradients increase as well. The increase in gradients is not representative of a change in valve area, but of a change in hemodynamics. Thus, reliance on peak and mean aortic valve gradients to assess severity of aortic stenosis is not recommended.

6. Ejection Fraction

The changes in cardiac size, cardiac function, and valvular function have been defined in the pregnant and nonpregnant states (3–5). One of the most frequently requested measurements in pregnant women with known or suspected cardiac disease is systemic arterial ventricular ejection fraction. The ejection fraction is calculated as the quotient of stroke volume divided by end-diastolic volume. Stroke volume can be calculated by determining the difference between end-diastolic volume and end-systolic volume.

7. Technique(s) of Ejection Fraction Measurement

One of the simplest methods that can be used to assess left ventricular ejection fraction is that of Tortoledo and associates (6). In this technique the ejection fraction (EF) is regarded as the quotient of the stroke volume (SV) divided by the end-diastolic volume (EDV) expressed as a percentage: i.e., EF = SV/EDV × 100. The EDV is calculated by using the formula of Tortoledo and associates (6), where EDV = (LV short axis × LV long axis × 3.42) − 6.44. The long axis is measured from the epicardial surface of the apex to the insertion of the mitral valve leaflet (Figure 16). The left ventricular diameter is measured in the short-axis view using M-mode echocardiography at the level of the papillary muscle. Both measure-

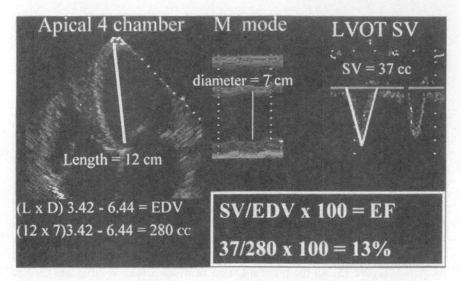

Figure 16 Calculation of LVEF using a two-dimensional estimate of EDV and a Doppler estimate of SV. End-diastolic volume can be obtained manually by using the formula EDV = (L × D) 3.42 − 6.44, where L = end-diastolic length of the left ventricle from the apex to the insertion of the mitral valve in the four-chamber view, and D = end-diastolic diameter of the left ventricle obtained in the parasternal short axis view by M-mode or two-dimensional echocardiography. Using the EDV and SV calculations, the LVEF is calculated as LVEF = SV/EDV × 100. In this patient with cardiomyopathy, the apical four-chamber is depicted in the left panel, the M-mode is in the center, and the LVOT SV is at the right. Using data from these three measurements, the LVEF is calculated at 13%. Abbreviations as in text and previous figures.

ments should be made at end-diastole. Common errors using this technique are failure to acquire a true apical four-chamber view with foreshortening of the left ventricle and acquisition of oblique short-axis views of the heart that result in over- or underestimation of ventricular length. As with estimates of stroke volume during pregnancy, left ventricular EF can vary. However, an ejection fraction of less that 50% is considered abnormal.

The technique described is not the only one that can be used. We have chosen it because of its ease of use and the minimal technical knowhow required to estimate the EF this way. Another useful technique for estimation of EF is the disk-summation method. This is also a relatively simple way to estimate ejection fraction. Two-dimensional images are acquired in diastole and systole. The endocardial borders are outlined by using commercially available software available in most ultrasound machines. The end-diastolic and end-systolic volumes are calculated and the difference representing stroke volume is calculated (Figure 17). Division of stroke volume by the end-diastolic volume yields ejection fraction.

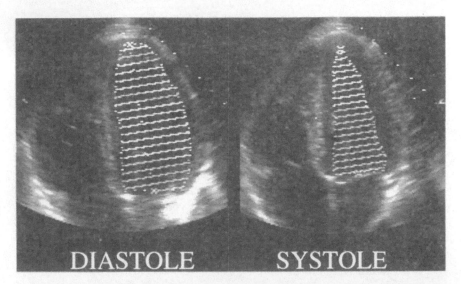

Figure 17 Left ventricular ejection fraction is calculated by the formula LVEF = [(EDV − ESV)/EDV] or SV/EDV since SV = EDV − ESV. Estimation of left ventricular ejection fraction based on the disk summation method (Simpson's rule) is shown in this figure. By using commercially available software, the left ventricular EDV and ESV can be calculated by the disk summation method, as shown in panels A and B. The LVEF is 69%. LVEF = left ventricular ejection fraction; EDV = end-diastolic volume; ESV = end-systolic volume; SV = stroke volume.

Common errors that occur in using this technique include tracing borders with inadequate resolution and calculating data in images that are foreshortened or "off-axis."

Numerous other echocardiographic techniques can be used to estimate ejection fraction accurately. These include use of M-mode echocardiography, two-dimensional echocardiography, or a combination of Doppler and two-dimensional echocardiography. These techniques are beyond the scope of this chapter.

IV. HEMODYNAMIC MONITORING FOR PREECLAMPSIA

A. Invasive Hemodynamic Monitoring

The pulmonary artery catheter, introduced nearly 30 years ago, has been very useful in the management of critically ill patients (7). In cases of severe preeclampsia, most clinicians have obtained excellent results without invasive monitoring (8). Invasive hemodynamic monitoring was initially recommended for patients with severe preeclampsia complicated by profound oliguria, pulmonary edema of uncertain cause, hypertension unresponsive to conventional therapy, and medical conditions that would normally require such monitoring (9). Protocols developed to study the central hemodynamic parameters of severe preeclampsia have revealed interesting data, which are sometimes confounded by differences in clinical patient management prior to and at the time of catheterization (10). Current indications for the use of pulmonary artery catheter in preeclampsia (11,12) include the following:

1. Complications related to central volume status such as pulmonary edema of uncertain cause, pulmonary edema unresponsive to conventional therapy, hypertension unresponsive to conventional therapy, and persistent oliguria despite aggressive volume expansion
2. Induction of conduction anesthesia in hemodynamically unstable patients
3. Medical complication that would otherwise require invasive monitoring

The routine use of a pulmonary artery catheter in uncomplicated severe preeclampsia is no longer recommended. The potential morbidity of pulmonary artery catheterization is not justified. Known complications of invasive monitoring at the time of insertion include cardiac arrhythmias, pneumothorax, hemothorax, injury to vascular and neurological structures, pulmonary infarction, and pulmonary hemorrhage. Later complications include balloon rupture, thromboembolism, catheter knotting, pulmonary valve rupture, and catheter migration into the pericardial and pleural spaces, with subsequent cardiac tamponade and hydrothorax (13). However, it should be noted that Clark and associates (11) observed no significant complications of pulmonary artery catheterization in a series of 90 patients who had the procedure in an obstetrics-gynecology practice.

B. Noninvasive Hemodynamic Monitoring

We now suggest that most of the important hemodynamic information required for initial management of patients with complicated severe preeclampsia can be acquired by the use of noninvasive two-dimensional echocardiography and Doppler ultrasound. Belfort and coworkers (1) prospectively studied 11 critically ill obstetrical patients (4 patients with sepsis/ARDS, 2 patients with preeclampsia, 2 patients with cardiomyopathy, and 1 patient each with aortic valve disease, massive pulmonary embolus, and renal artery stenosis) requiring invasive monitoring for clinical management. The techniques employed in the measurement of cardiac output, left ventricular filling pressure, right atrial pressure, and ejection fraction have been reported above and the reader is referred to recent publications for further technical information and methodology (1,4). Simultaneous Doppler echocardiography and pulmonary artery catheterization readings of cardiac index, left ventricular filling pressure, pulmonary arterial systolic pressure, and right atrial pressure were acquired and compared by using regression analysis. There was no significant difference between the two techniques in the estimation of cardiac index or intracardiac filling pressures. There was a good correlation between the two methods for cardiac index ($R = 0.99$), left ventricular filling pressure ($R = 0.86$), pulmonary arterial systolic pressure ($R = 0.92$), and right atrial pressure ($R = 0.87$). These authors concluded that two-dimensional and Doppler echocardiography allow rapid, reliable, noninvasive assessment of hemodynamic parameters in critically ill obstetrical patients. They then went on to test their hypothesis in a group of 14 patients with oliguria unresponsive to crystalloid boluses, hypertension unresponsive to hydralazine, and in women at high risk for pulmonary edema (14). All of these patients were potential candidates for invasive monitoring. They were studied with two-dimensional echocardiography and Doppler ultrasound without a pulmonary artery catheter. They included women with intractable hypertension ($n = 1$), pulmonary edema ($n = 2$), complex cardiac lesions ($n = 2$), oliguria ($n = 5$), intractable hypertension and oliguria ($n = 1$), and unexplained dyspnea with peripheral arterial oxygen desaturation ($n = 1$). Although some patients received as much as 8 L of crystalloid, none experienced pulmonary edema or left ventricular failure, and none had seizures. In all 12 cases the ultrasound monitoring allowed successful noninvasive management of the patient. These authors (14) concluded that two-dimensional echocardiography and Doppler examination may be an effective alternative to invasive monitoring in the management of selected pregnant patients. There are obvious difficulties in instituting a program of noninvasive monitoring in a busy labor and delivery unit. There should ideally be someone capable of performing the monitoring available at all times. In practice, however, it is very infrequent that more than evaluation will be needed and in most situations in which this may be required it would be advisable to have a pulmonary artery catheter in situ. In the most common situation a patient with oliguria has not responded to what is deemed to be an adequate fluid challenge. Under these circumstances the physician is fearful of precipitating pulmonary edema and requests invasive monitoring. If there were a way to reassure the physician that the patient has a good ejection fraction, is not in incipient cardiac failure, is centrally volume depleted, and could easily tolerate another 2 L of fluid, most physicians would forgo the pulmonary artery catheter. In many situations two-dimensional echocardiography and Doppler assessment can provide this reassurance. Most young pregnant women have a healthy heart and tolerate volume infusion easily. Even in cases in which a preeclamptic patient experiences pulmonary edema it is possible to manage her without invasive monitoring. In many of these cases the preterm patient has received steroids and magnesium sulfate therapy and edema is not due to cardiac failure but noncardiogenic pulmonary capillary leakage. In such a case, noninvasive monitoring quickly shows an adequate cardiac output and ejection fraction, and a low capillary wedge pressure. The information gained from invasive monitoring under these circumstances does not justify the risks of the procedure.

In women with hypertension that is unresponsive to standard hydralazine therapy noninvasive echocardiographic studies may help in the choice of the most suitable alternative antihypertensive agent. In using hemodynamic information the selection of therapy can be based on a knowledge of the underlying pathophysiological condition and the expected mechanism of action of the drug, rather than on empiricism. Some patients with severe preeclampsia have underlying chronic hypertension and are at risk for hypertensive cardiomyopathy with systolic dysfunction. In a large number of patients unsuspected diastolic dysfunction is also present (15). A knowledge of chamber dimensions, ejection fraction, fractional shortening, intracardiac pressures, and cardiac output allows a much more informed decision regarding the choice of a preferential vasodilator (calcium channel blocker, arterial vasodilator) versus an agent with a predominantly negative inotropic effect (beta-blocker). The ability to calculate the systemic vascular resistance is also helpful when choosing an antihypertensive agent. Echocardiographic measurements can also allow the physician to estimate systemic vascular resistance and cardiac output after any intervention. Thus, the hemodynamic consequences of volume expansion and/or antihypertensive therapy can be assessed almost immediately without the need for invasive monitoring.

Frequently, once it has been determined that cardiac function is normal, volume expansion can be carried out, using only evaluation of the central venous pressure. Imaging of the inferior vena cava is easily accomplished with standard equipment, requires little training or special expertise, and is well accepted by patients. This technique represents a practical way for the clinician to evaluate central venous pressure without the need for sophisticated hemodynamic monitoring equipment and without exposure of the patient to added risk. The ability to visualize right atrial and ventricular wall motion, and simultaneously to estimate right atrial pressure from the inferior vena cava allows a more informed estimate of the state of filling of the central veins than the pulmonary artery catheter, in our opinion.

Although estimation of cardiac output requires more expertise than that needed for visualization of the inferior vena cava, this technique is easily acquired and can be taught to people with little or no previous ultrasound experience. The additional information regarding chamber dimensions, ejection fraction, and fractional shortening may also be very useful in gaining a better indication of the patient's true cardiac function and status. There is no reason why the noninvasive techniques cannot be performed on patients with a pulmonary artery catheter in situ to gain additional information. Such situations may include those in which there is disparity between left and right ventricular output, systolic or diastolic dysfunction, or impaired ventricular relaxation.

V. SUMMARY

Two-dimensional and Doppler echocardiography allow reliable noninvasive assessment of cardiac morphological characteristics, function, and hemodynamics in pregnant women. When appropriately obtained and interpreted, this information can be invaluable in their management during gestation, labor, delivery and post partum.

REFERENCES

1. Belfort MA, Rokey R, Saade GR, Moise KJ Jr. Rapid echocardiographic assessment of left and right heart hemodynamics in critically ill obstetric patients. Am J Obstet Gynecol 1994; 171:884–892.
2. Hoffmann R, Flachskampf FA, Hanrath P. Planimetry of orifice area in aortic stenosis using multiplane transesophageal echocardiography. J Am Coll Cardiol 1993; 22: 529–534.
3. Young P, Johanson R. Haemodynamic, invasive and echocardiographic monitoring in the hypertensive parturient. Best Pract Res Clin Obstet Gynaecol 2001; 15:605–622.
4. Rokey R, Belfort MA, Saade GR: Quantitative echocardiographic assessment of left ventricular function in critically ill obstetric patients: a comparative study. Am J Obstet Gynecol 1995; 173:1148–1152.
5. Dabaghi SF, Rokey R, Rivera JM, Saliba WI, Majid PA. Comparison of echocardiographic assessment of cardiac hemodynamics in the intensive care unit with right-sided cardiac catheterization. Am J Cardiol 1996; 76:392–395.
6. Tortoledo FA, Quinones MA, Fernandez GC, Waggoner AD, Winters WL Jr. Quantification of left ventricular volumes by two-dimensional echocardiography: a simplified and accurate approach. Circulation 1983; 67:579–584.
7. Phillips SJ, Krakauer J. Percutaneous pulmonary artery cannulation. J Thorac Cardiovasc Surg 1971; 61:490–491.
8. Cunningham FG, Pritchard JA. How should hypertension during pregnancy be managed? Experience at Parkland Memorial Hospital. Med Clin North Am 1984; 68: 505–526.
9. Clark SL, Cotton DB. Clinical indications for pulmonary artery catheterization in the patient with severe preeclampsia. Am J Obstet Gynecol 1988; 158:453–458.
10. Wasserstrum N, Cotton DB. Hemodynamic monitoring in severe pregnancy-induced hypertension. Clin Perinatol 1986; 13:781–799.
11. Clark SL, Horenstein JM, Phelan JP, Montag TW, Paul RH. Experience with the pulmonary artery catheter in obstetrics and gynecology. Am J Obstet Gynecol 1985; 152:374–378.
12. Cotton DB, Lee W, Huhta JC, Dorman KF. Hemodynamic profile of severe pregnancy-induced hypertension. Am J Obstet Gynecol 1988; 158:523–529.
13. Kirshon B, Cotton DB. Invasive hemodynamic monitoring in the obstetric patient. Clin Obstet Gynecol 1987; 30:579–590.

14. Belfort MA, Mares A, Saade G, Wen TS, Rokey R. The use of two-dimensional echocardiography and Doppler ultrasound in managing obstetric patients. Obstet Gynecol 1997; 90(3):326–330.
15. Mabie WC, Hackman BB, Sibai BM. Pulmonary edema associated with pregnancy: echocardiographic insights and implications for treatment. Obstet Gynecol 1993; 81:227–234.
16. Zoghbi WA, Farmer KL, Soto JG, Nelson JG, Quinones MA. Accurate noninvasive quantitation of stenotic aortic valve area by Doppler echocardiography. Circulation 1986; 73:452–459.

14

Anesthesia for the Patient with Severe Preeclampsia

Usha Singh, Pragasan Dean Gopalan, and D. A. Rocke
Nelson R. Mandela School of Medicine, University of Natal, Durban,
South Africa

I. INTRODUCTION

Despite the many advances in the management of preeclampsia-eclampsia syndrome over the past 25 years, it continues to be a major direct cause of maternal deaths in many parts of the world (1–3). Although this disorder affects only a small percentage of all pregnancies in developed countries, it still accounts for a considerable proportion of the maternal morbidity and mortality rates (4). Efforts in prevention have been disappointing principally because of a failure to understand the underlying pathophysiological characteristics. Poor maternal outcome has been largely linked to inappropriate or substandard care (1,5). This may be overcome if caregivers vigilantly address the complications of severe preeclampsia. The severity of preeclampsia-eclampsia syndrome should not be underestimated. Teamwork between obstetrician and anesthesiologist is crucial. The expertise of the latter in cardiovascular and respiratory complications, combined with sound obstetrical principles, facilitates management of these often-difficult conditions. There is a wide interindividual variation in the effects on specific organs and the severity of the disease. The pattern of disease ranges from a low-grade condition with slow progression to a fulminant acute multiorgan dysfunction syndrome. The latter represents the final phase of the disorder, in which there are multiorgan ischemia and a poor prognosis. Hence, anesthesia must be tailored to each patient, based on the clinical context of the condition. This chapter is an attempt to highlight the recent advances, and the controversial aspects, of anesthetic intervention strategies in severe preeclampsia.

II. ANESTHESIA FOR SEVERE PREECLAMPSIA

The involvement of the anesthesiologist in the management of the severely preeclamptic woman should begin as soon as the provisional diagnosis is made. There is a distinct advantage to early consultation with the anesthesiologist since it allows a timely baseline assessment. Early recognition of potential anesthetic problems, such as poor blood pressure control, airway difficulties, need for special investigations or equipment, or insertion of invasive monitoring lines, is possible. Furthermore, early involvement enables the anesthesiologist to participate actively and advise in cases in which immediate and urgent action is required.

III. PREOPERATIVE EVALUATION

A. General Principles of Prenatal Management

Screening and early detection of problems in the prenatal period are essential to circumvent the possible devastating sequelae of this condition. The anesthesiologist may be involved in cases in which delivery is delayed in early onset preeclampsia to allow steroid administration for fetal lung development. Bed rest with frequent measurement of blood pressure, daily body mass, creatinine clearance estimation, total urinary protein excretion, serum uric acid, liver function, coagulopathy screening, hematocrit, and platelet count form the basic in-patient maternal management (6). Ultrasound examination with measurement of biometric parameters and biophysical profile, as well as frequent or continuous fetal heart monitoring, may provide the obstetrician with important information regarding fetal well-being. These investigations may be crucial in determining the time of delivery. The decision to terminate the pregnancy depends on a combination of maternal and fetal indications. The indications for immediate delivery in severe preeclampsia are summarized in Table 1 (7). The anesthesiologist must be aware of the current fetal condition and, just as importantly, the reserve of the fetoplacental unit, since measures to reduce anesthesia-induced stress on the fetus may be important considerations for the anesthetic technique.

Table 1 Indications for Delivery in Preeclampsia

1. Severe hypertension unresponsive to therapy
2. Progressive thrombocytopenia, especially if the platelet count drops below 50,000/mL
3. Liver dysfunction (aspartate aminotransferase [AST] and alanine aminotransferase [ALT] levels > 70 IU/mL)
4. Progressive renal dysfunction (including sudden oliguria)
5. Premonitory signs of eclampsia (visual disturbances, severe headache, clonus)
6. Evidence of fetal distress

B. Assessment of Risk

The early recognition of preeclampsia is often difficult. The prodromal phase of the disease is subclinical, and some cardinal signs may be overlooked unless specifically sought. Subsequent to the diagnosis of severe preeclampsia, the risk should be stratified and correlated with the preanesthetic functional status. The American Society of Anesthesiologists (ASA) physical status findings and inherent surgical risk factors are collectively used. The spectrum of clinical presentation is broad and, accordingly, patients with severe preeclampsia may fulfill criteria ranging from grade III of the ASA classification at one end of the spectrum, to life-threatening grade V risk conditions (such as hepatic rupture) at the other end. Clinical evidence of organ dysfunction or failure must be actively excluded (Table 2). If these features are present, the anesthesiologist should be aware of the potential for serious complications. Martin and associates (8) in 1999 focused on symptoms such as nausea, vomiting, and epigastric pain in conjunction with elevated lactate dehyrogenase, aspartate aminotransferase, and uric acid levels in an attempt to predict the risk of morbidity in severe preeclampsia. Their conclusions were that such symptoms and laboratory findings were indicative of a high morbidity risk. They further stated that a decreasing platelet count, although an independent marker of maternal risk, was additive to the other features.

The anesthetic technique must take into account the organs affected by the disease process. In addition, appropriate postoperative care should be preplanned. Basic history taking and clinical examination are invaluable. It is well substantiated that early recognition of the symptomless phase of the syndrome of pre-

Table 2 Features of Severe Preeclampsia

Maternal

    Blood pressure: ≥ 160 mmHg systolic or ≥ 110 mmHg diastolic while at bed rest, on two occasions at least 6 hours apart; diagnosis not delayed if the diastolic blood pressure exceeds 110 mmHg

    Proteinuria: > 5 g in a 24-hour urine specimen (or 3+ to 4+ on a semiquantitative analysis)

    Oliguria: Urine output < 400 mL in 24 hours)

    Cerebral or visual disturbances: headache, blurred vision, or altered consciousness

    Grand mal seizure (eclampsia)

    Pulmonary edema or, pending its diagnosis, cyanosis

    Epigastric or upper right quadrant pain

    Impaired liver function

    Thrombocytopenia-HELLP syndrome

Fetal

    Intrauterine growth restriction

    Oligohydramnios

---

eclampsia is important for optimal patient care (9). Special attention should be paid to the symptoms of severe preeclampsia, which include headache, blurred vision, visual field loss, visual disturbances (such as flashes of light), ready bruising or bleeding, shortness of breath, and right upper quadrant or epigastric pain. A strong association between headache and abnormal cerebral perfusion has been demonstrated in women with this disorder (10). Severe hypertension (≥160/110 mmHg) and proteinuria (3+ or more on a semiquantitative urine analysis) consistently indicate severe disease (11). Mildly elevated blood pressure (>140/90 mmHg) and proteinuria associated with symptoms, intrauterine growth restriction, hematological (hemolysis or thrombocytopenia) abnormalities, or biochemical (abnormally high liver enzyme or creatinine level) disturbances should lead to the diagnosis of severe preeclampsia. Generalized edema is not used to categorize severity, although excessive, nondependant facial and hand edema should be noted since it is occasionally a harbinger of life-threatening laryngeal or epiglottal edema. Eclampsia, presumed to be most commonly a manifestation of cerebral autoregulatory dysfunction and hypertensive encephalopathy, but occasionally associated with cerebral vasospasm, is one of the most severe representations of the disease. Patients who have a diagnosis of severe preeclampsia require complete preoperative testing that should include a complete blood count (including platelets), liver and renal function tests, coagulation profile (may include prothrombin time/partial thromboplastin time [PT/PTT], d-dimer/fibrin split products, and fibrinogen), and blood typing or cross match as appropriate. Depending on symptoms and signs, a chest radiograph, electrocardiogram (EKG), echocardiogram, and arterial blood gas evaluation may be indicated. If there is suspicion of a liver hematoma, appropriate diagnostic testing (magnetic resonance imaging [MRI] or computed tomography [CT] scan) may be required. When liver hemorrhage is suspected, rapid preparation for massive blood transfusion, emergency surgery, invasive intraoperative monitoring, and postoperative intensive care unit (ICU) care are paramount. These are often the responsibility of the anesthesiology team.

IV. FLUID MANAGEMENT AND ANESTHESIA

Fluid management continues to generate controversy especially in terms of the discussion of volume restriction versus volume expansion, and the use of crystalloid versus colloid as the fluid of choice. In recent years, there has been a shift away from routine fluid restriction. Fluid therapy must be directed to optimizing global perfusion in order to improve oxygen delivery in the setting of severe vasoconstriction. Such therapy should simultaneously aim to prevent iatrogenic pulmonary edema and circumvent acute blood pressure instability after vasodilator therapy or epidural anesthesia.

Pritchard and colleagues (12) in their evaluation of 245 cases advocated fluid restriction and recommended crystalloid infusions of 60–150 mL/h without invasive monitoring. Work by Belfort and coworkers (13) suggested that plasma volume expansion with colloid to achieve a normal pulmonary capillary wedge pressure (PCWP) was advantageous to restore and maintain cardiac output and oxygen consumption, while reducing peripheral vascular resistance. Although Kirshon and associates (14) suggested that colloid oncotic pressure (COP) was a useful endpoint to guide fluid expansion with albumin, this is no longer advocated or practiced. In situations in which albumin was infused to increase oncotic pressure, excessively high postpartum PCWP often necessitated aggressive diuretic therapy (14). The diversity of the clinical presentation of preeclampsia precludes the universal application of a single "restriction" or "expansion" strategy (15); in practice, there are situations in which either of these strategies may be appropriate. The volume and type of fluid remain a source of contention. Robson and colleagues (16) described rational guidelines for selective fluid therapy. They proposed accurate monitoring of fluid balance and suggested that the urine output provides vital information regarding fluid requirement. Delivery and postpartum blood losses must be taken into consideration when the fluid balance is calculated. Maintenance crystalloid infusion of Ringer's lactate or other balanced salt solutions such as 0.9% saline solution (16) is advisable at a rate of 125–150 mL/h, but the infusion rate depends on the presence or absence of underlying renal impairment and electrolyte disturbances. Dextrose in water carries a risk of water intoxication, and its use is discouraged. In some cases the short intravascular half-life of crystalloids renders them unsuitable for volume expansion, and colloidal solutions such as hetastarch, fresh frozen plasma, and packed red cells may be more useful. Selective colloid volume expansion is an option in cases of significant intravascular volume contraction that require aggressive vasodilator therapy. Central venous pressure (CVP) monitoring is thought to be unreliable in preeclampsia (43), and in situations in which reliable and frequent measurement of central hemodynamics is required, a pulmonary artery catheter (PAC) may be necessary.

Belfort and coworkers have described a noninvasive method of assessing central hemodynamics using two-dimensional and Doppler echocardiography (16a,16b). This technique allows rapid evaluation of ejection fraction, chamber size and motion, cardiac output, and central venous pressure. Estimates of peripheral vascular resistance can then be made. Noninvasive investigation can be used if continuous monitoring is unnecessary, the heart is healthy, and instantaneous decisions can be made for fluid or drug therapy. Most women with severe preeclampsia who do not respond to vasodilators or who have oliguria unresponsive to fluid challenges can be managed in this way. Occasionally the echocardiogram reveals a need for invasive monitoring, most commonly when poor cardiac function or hypertensive cardiomyopathy is recognized.

Diuretics should be used with caution in severe preeclampsia because most of these patients have some degree of plasma volume constriction and further volume reduction may exacerbate the condition. In general, diuretics are reserved for those women with a confirmed diagnosis of pulmonary edema or early renal failure thought to be responsive to diuresis.

Fluid restriction becomes necessary in established cases of pulmonary edema and acute tubular necrosis. In a series of 37 severely preeclamptic women published by Sibai and coworkers (17), the majority of cases (70%) of pulmonary edema occurred in the early puerperium. This coincides with a nadir in the COP. Pulmonary edema is more likely when the COP value is low. The COP may drop to less than 15 mmHg in severe preeclampsia. Edema is also associated with large volume infusions of intravenous fluids (usually > 5 L) and a negative COP-PCWP gradient (18). Some authorities believe that the increased maternal mortality rate of respiratory complications in preeclamptic women may be directly linked to aggressive fluid administration and subsequent pulmonary edema (19). As mentioned, CVP monitoring alone can often be misleading and pulmonary edema can occur with seemingly innocuous CVP values. Although the pulmonary artery catheter (PAC) is useful in providing further cardiovascular information, it is invasive and has associated morbidity and mortality risks. Although Yeast and associates (20) suggested that the risk of pulmonary edema may be simply and inexpensively ascertained by serial COP measurements, this method has not gained popularity and is not recommended given the more efficient alternate methods available for the determination of pulmonary function.

Fluid expansion may be necessary in a few clinical situations such as prior to regional analgesia and/or vasodilator therapy. Most fluid regimens advocate crystalloid maintenance therapy at 75–150 mL/h, and hypovolemia should be corrected with crystalloid or colloid, using noninvasive or invasive monitoring as appropriate.

In cases in which severe intravascular depletion is suspected, some estimate of intracardiac filling pressures is advised before the institution of regional blockade or vasodilator drugs. In this situation, noninvasive evaluation of the state of distention and degree of collapse of the inferior vena cava may be beneficial. The patient may then have volume expansion without invasive monitoring. In cases in which noninvasive monitoring is not available and there is good evidence of low filling pressures (oliguria, labile blood pressure, significant edema), cardiac function should be assessed before volume expansion. In most mildly preeclamptic patients this is not an issue and cardiac function is assumed to be adequate. These women usually tolerate volume expansion without difficulty. Clinical evaluation consistent with a central venous pressure of 4–6 cmH$_2$O is regarded as safe for the institution of regional analgesia or judicious vasodilation. In some cases, however, there are symptoms and signs of malignant hypertension, prior chronic hypertension, renal disease, preexisting heart disease, or new onset cardiac decompensation. These women need much more careful testing and evaluation prior to volume expansion or use of regional blockade. This may involve echocardiography, evaluation by a cardiologist, or insertion of a pulmonary artery catheter. The drug and infusion volumes should be amended as appropriate.

Oliguria (defined as urine output < 100 mL/4h or < 30 mL/h for consecutive 3 hours) is an indication for volume expansion. The classic renal lesion of preeclampsia, glomeruloendotheliosis, is usually reversible and does not result in long-term sequelae, but in some cases of protracted oliguria with uncorrected hypovolemia, acute tubular necrosis may result. This can cause cortical necrosis and permanent renal damage. Patients at highest risk of permanent renal damage are those with underlying chronic hypertension, especially if it is secondary to renal disease. Monitoring of the central volume status is useful if volume expansion is needed to treat oliguria. Noninvasive evaluation is ideal in this circumstance since continuous monitoring is usually not needed and management can be guided by a single (or a few) evaluations(s). Although crystalloid solutions are almost always employed for volume expansion, colloidal solutions may be more useful in severe preeclampsia when rapid infusion is needed because of the prompt increase in the PCWP and COP values. Further advantages of colloidal solutions include a less dramatic decrease in puerperial COP (21), hence less risk of pulmonary edema. Patients with mild to moderate preeclampsia are better managed with a more flexible approach to fluid strategies.

Atrial natriuretic peptide (ANP) levels have been demonstrated to be higher in preeclamptic women than in their normotensive counterparts. Furthermore, an exaggerated increase in ANP level has been elicited in response to volume preloading (22). This may assist preeclamptic patients to accommodate intravascular volume expansion. Oxytocin in high doses or during prolonged infusion may produce an antidiuretic effect that may complicate fluid management. In short, most authorities agree that it is best to approach fluid therapy with moderation and attention to the individual need of the patient (23).

V. ANTIHYPERTENSIVE THERAPY

Numerous antihypertensive agents have been used since the 1980s, but the ideal agent remains elusive. Antihypertensive treatment has a definitive role in reducing maternal morbidity and mortality rates but must be individualized to balance the maternal and fetal needs.

The different hemodynamic subsets of severe preeclampsia must be understood in order to utilize these antihypertensive agents rationally. There are two distinct hemodynamic variants. The majority of severe preeclamptic patients demonstrate normal to moderately elevated systemic vascular resistance (SVR) in association with hyperdynamic left ventricular performance. A smaller group of patients with a higher risk are noted to have a markedly elevated SVR with a concomitant decrease in cardiac output. It is not uncommon for the anesthesiologist to be faced with the need to lower the blood pressure acutely with rapidly acting antihypertensives prior to anesthesia. The primary maternal objective in antihypertensive therapy is to prevent complications such as cerebral hemorrhage and encephalopathy (19). Myocardial ischemia must be prevented, and perfusion of vital organs should be maintained to provide adequate oxygen delivery. As recommended in 1996 by Sibai (24), urgent pharmacological therapy is necessary when the diastolic pressure is greater than 110 mmHg and mean arterial pressures is more than 125 mmHg. The fetal implications of severe maternal hypertension include disturbances in uteroplacental perfusion with resultant acidosis/asphyxia and abruptio placentae. Drug interactions may occur and care should be taken to check for such complications when using additive therapy for antihypertensive management.

VI. HYDRALAZINE

Hydralazine remains the most commonly used antihypertensive drug. In most instances, it is successful in controlling the blood pressure, and it is considered by many to be the drug of choice (25). There are, however, several caveats to its usage. Although hydralazine, given in 5-mg boluses, has been shown to be a safe and effective method of treating severe hypertension in preeclampsia (26), it has several undesirable side effects, including symptoms that mimic imminent eclampsia. Furthermore, information about the filling pressure in the right side of the heart is useful prior to the administration of hydralazine to identify those women who have "relative hypovolemia" and intravascular volume contraction. These individuals may require volume expansion guided by some form of monitoring (as discussed previously), since hydralazine frequently precipitates severe hypotension in the face of hypovolemia. This can result in fetal compromise caused by shunting of blood from the uteroplacental circulation. Repeat doses of hydralazine should be judiciously delayed and sufficient time should be allowed for the drug to take effect, since the onset of action may be as long as 15–20 minutes after injection, with a peak effect 1 hour after administration. Continuous infusion should be discouraged because of difficulties with titration and a susceptibility to overdosage (27). Although reviews in 1997 and 1998 emphasized the benefits and reliability of hydralazine (28,29), new treatments continue to be introduced. One such example is ketanserin, a serotonin antagonist, which may be an attractive alternative to hydralazine in the management of early onset preeclampsia (30) but requires further study before its use can be recommended.

VII. LABETALOL

Labetalol is a nonselective β-adrenergic antagonist with some α-adrenergic blocking properties (β/α, 7: 1 with intravenous administration). These properties make labetalol a suitable agent in patients with hyperdynamic left ventricular function. However, in preeclamptic patients with depressed cardiac performance the β-antagonist properties may adversely affect cardiac output. Hydralazine is then the preferred agent. The individual response to labetalol is inconsistent, and in approximately 10% of severe preeclamptic patients tachyphylaxis develops, mandating larger doses or causing a shorter duration of effect (31). On the basis of individual clinical experience, many workers have suggested alternate regimens. Labetalol is safe when given intravenously in 5- to 20-mg increments, and it may be titrated to a maximal single-dose of 1 mg/kg. A commonly used regimen employs labetalol in an initial dose of 20-mg followed by 20-mg incremental increases every 15–20 minutes (as needed) up to a maximum of 100 mg, with a maximal cumulative dose of 300 mg (32). Alternatively labetalol can be given as an infusion in a dosage of 1 mg/min until the blood pressure begins to fall, at which time the infusion should be stopped. This form of therapy is best carried out with an arterial line so that the blood pressure can be continuously measured, and the infusion can be accurately titrated. Labetalol is also useful in controlling ventricular dysrhythmias that may occur in eclampsia (33), and it has also been used to obtund the intubation response in general anesthesia in patients with preeclampsia (34). Caution should be exercised since excessive beta-adrenergic blockade after a single intravenous dose of labetalol in preterm twins has been described (35).

VIII. NIFEDIPINE

Despite considerable success and widespread use, nifedipine and the other calcium channel antagonists are not favored as first-line agents in blood pressure control in preeclampsia (36). Sublingual nifedipine, 10 mg, was popular in the past because of ease of administration and rapid effect. A major drawback, however, is the lack of control of the anytihypertensive response, which may lead to precipitous hypotension, myocardial ischemia, and fetal compromise. Although sublingual administration is now strongly discouraged, swallowed nifedipine may be used orally for the control of antepartum and postpartum hypertension. It is an effective agent for the long-term control of patients with severe preeclampsia who are undergoing an aggressive conservative protocol to prolong the pregnancy to improve fetal lung maturation. Because of the potential deleterious effect on myocardial perfusion in cases in which there is a precipitous reduction in blood pressure, nifedipine is no longer recommended for the acute treatment of severe hypertension in the United States. Its use is still sanctioned in women with gestational and chronic hypertension to maintain the blood pressure within an acceptable range once the hypertension has been acutely controlled. This has resulted in a decline in its use in severe preeclampsia.

The potentiation of the effect of magnesium by calcium channel blockers has been addressed by Waisman and colleagues (37). Concern regarding profound hypotension and uterine atony has not been shown in clinical use, and in some U.S. centers nifedipine and magnesium sulfate are routinely given together for preeclamptic women. Nevertheless, if this is done, the clinician should monitor blood pressure and heart rate closely.

IX. NITROGLYCERIN

Nitroglycerin is a potent, rapidly acting antihypertensive agent that generates nitric oxide, leading to vasodilatation. It predominantly relaxes venous vascular smooth muscle but also affects the arterial musculature. It decreases preload at low doses and afterload in high doses (37a). Nitroglycerin has a very short hemodynamic half-life and is therefore administered by infusion pump. The initial rate is 5 μg/min, and this dose can be doubled every 5 minutes until control is achieved. Methemoglobinemia may result from high doses (> 7 μg/kg/min) given by intravenous (IV) infusion, and this side effect is more important in pregnancy because of the presence of the fetus. Since the vasospasm of preeclampsia predominantly occurs in the arterial vascular beds, nitroglycerin should be reserved for cases in which specific venodilation is required, such as pulmonary edema complicating hypertensive cardiomyopathy.

Invasive arterial pressure monitoring is desirable when using nitroglycerin in order to detect rapid and dramatic decreases in blood pressure. Patients with marked volume contraction are particularly susceptible and require preemptive volume expansion. However, expansion of the intravascular volume in such cases should be guided by monitoring of central hemodynamic indices so that overzealous fluid administration does not nullify the effect of the nitroglycerin or lead to pulmonary edema. Nitroglycerin may also have unanticipated and undesirable side effects such as a decrease in preload without any afterload reduction. This can cause a decrease in oxygen delivery and consumption.

X. NITROPRUSSIDE

Sodium nitroprusside is a potent antihypertensive that produces nitric oxide–mediated smooth muscle relaxation. When first-line drugs such as labetalol and hydralazine do not adequately lower blood pressure, this agent may be of use in patients with severe preeclampsia. Sodium nitroprusside is mainly used in the operating room when severe hypertension must be controlled prior to general anesthesia. Invasive blood pressure and central hemodynamic monitoring is desirable since sodium nitroprusside may dramatically lower blood pressure (29). The recommended intravenous infusion dose, 0.5–5.0 μg/kg/min in nongravid individuals should be modified in pregnant patients (32). The initial infusion in gravid women should be 0.2 μg/kg/min. This drug should be reserved for extreme emergencies because of concerns regarding thiocyanate toxicity in the neonate. The solution is light sensitive and should be covered in foil and changed every 24 hours (37b). Arterial blood gases should be monitored to exclude metabolic acidosis, which may be an early sign of cyanide toxicity. Antepartum therapy should be limited because of the potential for fetal cyanide toxicity (37c). The hemodynamic effect of nitroprusside suggests that its effect is mediated by a cardiopulmonary baroreceptor reflex. This is presumably the result of the prominent venodilator action of nitroprusside in conditions of reduced blood volume such as that seen in severe preeclampsia.

XI. HEMODYNAMIC MONITORING

There is an abundance of literature pertaining to the usefulness of invasive monitoring in the peripartum and perioperative periods in the severely preeclamptic patient. Despite this, a clear benefit of the routine use of such monitoring in uncomplicated severe preeclampsia has not been demonstrated, and most clinicians only resort to invasive monitoring when the patient's condition is so unstable that continuous data are required.

The use of invasive monitoring has allowed the description of a number of different hemodynamic subsets in women with preeclampsia. The majority of patients, however, have increased peripheral vascular resistance and normal to high cardiac output. The decision to utilize invasive monitors requires serious consideration by the anesthesiologist, and issues such as potential complications, individual expertise with insertion and interpretation, and possible need for admission to the ICU are important. In the obstetrical population, complicated severe preeclampsia is the single most frequent cause of admission to the ICU (38,39) and the most common system affected is the respiratory system (40). The role of central venous pressure (CVP) and the PAC is briefly reviewed in the section that follows.

XII. CENTRAL VENOUS PRESSURE

The value of CVP measurement has been extensively debated. In many obstetrical suites where CVP is measured, the antecubital approach is popular since it is less invasive than the internal jugular and subclavian routes. Furthermore, obstetrical personnel believe that the information it provides is reliable. The internal jugular is the next most preferred route. This approach must be utilized only by those familiar with the technique, so that the risks of inadvertent carotid artery cannulation or pneumothorax are minimal. In the operating room, the anesthesiologist may elect to use a CVP monitor to obtain an estimate of intravascular volume prior to anesthesia and vasodilator therapy. It may also help to guide volume expansion during anesthesia. Furthermore, the use of the CVP monitor in the post-partum period may help to elucidate postoperative fluid requirements until the patient experiences a diuresis after delivery. Cotton and coworkers (41) showed poor correlation between the CVP and PWCP in women with preeclampsia, and this finding led several investigators to recommend pulmonary artery catheterization over CVP measurement in severe preeclamptic patients (42,43). The CVP is a poor reflection of left ventricular function in the presence of myocardial dysfunction and hence an unreliable guide to fluid management in such cases. Fortunately the majority of severe preeclamptic patients have normal to high cardiac performance indices due to hyperdynamic left ventricular function even when systemic vascular resistance is markedly elevated (43). This tendency has caused many obstetricians and anesthesiologists to treat patients without invasive monitoring until such time as it becomes clear that the patient is not responding to usual therapy.

XIII. PULMONARY ARTERY CATHETER

The value of the pulmonary artery catheter (PAC) in acutely ill patients (including those with severe preeclampsia) is still debated. This catheter was first described more than 20 years ago, and although the PAC has definitely contributed to our understanding of severe preeclampsia, its therapeutic benefit is less clear. Recommendations in 1988 confine the anesthetic indications for a PAC to a few conditions (Table 3). The American College of Obstetricians and Gynecologists has outlined the circumstances in which the use of a PAC is recommended in pregnancy (44). They state that the PAC does not form part of routine management of severe preeclampsia. Many patients who satisfy the ACOG criteria for invasive monitoring can be safely treated by noninvasive techniques (16a,16b), and in general only those women who may require long-term or very frequent estimates of central pressures and cardiac output need be subjected to the risks of a PAC.

The characterization and treatment of oliguria warrant discussion. They have been described in three distinct hemodynamic groups (45). The majority of women had volume depletion, as indicated by low PCWP, hyperdynamic ventricular function, and moderately elevated SVR. Volume expansion was recommended in this group. In a second group, oliguria secondary to severe renal artery

Table 3 Conditions That May Indicate a Need for Pulmonary Artery Catheterization in Severe Preeclampsia or Eclampsia—in Many of These Situations Noninvasive Assessment with Echocardiography May Preclude the Need for Invasive Monitoring

1. Pulmonary edema with
   a. Cardiogenic or left ventricular failure
   b. Increased systemic vascular resistance
   c. Noncardiogenic volume overload
   d. Decreased colloid oncotic pressure
2. Oliguria unresponsive to modest fluid load (500–1000 mL)[a]
   a. Low preload
   b. High systemic vascular resistance with low cardiac output
   c. Selective renal artery vasoconstriction
3. Severe hypertension unresponsive or refractory to therapy[a]
   a. High systemic vascular resistance
   b. Increased cardiac output
4. Persistent arterial desaturation; inability to distinguish between cardiac and noncardiac origin

[a]In patients who are in labor, temporization in anticipation of improvement following delivery is an acceptable alternative to pulmonary artery catheterization.
Source: Ref. 43.

vasospasm was present in women who had normal or increased PCWP and normal CO and SVR values. These patients were treated with low-dose dopamine and mild afterload reduction. In a third group, depressed ventricular function and elevated PCWP and SVR were present, and oliguria was attributed to volume overload and excessive systemic afterload. Treatment in these women consisted of volume restriction and aggressive afterload reduction. In clinical practice, the PAC is not very helpful in oliguric patients who do not respond to volume therapy. As mentioned, some authorities (43) advocate the placement of a PAC in all women with severe preeclampsia. Others have highlighted that not only is the insertion and use of a PAC not innocuous, but there is a paucity of data to support improved outcome with its use. There are valid concerns regarding the morbidity and even mortality rates associated with the PAC, and placement must be carefully considered by the anesthesiologist and obstetrician.

XIV. INVASIVE BLOOD PRESSURE MONITORING

Radial artery cannulation for invasive monitoring of blood pressure is largely confined to situations in which rapidly acting antihypertensive agents are employed to control blood pressure. In the obese patient invasive blood pressure monitoring is indicated when noninvasive blood pressure measurement proves difficult. Severe preeclamptic conditions are said to be prone to wide fluctuations in blood pressure, especially after regional anesthesia, but there is little evidence for this assertion in the literature. Arterial cannulae offer the further advantage of allowing frequent blood gas and acid-base analysis.

XV. COAGULATION AND ANESTHESIA

It is not uncommon for the clinician to be faced with the dilemma of planning anesthesia and labor analgesia in a preeclamptic patient with abnormal coagulation studies. Approximately 15% of severely preeclamptic patients (but less than 5% of mild preeclamptic patients) have a clinically significant coagulopathy (6). The most common aberration in coagulation is a platelet defect that may be quantitative or qualitative (46). Consequently a platelet count is essential to assess the suitability for regional blockade (47). In an observational study of 40 preeclamptic patients by Schindler and associates (47), the bleeding time was prolonged in 2.5% of patients and there was a slightly decreased availability of platelet factor 3 (PF3). In addition, 21% had evidence of fibrinolysis and elevated monoclonal D-dimer. They concluded that the platelet count is an adequate screening test, and that a count between 50 and 100×10^9/L requires the determination of a bleeding time. Ramanathan and colleagues (48) concurred with this opinion. Whereas some authorities accept that the bleeding time is a useful and reliable method of assessing platelet function, most support the opposite view of Rodgers and Levin (49), who state that it does not accurately predict the risk of bleeding and is a poor diagnostic test prior to regional analgesia.

Despite the introduction of the thromboelastogram (TEG) more than a decade ago, its role still remains a source of contention. Some believe that this device has a well-established place in measuring whole blood clotting time (50). Orlikowski and Rocke have addressed the potential benefit of the use of the TEG in the labor suite (51). They suggest that the TEG may be a valuable guide to diagnosis and monitoring of hemostatic abnormalities in preeclamptic patients. They reported a strong correlation between the platelet count and the maximal amplitude of the TEG. In contrast, in 1995 Wong and coworkers (52) compared the TEG with routine coagulation screening tests and showed that the TEG was less effective. They also demonstrated that an abnormal maximal amplitude from TEG correlated with a prolonged bleeding time. In a study pertaining to severe preeclampsia, Sharma and associates (53) showed that a platelet count less than 100,000/mm³ was associated with hypocoaguability on the TEG. Nevertheless, TEG parameters that would allow safe epidural placement remain unclear. The availability of the TEG and the familiarity of the anesthesiologist with its use, rather than any defined benefit, currently determine the popularity of this technique in assessing hemostasis in preeclampsia.

XVI. MAGNESIUM AND ANESTHESIA

Eclamptic patients receiving magnesium sulfate frequently consult the obstetrical anesthesiologist for anesthesia. In 1995 the Collaborative Eclampsia Trial (54) provided definitive evidence that $MgSO_4$ is a superior anticonvulsant to phenytoin and diazepam in the prevention of recurrent seizures in women with eclampsia. There is some debate as to whether magnesium is beneficial for the prophylaxis of eclampsia in women who have preeclampsia. A large multicenter trial (MAGPIE trial) is currently addressing this question.

The underlying abnormality of convulsions in eclampsia is unknown but is thought to involve, at least in some cases, cerebral ischemia secondary to vasospasm. Magnesium is thought to alleviate cerebral vasospasm (55,56). In obstetrical practice magnesium sulfate has also been used as a tocolytic agent. For some unknown reason, the hemodynamic effects of magnesium sulfate appear to be more significant in women with preeclampsia. Scardo and colleagues (57) demonstrated in 1995 that women receiving magnesium sulfate for the treatment of preeclampsia experienced a more pronounced increase in cardiac output and reduction in systemic vascular resistance than women given magnesium in preterm labor.

Magnesium has catecholamine antagonist effects and a bolus (40–60 mg/kg) is often used at induction of general anesthesia to obtund the hemodynamic response to intubation (58). Combination of 30 mg/kg magnesium sulfate and alfentanil 7.5 µg/kg offers superior blood pressure control at intubation when compared to use of either agent alone (59). Magnesium is not recommended for the attenuation of the extubation response because of its postoperative neuromuscular depressant effect (60).

At therapeutic serum concentrations, magnesium sulfate potentiates the effect of nondepolarizing muscle relaxants. Hence, competitive neuromuscular blockers must be used in reduced doses and supplemental doses should be administered less frequently. Some investigators recommend the use of mivacurium chloride as an appropriate nondepolarizing muscle relaxant (61), despite its prolonged duration of action in the presence of magnesium (62). Although the interaction between suxamethonium and magnesium sulfate is less clear, some authors believe that suxamethonium chloride should be used for muscle relaxation after magnesium administration (6). In preeclampsia, there is a reduction in the normal plasma cholinesterase concentration so that suxamethonium chloride may have a prolonged effect in conjunction with magnesium.

The simultaneous use of nifedipine and magnesium sulfate has been shown to cause neuromuscular blockade (63). The question of whether there is greater hypotension and subsequent refractoriness to treatment when regional anesthesia is simultaneously employed with magnesium sulfate is confined to animal studies and remains speculative. Despite the fact that most of our knowledge in this regard has been derived from work in gravid ewes, some authors have extrapolated these data and suggest that because of the mechanism of action of magnesium sulfate, ephedrine should be used as a vasopressor rather than phenylephrine (64).

The possible interaction of calcium channel antagonists and magnesium requires discussion. Opinions differ regarding the effect of this drug combination on the cardiovascular system. Scardo and coworkers (65) in their analysis of 10 patients with severe preeclampsia demonstrated a decrease in systemic vascular resistance and an increase in the cardiac index during hypertensive emergencies. Other workers suggest that the combination can be used with caution (66). Although there remains no conclusive answer, the risks may have been exaggerated by poorly controlled in vitro studies.

Magnesium-related antiplatelet and antithrombotic properties have been described, leading to concerns regarding the placement of an epidural catheter. To date there are no definitive investigations that determine whether the platelet-magnesium interaction is clinically significant. One study showed that magnesium serum concentrations greater than 7 mmol/L produced statistically, but not clinically, significant TEG changes (67). One group observed an increase in blood loss at delivery in preeclamptic women with a prolonged bleeding time who received magnesium (68). This finding has not been independently confirmed.

XVII. LABOR ANALGESIA

A. Epidural Analgesia

It is widely accepted that epidural analgesia is usually the preferred method for labor analgesia and vaginal delivery in the severely preeclamptic parturient (5,6,69). One of the most important benefits of the epidural technique is the high-quality analgesia provided. Patient comfort and restful labor are characteristics of epidural analgesia that ensure maintenance of cardiovascular stability and a reduced need for antihypertensive medications. There is also a suggestion of a beneficial effect on placental blood flow. Joupilla and associates (70) showed that lumbar epidural analgesia produced a definite, albeit modest, improvement in the intervillous blood flow during labor in severe preeclamptic conditions. More recent evidence by Ramos-Santos and colleagues (71) supports this view. They compared Doppler resistance indices in the umbilical and uterine arteries of normal, chronic hypertensive, and preeclamptic patients. There was a reduction in resistance in the uterine arteries of preeclamptic women during epidural analgesia initiated for active term labor. They speculated that the fetus might benefit from this. Another advantage of the epidural technique is the provision of excellent analgesia for operative vaginal or abdominal delivery. Thus in cases of severe preeclampsia insertion of an epidural should be considered when the obstetrician has committed the patient to delivery. There is no benefit in waiting for the development of painful contractions and established labor. It has been suggested that preeclamptic women are more likely to have a successful induction of labor than nonpreeclamptic patients, but this was questioned in 1997 by Xenakis and coworkers (72). In their prospective study of 183 preeclamptic women requiring induction, they noted a higher risk of failed induction and a higher incidence of cesarean section in the preeclamptic than in the normal patients.

Another controversial area is the volume of fluid preload that can be safely given to the severely preeclamptic parturient. The incidence of hypotension in Moore and coworkers' retrospective review (73) of 185 preeclamptic gravidas was shown to be 7%, which compared favorably to the 6% incidence in women who received local anesthesia. Clinical experience shows that supplemental fluids and vasoconstrictors are often not required (5) prior to epidural blockade. It is likely that the introduction of the low-dose and low-concentration epidural technique has appreciably reduced the incidence of hypotension. Nonetheless, the anesthesiologist should not to be complacent and should be prepared for hypotension. Fluid therapy should be administered with due consideration of factors such as the severity of the disease, the presence of renal compromise and/or oliguria, and indicators of central hemodynamic status. A modest preload volume of 500–1000 mL of a balanced salt solution may be safely infused prior to epidural insertion (6) in the majority of preeclamptic patients.

Most obstetrical anesthesiologists are concerned about the development of an epidural hematoma in a severely preeclamptic woman with thrombocytopenia. Therefore, an absence of bleeding diatheses (as evidenced by petechiae and excessive bleeding from mucosal and puncture sites) must be confirmed. The withholding of an epidural anesthetic because of thrombocytopenia (defined as a platelet count of 50–100,000/mm^3) in this regard has been challenged by Beilin and associates (74), who looked retrospectively at 30 thrombocytopenic patients (platelet count of 69–98,000 mm^3) who had received epidural analgesia. Neurological complications developed in none. They concluded that epidural analgesia should not necessarily be contraindicated in this circumstance. In most patients with preeclampsia, a complete blood count including platelet count suffices as a screening investigation. Fitzgerald and colleagues (75), however, still recommend that fibrinogen, prothrombin time, and partial thromboplastin time be determined in those patients with severe preeclampsia in whom an operative delivery under regional anesthesia is contemplated. This recommendation was based on minor abnormalities detected in their study. In milder forms of the disease, laboratory investigations may be unnecessary (76).

With regard to the addition of epinephrine to the local anesthetic solution, opinions remain polarized. The potential for exacerbation of hypertension is frequently cited (77), even though β-2 effects are predominant with epidural doses of epinephrine (78). Thus the dangers of iatrogenic hypertension with simultaneous epinephrine and local anesthetic are mainly theoretical. In one study of epinephrine-containing local anesthetics in women with mild preeclampsia, there was no evidence of cardiovascular instability or dysrhythmias (79). Some authorities still believe that the potential dangers of systemic absorption contraindicate the use of epinephrine in both the test dose and the infusion (5). They maintain that the uterine vasculature in patients with preeclampsia is hyperreactive to cate-cholamines and any worsening of the preexisting hypertension could have delete-rious effects on both mother and fetus (80). A 1995 report (81) described exacerba-tion of the hypertension in a preeclamptic parturient after the administration of epinephrine-containing local anesthetic solution. However, the pathophysiologi-cal mechanism for this reaction was not clear and there is no obvious association between the reaction and epidural epinephrine administration. Nevertheless, there are a number of cautionary reports describing adverse effects of epidural epi-nephrine on the uteroplacental and fetal circulations (82,83). We therefore advise that epinephrine containing solutions should not be used in epidural anesthesia of preeclamptic women.

XVIII. SUBARACHNOID ANALGESIA

In 1966 direct injection of local anesthetic into the subarachnoid space was shown to be a safe alternative to other methods of analgesia for pain control in labor (84). Important cautionary measures included judicious volume preload and ensuring of uterine displacement. In modern day practice, the combined spinal-epidural tech-nique has replaced the "single-shot" subarachnoid method, and so the role of the latter is limited. The shortcomings of this technique include the inability to extend both the duration and the extent of the block. Additionally, intrathecal local anesthetics may be associated with a dense motor block, which is undesirable during labor.

XIX. PARENTERAL OPIOIDS

Parenteral opioids for labor analgesia may be used when neuraxial blockade is contraindicated, as in cases of uncorrected coagulopathy or patient refusal. Al-though the quality of analgesia may be acceptable to some, supplementation of analgesia with inhalational agents such as nitrous oxide in oxygen is often neces-sary as labor advances. Incomplete analgesia may exacerbate hypertension (6) and not uncommonly necessitates pharmacological intervention. More recently many anesthesiologists have used alfentanil, which in the author's experience is a useful alternative to the longer-acting opioids.

XX. CESAREAN SECTION ANESTHESIA

Perspectives regarding the safety as well as the advantages and disadvantages of various anesthetic methods used for cesarean section have significantly changed in recent years. Some authors have demonstrated the superiority of certain regional techniques (85,86), whereas others have shown both regional and general anesthetic techniques are equally acceptable if appropriately performed (87,88). It is important to remember that none of the methods of anesthesia is without complications and that the choice of anesthesia must reflect the balance between risk and benefit.

A. Epidural Anesthesia

Hodgkinson and coworkers (85) in their landmark study showed stable hemodynamic variables i.e., pulmonary artery pressures (PAPs), pulmonary capillary wedge pressures, and mean arterial pressures in women receiving epidural analgesia for cesarean section. Women who had general anesthesia displayed dramatic, albeit transient, changes in hemodynamic variables at endotracheal intubation and extubation. The potential for morbidity is difficult to estimate. Ramanathan and associates (89) showed that epidural anesthesia is associated with a suppression of the neuroendocrine stress response in severe preeclampsia. In this important study, it was evident that obliteration of the catecholamine response was the most likely reason for the stable intraoperative hemodynamic variables in patients who received epidural anesthesia. In the general anesthetic group, there was evidence of a neuroendocrine stress response, as evidenced by a rise in the mean arterial pressure (MAP), initially apparent at the time of the skin incision but subsequently maintained throughout the study period. The authors claimed a short-term benefit to neonates of severely preeclamptic women who were given epidural anesthesia, since these babies had a higher 1-minute Apgar score (89). A poor 1-minute Apgar score is, however, not known to be strongly related to the long-term outcome of a neonate with a normal 5-minutes score; thus the significance of this finding is questionable.

The fetal outcome in severe preeclampsia, especially in the low- and very-low-birth-weight groups, may be improved by epidural anesthesia. Extremely immature infants do not tolerate well the hypotension induced by subarachnoid block; nor do they tolerate the central nervous system (CNS)-depressant anesthetic drugs required for general anesthesia. There is a need for comprehensive long-term outcome studies to define the potential advantages of epidural analgesia in neonates delivered of mothers with severe preeclampsia. Alexander and colleagues (90) showed no detrimental neonatal effects of induction of labor compared with cesarean delivery in very-low-birth-weight infants of women with severe preeclampsia. Unfortunately these authors did not include in their findings a specific evaluation of labor analgesia and anesthetic management.

Airway management in women with severe preeclampsia can be complicated by difficult intubation or aspiration of gastric contents, and epidural anesthesia may be a significant factor in reducing anesthetic morbidity and mortality rates. Epidural anesthesia is the technique of choice in appropriately screened severely preeclamptic women, and the method was substantially refined in the 1990s (5,6,91–93). Pritchard and colleagues (12) in a study of 245 patients urged caution in the use of regional anesthesia for severe preeclampsia-eclampsia. It was suggested that hypotension was associated with sympathetic blockade and that there was a need to treat this with large volumes of intravenous fluids and vasopressor agents that could increase the risk of pulmonary edema. Further reservations were related to the safety of the fetus. Nonreassuring changes in the intrapartum fetal heart rate pattern have been associated with decreased uteroplacental blood flow, possibly mediated by epidurally induced hypotension (94). The American College of Obstetricians and Gynecologists recommends that epidural blockade in the severely preeclamptic parturient requires an experienced obstetrical anesthesiologist but does not contraindicate the practice (95).

Whether the local anesthetic agent lidocaine should still be used for the establishment of epidural blockade is debatable. Some authorities choose other agents (5) because of the perceived unfavorable pharmacokinetic properties of lidocaine, which include fetal acidosis, maternal and fetal toxicity, and a narrow therapeutic range (96). It is our contention that lidocaine may be used without serious risk to mother and fetus, with the caveats that the correct dose and concentration must be ensured and that the placement of the epidural catheter should be routinely tested.

B. Epidural Anesthesia for Emergency Cesarean Section

Most laboring patients with severe preeclampsia have in situ epidural analgesia. Usually this enables emergency cesarean section to be undertaken. The convenience and safety of this method have led to the widespread acceptance of epidural analgesia. The most frequent indication for emergency cesarean section in the severely preeclamptic patient is presumed fetal distress during labor. Chronic fetal compromise is not necessarily a contraindication to epidural analgesia for cesarean section, although one should realize that a growth restricted baby is less able to tolerate maternal hypotension than a normally grown one. In most circumstances spinal anesthesia is not recommended when immediate delivery is required (discussed later). Obviously in an acute emergency the safest technique for both mother and baby should be used and consultation between obstetrician and anesthesiologist is essential. There is ongoing controversy regarding the anesthetic technique when urgent delivery is necessary.

C. Spinal Anesthesia for Cesarean Section

Many anesthesiologists and obstetricians believe that spinal anesthesia is contraindicated in severe preeclampsia. This idea was challenged in the 1990s. In fact, in some institutions, spinal anesthesia is becoming increasingly popular for cesarean section in severely preeclamptic women (5). The traditionalists believe that the danger of precipitous hypotension that necessitates intravenous fluids and vasopressor agents pose a threat to both the mother and the fetus. This idea has not been substantiated by well-conducted clinical trials. Since 1990 there has been evidence presented to suggest that spinal anesthesia is acceptable in severe preeclampsia (87,97) and in some cases is preferable to epidural analgesia (86). A 1999 retrospective review of 103 patients with severe preeclampsia indicated that the reductions in blood pressure in women with epidural or spinal analgesia were comparable (97) and that both maternal and fetal outcomes were similar. Intravenous fluid requirements were appreciably greater after spinal as opposed to epidural analgesia, although there was no increase in the rate of serious complications. A comparison of hemodynamic variables in women with spinal versus general anesthesia for cesarean section showed no significant differences in blood pressure, although heart rate variability increased in the severely preeclamptic women treated with spinal analgesia (88). Assessment of Apgar scores suggests that the uteroplacental changes caused by spinal hypotension do not have a major impact on the immediate neonatal outcome (98). Although preeclampsia and spinal anesthesia are both independently associated with umbilical arterial acidemia (77,99), poor fetal/neonatal outcome does not necessarily result. The role of continuous spinal anesthesia in the management of parturients with severe preeclampsia requires further investigation before it can be recommended (100).

D. General Anesthesia for Severe Preeclampsia

The potential for complications of general anesthesia in severe preeclampsia is well recognized. The neuraxial route of anesthesia, principally the epidural technique, boasts a better safety record than and has largely replaced general anesthesia in the uncomplicated severe preeclamptic population. The hypertensive and neuroendocrine stress response associated with tracheal intubation in severe preeclampsia increases the risk of cerebral hemorrhage and cerebral edema (89,101). In Ramanathan and colleagues' study of eight patients with severe preeclampsia (102), a significant, albeit transient, rise in mean arterial pressure was matched by concomitant increase in maternal cerebral blood flow velocity. This remained increased for 6 minutes after rapid-sequence induction-intubation. Whether these findings indicate a predisposition of the severe preeclamptic to cerebral edema and hemorrhage is uncertain at this stage. Regardless, this study does show significant and prolonged cerebral hemodynamic perturbation after induction of general anesthesia, and avoidance of such a hemodynamic effect may well be in the best interests of the mother. Cerebrovascular autoregulation is impaired in preeclampsia, and forced overdistention of small intracranial arteries and subsequent vasogenic edema has been described (103). The pharmacological blunting of the hypertensive response to intubation is thus mandatory when performing general anesthesia in these patients, and there are many therapeutic options available to the anesthesiologist. Labetalol (20-mg bolus), increased in 10-mg increments to a total of 1 mg/kg before induction, reliably controls blood pressure prior to induction of general anesthesia (104). This technique does not appear to cause neonatal hypotension, bradycardia, or hypoglycemia, although there is a report (35) of fetal heart rate effects with similar doses. The use of the β_1 selective antagonist esmolol is discouraged for several reasons. The negative chronotropic effect is associated with an undesirable decrease in maternal cardiac output, and unopposed α-agonism may cause an increase in SVR and exacerbate hypertension. Several case reports suggest an added risk of fetal bradycardia from transplacental transfer of this drug (106,107). Nitroglycerin has been used by Hood and colleagues (105) in patients with severe preeclampsia and may be useful, but as outlined previously there are better alternatives to this drug for preeclampsia.

A comparison of currently used agents by Allen and coworkers (108) showed that in 69 parturients with moderate to severe hypertension magnesium sulfate (40 mg/kg), given immediately after induction of anesthesia, was as effective as alfentanil (10 μg/kg) and superior to lignocaine (1.5 mg/kg) in attenuating the hypertensive response to intubation. A subsequent study (59) illustrated that the combination of alfentanil (7.5 μg/kg) and magnesium (30 mg/kg) may be even more effective than either drug used alone. Neither of the latter two agents however, is suitable for blunting the extubation response.

Edema of the upper airway is not an unusual finding in women with severe preeclampsia and can coexist with facial or generalized edema (109). Its presence may pose a challenge to the management of the airway. Endotracheal intubation may be difficult, and trauma and subsequent hemorrhage, hypoxemia, or aspiration may occur. Preoperative airway examination must therefore be complete and preparation for specialized methods of endotracheal intubation is essential. Laryngeal edema may develop rapidly at any stage in the peripartum period and usually manifests as acute respiratory decompensation (109). The anesthesiologist must also exercise caution when attempting extubation of preeclamptic patients after cesarean section, and the cuff test (described by Potgeiter and Hammond) is recommended (110). The presence of laryngeal edema is an indication for continued postoperative ventilation.

XXI. HEMOLYSIS, ELEVATED LIVER ENZYME LEVEL, LOW PLATELET COUNT SYNDROME

The HELLP syndrome is characterized by *h*emolysis, *e*levated *l*iver enzyme levels and a *l*ow *p*latelet count (HELLP) and is an indicator of hepatic ischemia that is causing periportal hemorrhage and necrosis. Since its first description in 1982, there remains debate regarding whether it is an independent disease entity (111) or a subset of severe preeclampsia. In up to 70% of affected patients HELLP syndrome develops in the antepartum period, most often before 36 weeks gestation (112). In some, the laboratory evidence of HELLP syndrome may precede the development of hypertension and proteinuria, and in up to 15% of patients with HELLP syndrome there is no hypertension or proteinuria. Although the presence of the syndrome suggests a severe form of preeclampsia, the clinical presentation is variable (113). This may cause problems for the anesthesiologist as the syndrome may be misdiagnosed. Parturients with HELLP syndrome are at particular risk for hemorrhage, rupture of a subcapsular hepatic hematoma, acute renal failure, and acute respiratory distress syndrome (ARDS). The anesthesiologist should therefore identify which organ systems are affected and plan the anesthetic intervention accordingly. Thrombocytopenia may be sufficient to preclude epidural analgesia. Attention must be paid to the possibility of postpartum hemorrhage as the nadir of the thrombocytopenia may occur up to 72 hours after delivery (114). Clinicians involved in the management of patients with HELLP syndrome should always consider other diagnoses, such as thrombotic thrombocytopenic purpura (TTP), hemolytic uremic syndrome (HUS), acute hepatorenal failure, fatty metamorphosis of pregnancy ("fatty liver"), and acute liver failure from other causes. This analysis becomes especially important in postpartum thrombocytopenia that does not resolve despite platelet transfusion. In these cases TTP should be ruled out by peripheral smear analysis, and hematological consultation should be sought since platelet transfusion may significantly worsen the prognosis. In acute idiopathic TTP, plasma exchange and high-dose steroid therapy are indicated.

XXII. ECLAMPSIA

The development of generalized tonic-clonic epileptiform seizures during pregnancy in conjunction with proteinuric hypertension is defined as *eclampsia* (115). The anesthesiologist may be involved early in the management of such patients for basic cardiopulmonary resuscitation and airway control. Postictal confusion and sedation from anticonvulsant therapy may complicate the assessment of the neurological status prior to anesthetic intervention. The anesthesiologist should prevent further seizures with magnesium sulfate (occasionally in combination with short-acting benzodiazepines), control the blood pressure, and order appropriate blood tests to exclude the other complications of severe preeclampsia. Although acute severe hypertension may not always be present (116), it is imperative that the mean arterial blood pressure be maintained above 90 mmHg in order to ensure adequate cerebral and uteroplacental perfusion. When rapid-acting intravenous agents are required to control the blood pressure, central venous access is useful.

The definitive treatment of eclampsia is delivery of the fetus. However, optimization of maternal condition is imperative for the good outcome of both mother and baby. Both an ill-prepared mother and the fetus are exposed to obstetrical and anesthetic risk. Anesthesia may be hazardous in those with severe hypertension as they are at risk of cerebrovascular hemorrhage (117). Most authors support the recommendation by Sibai and associates (118) that a minimum of 2 hours be taken to effect maternal stabilization. In addition, eclampsia should not be regarded as an automatic indication for cesarean delivery. In most cases fetal condition mirrors that of the mother, and once convulsions cease and maternal oxygenation is optimized, the fetal condition rapidly improves. Induction of labor is often safest.

XXIII. CONCLUSION

Maternal mortality due to preeclampsia has declined in the United States (119). This decline may in part reflect improved intensive care services (120) but also suggests that modern antenatal and intrapartum care has evolved to a higher level. The role of the anesthesiologist in the management of severe preeclampsia is vital, and adherence to the principles of management discussed here will go a long way to helping ensure a good outcome.

REFERENCES

1. Department of Health and others. Report on Confidential Enquiries into Maternal Deaths in the United Kingdom 1991–1993. London: HMSO, 1996.
2. Department of Health. Report on Confidential Enquiries into Maternal Deaths in the United Kingdom 1994–1996. London: HMSO, 1998: 36–46.
3. National Committee on Confidential Enquiries into Maternal Deaths. A review of maternal deaths in South Africa during 1998. S Afr Med J 2000; 90:367–373.
4. Brodie H, Manilow M. Anesthetic management of preeclampsia/eclampsia. Int J Obstet Anesth 1999; 8:110–124.
5. Hood DD. Preeclampsia. In: Dewan DM, Hood DD, ed. Practical Obstetric Anesthesia, 1st ed. Philadelphia: W.B. Saunders, 1997:211–237.
6. Cheek TG, Samuel P. Pregnancy-induced hypertension. In: Datta S, ed. Anesthesia and Obstetric Management of High-Risk Pregnancy. St Louis: Mosby-Year Book, 1996:386–411.
7. Desmond Writer. Hypertensive Disorders. In: Chestnut DH, ed. Obstetric Anesthesia—Principles and Practice. St. Louis: Mosby-Year Book, 1994: 846.
8. Martin JN Jr, May WL, Magann EF et al. Early risk assessment of severe preeclampsia: admission battery of symptoms and laboratory tests to predict likelihood of subsequent maternal morbidity. Am J Obstet Gynecol 1999; 180:1407–1414.

9. Redman CWG, Roberts JM. Management of preeclampsia. Lancet 1993; 341:1451–1454.
10. Belfort MA, Saade GR, Grunewalde C et al. Association of cerebral perfusion pressure with headache in women with preeclampsia. Br J Obstet Gynaecol 1999; 106(8):814–821.
11. Sibai BM et al. Pregnancy outcome in 303 cases with severe pre-eclampsia. Obstet Gynecol 1984; 64:319–325.
12. Pritchard JA, Cunningham FG, Pritchard SA. The Parkland Memorial Hospital protocol for the treatment of eclampsia: evaluation of 245 cases. Am J Obstet Gynecol 1984; 148:951–963.
13. Belfort MA, Uys P, Dommisse J, Davey DA. Hamodynamic changes in gestational proteinuric hypertension: the effects of rapid volume expansion and vasodilator therapy. Br J Obstet Gynaecol 1989; 96:634–641.
14. Kirshon B, Moise KJ, Cotton DB et al. Role of volume expansion in severe preeclampsia. Surg Gynecol Obstet 1988; 167:367
15. Robson SC, Pearson JF. Fluid restriction policies in preeclampsia are obsolete. Int J Obstet Anesth 1999; 8:49–55.
16. Robson SC, Thomas DG. Hypertensive disease in pregnancy. Monitoring and fluid management. In: Goldstone JC, Pollard BJ, eds. Handbook of Clinical Anaesthesia. London: Churchill Livingstone, 1996: 414–416.
16a. Belfort MA, Rokey R, Saade GR, Moise KJ. Rapid echocardiographic assessment of left and right heart hemodynamics in critically ill obstetric patients. Am J Obstet Gynecol 1994; 171(4):884–892.
16b. Belfort MA, Mares A, Saade G, Wen T, Rokey R. Two-dimensional echocardiography and Doppler ultrasound in managing obstetric patients. Obstet Gynecol 1997; 90(3):326–330.
17. Sibai BM, Mabie WC, Harvey CJ, Gonzales AR. Pulmonary edema in severe preeclampsia-eclampsia: analysis of thirty-seven consecutive cases. Am J Obstet Gynecol 1987; 156:1174–1179.
18. Benedetti TJ, Kates R, Williams V. Hemodynamic observations in severe pre-eclampsia complicated by pulmonary edema. Am J Obstet Gynecol 1985; 152:330.
19. Mortl MG, Schneider MC. Key issues in assessing, managing and treating patients presenting with severe preeclampsia. Int J Obstet Anesthesia 2000; 9:39–44.
20. Yeast JD, Halberstadt C, Meyer BA et al. The risk of pulmonary edema and colloid oncotic pressure changes during magnesium therapy. Am J Obstet Gynecol 1993; 169:1566.
21. Sibai BM, Villar MA, Mabie BC. Acute renal failure in hypertensive disorders of pregnancy. Am J Obstet Gynecol 1990; 162:777–783.
22. Pouta A, Karinen J, Vuolteenahoo O, Laatikainen T. Preeclampsia: the effect of intravenous fluid preload on atrial natriuretic peptide secretion during Caeserean section under spinal anaesthesia. Acta Anesthesiol Scand 1996; 40(10):1203–1209.
23. Engelhardt T, MacLennan FM. Fluid management in preeclampsia. Int J Obstet Anesth 1999; 8:253–259.
24. Sibai BM. Treatment of hypertension in pregnant women. N Engl J Med 1996; 335:257–265.
25. Cunningham FG, Lindheimer MD. Hypertension in pregnancy. N Engl J Med 1992; 326(14):927–932.

26. Paterson-Brown S, Robson SC, Redfern N et al. Hydralazine boluses for the treatment of severe hypertension in preeclampsia. Br J Obstet Gynaecol 1994; 101: 409–413.

27. Kirshon B, Wasserstrum N, Cotton DB: Should continuous hydralazine infusions be utilized in severe pregnancy-induced hypertension? Am J Perinatol 1991; 8:206–208.

28. Powers DR, Papadakos PJ, Wallin JD. Parenteral hydralazine revisited. J Emerg Med 1998; 16:191–196.

29. Khedun SM, Moodley J, Naicker T, Maharaj B. Drug management of hypertensive disorders of pregnancy. Pharmacol Ther 1997; 74:221–258.

30. Bolte AC, van Eyck J, Kanhai HH et al. Ketanserin versus dihydralazine in the management of severe early onset preeclampsia: maternal outcome. Am J Obstet Gynecol 1999; 180:371–377.

31. Mabie WC, Gonzalez AR, Sibai BM, Amon E. A comparative trial of labetalol and hydralazine in the acute management of severe hypertension complicating pregnancy. Obstet Gynecol 1987; 70:328–333.

32. Chari S, Friedman SA, Sibai BM. Anti-hypertensive therapy during pregnancy. Fetal Matern Med Rev 1995; 7:61–75.

33. Bhorat IE, Naidoo DP, Rout CC, Moodley J. Malignant ventricular arrhythmias in eclampsia: a comparison of labetalol and dihydralazine. Am J Obstet Gynecol 1993; 168:1292–1296.

34. Ramanathan J, Sibai BM, Mabie WC et al. The use of labetalol for the attenuation of the hypertensive response to endotracheal intubation in preeclampsia. Am J Obstet Gynecol 1988; 159:650–654.

35. Klarr JM, Bhatt-Metha V, Donn SM. Neonatal adrenergic blockade following single dose intravenous maternal labetalol administration. Am J Perinatol 1994; 11:91–93.

36. Levin AC, Doering PL, Hatton RC. Use of nifedipine in the hypertensive diseases of pregnancy. Ann Pharmacother 1994; 28:1371–1378.

37. Waisman DG, Mayorga LM, Camera MI et al. Magnesium plus nifedipine: potentiation of hypotensive effect in preeclampsia. Am J Obstet Gynecol 1988; 159: 308–309.

37a. Herling IM. Intravenous nitroglycerin: clinical pharmacology and therapeutic considerations. Am Heart J 1984; 108:141–149.

37b. Pasch T, Schulz V, Hoppelshauser G. Nitroprusside-induced formation of cyanide and its detoxification with thiosulfate during deliberate hypotension. J Cardiovasc Pharmacol 1983; 5:77–85.

37c. Shoemaker CT, Meyers M. Sodium nitroprusside for control of severe hypertensive disease of pregnancy: a case report and discussion of potential toxicity. Am J Obstet Gynecol 1984; 14:171–173.

38. Mabie WC, Sibai BM. Treatment in an obstetric intensive care unit. Am J Obstet Gynecol 1990; 162:1–4.

39. Kilpatrick SJ, Matthay MA. Obstetric patients requiring critical care: a five year review. Chest 1992; 101:1407–1412.

40. Collop NA, Sahn SA. Critical illness in pregnancy: an analysis of 20 patients admitted to a medical intensive care unit. Chest 1993; 103:1541–1552.

41. Cotton DB, Lee W, Huhta JC, Dorman KF. Hemodynamic profile of severe pregnancy-induced hypertension. Am J Obstet Gynecol 1988; 158:523–529.

42. Gibbs CP. Pulmonary artery catheterization in severe preeclampsia. Am J Obstet Gynecol 1989; 162:1089.
43. Clark SL, Cotton DB. Clinical indications for pulmonary artery catheterization in patients with severe preeclampsia. Am J Obstet Gynecol 1988; 158:453–458.
44. American College of Obstetricians and Gynecologists. Invasive hemodynamic monitoring in obstetrics and gynecology. ACOG Technical Bulletin No. 175, 1992.
45. Clark SL, Greenspoon JS, Aldahl D et al. Severe preeclampsia with persistent oliguria: Management of hemodynamic subsets. Am J Obstet Gynecol 1986; 154: 490–494.
46. Kelton JG, Hunter DJ, Neame PB. A platelet function defect in preeclampsia. Obstet Gynecol 1985; 65:107–109.
47. Schindler M, Gatt S, Isert P et al. Thrombocytopenia and platelet functional defects in pre-eclampsia: implications for regional anaesthesia. Anaesth Intensive Care 1990; 18:169–174.
48. Ramanathan J, Sibai BM, Vu T, Chauhan D. Correlation between bleeding times and platelet counts in women with preeclampsia undergoing cesarean section. Anesthesiology 1989; 71:188–191.
49. Rodgers RPC, Levin J. A critical reappraisal of the bleeding time. Semin Thromb Hemost 1990; 16:1–20.
50. Gorton H, Lyons G. Is it time to invest in a thromboelastograph? Int J Obstet Anesth 1999; 8:171–178.
51. Orlikowski CE, Rocke DA. Coagulation monitoring in the obstetric patient. Int Anesthesiol Clin 1994; 32(2):173–191.
52. Wong CA, Liu S, Glassenburg R. Comparison of thromboelastography with common coagulation tests in preeclamptic and normal parturients. Reg Anesth 1995; 20(6):521–527.
53. Sharma SK, Philip J, Whitten CW et al. Assessment of changes in coagualtion in parturients with preeclampsia using thromboelastography. Anesthesiology 1999; 90(2):385–390.
54. The Eclampsia Trial Collaborative Group. Which anticonvulsant for women with eclampsia? Evidence from the collaborative eclampsia trial. Lancet 1995; 345:1455–1463.
55. Naidu S, Payne AJ, Moodley J et al. Randomized study assessing the effect of phenytoin and magnesium sulphate on maternal cerebral circulation in eclampsia using transcranial Doppler ultrasound. Br J Obstet Gynaecol 1996; 103:111–116.
56. Naidu K, Moodley J, Corr P et al. Single photon emission and cerebral computerised tomographic scan and transcranial Doppler sonographic findings in eclampsia. Br J Obstet Gynaecol 1997; 104:1165–1172.
57. Scardo JA, Hogg BB, Newman RB. Favorable hemodynamic effects of magnesium sulfate in pre-eclampsia. Am J Obstet Gynecol 1995; 173:1249–1253.
58. James MFM, Beer RE, Esser JD. Intravenous magnesium sulphate inhibits catecholamine release associated with tracheal intubation. Anesth Analg 1989; 68: 772–776.
59. Ashton WB, James MFM, Janicki PK, Uys PC. The control of the hypertensive response to intubation in hypertensive pregnant patients with magnesium sulphate with and without alfentanil. Br J Anaesth 1991; 67:741–747.

60. James MFM. Magnesium in obstetric anesthesia. Int J Obstet Anesth 1998; 7(2): 115–123.

61. Hodgson RE, Rout CC, Rocke DA, Louw NJ. Mivacurium for caesarean section in hypertensive parturients receiving magnesium sulphate therapy. Int J Obstet Anesth 1998; 7(1):12–17

62. Ahn EK, Bai SJ, Cho BJ, Shin YS. The infusion rate of mivacurium and its spontaneous neuromuscular recovery in magnesium treated parturients. Anesth Analg 1998; 86(3):523–526.

63. Ben-Ami M, Giladi Y, Shalev E. The combination of magnesium sulphate and nifedipine: a cause of neuromuscular blockade. Br J Obstet Gynaecol 1994; 101: 262–263.

64. Sipes SL, Chestnut DH, Vincent RD et al. Which vasopressor should be used to treat hypotension during magnesium sulfate infusion and epidural anesthesia? Anesthesiology 1992; 77:101–108.

65. Scardo JA, Vermillion ST, Hogg BB, Newman RB. Hemodynamic effects of oral nifedipine in preeclamptic hypertensive emergencies. Am J Obstet Gynecol 1996; 175:336–338.

66. Davis WB, Wells SR, Kuller JA, Thorp JM Jr. Analysis of the risks associated with calcium channel blockade: implications for the obstetrician-gynecologist. Obstet Gynecol Survey 1993; 52:198–201.

67. James MFM, Neil G. Effect of magnesium on coagulation as measured by thrombo-elastography. Br J Anaesth 1995; 74:92–94.

68. Kynczl-Leisure M, Cibils LA. Increased bleeding time after magnesium sulfate infusion. Am J Obstet Gynecol 1996; 175:1293–1294.

69. Chadwick HS, Easterling T. Anesthetic concerns in the patient with preeclampsia. Semin Perinatol 1991; 15(5):397–409.

70. Joupilla P, Joupilla R, Holmen A, Koivula A. Lumbar epidural analgesia to improve intervillous blood flow during labor in severe preeclampsia. Obstet Gynecol 1982; 59:158–161.

71. Ramos-Santos E, Devoe LD, Wakefield ML et al. The effects of epidural anesthesia on the Doppler velocimetry of umbilical and uterine arteries in normal and hypertensive patients during active labor. Obstet Gynecol 1991; 77(1):20–26.

72. Xenakis EM, Piper JM, Field N et al. Preeclampsia: is induction more successful? Obstet Gynecol 1997; 89(4):600–603.

73. Moore TR, Key TC, Reisner LS et al. Evaluation of the use of continuous lumbar epidural anesthesia for hypertensive pregnant women in labor. Am J Obstet Gynecol 1985; 152:404.

74. Beilin Y, Zahn J, Comerford M. Safe epidural analgesia in thirty parturients with platelet counts between 69,000 and 98,000 mm^3. Anesth Analg 1997; 85(2):385–388

75. Fitzgerald MP, Floro C, Siegel J, Hernandez E. Laboratory findings in hypertensive disorders of pregnancy. J Natl Med Assoc 1996; 88(12):794–798.

76. Barron WM, Heckerling P, Hibbard JU, Fisher S. Reducing unnecessary coagulation testing in hypertensive disorders of pregnancy. Obstet Gynecol 1999; 94(3): 364–370.

77. Levy DM. Continuing controversy over the use of epidural adrenaline in pre-eclampsia. Br J Hosp Med 1993; 49:745.

78. Murphy TM, Mather LE, Stanton-Hicks MDA et al. The effects of adding adrenlaine to etidocaine and lignocaine in extradural anaesthesia. I. Block characteristics and cardiovascular effects. Br J Anaesth 1976; 48:893–898.

79. Dror A, Abboud TK, Moore T et al. Maternal hemodynamic responses to epinephrine containing local anesthetics in mild preeclampsia. Reg Anaesth 1988; 13:107.

80. Robinson DA. Epinephrine should not be used with local anesthetic for epidural anesthesia in preeclampsia. Anesthesia 1987; 66:578–579.

81. Hadzic A, Vloka J, Patel N, Birnbach D. Hypertensive crisis after successful placement of an epidural anesthetic in a hypertensive parturient. Case report. Reg Anesth 1995; 20:156–158.

82. Alahuta S, Rasanen J, Joupilla P et al. Uteroplacental and fetal circulation during extradural bupivacaine-adrenaline and bupivacaine for cesarean section in hypertensive pregnancies with chronic fetal asphyxia. Br J Anaesth 1993; 71:348.

83. Marx GF. Editorial comment. Obstet Anesth Dig 1994; 14:22.

84. Smith BE, Cavanaugh D, Moya F. Anesthesia for vaginal delivery in the patient with toxemia of pregnancy. Anesth Analg 1966; 45:853.

85. Hodgkinson R, Husain FJ, Hayashi RH. Systemic and pulmonary blood pressure during cesarean section in parturients with gestational hypertension. Can Anaesth Soc J 1980; 27:389–394.

86. Sharwood-Smith G, Clark VA, Watson EG. Regional anesthesia for Cesarean section for severe preeclampsia: spinal is the preferred choice. Int J Obstet Anesth 1999; 8:85–89.

87. Wallace DH, Leveno KJ, Cunningham FG et al. Randomized comparison of general and regional anesthesia for cesarean delivery in pregnancies complicated by severe preeclampsia. Obstet Gynecol 1995; 86:193–199.

88. Rout CC, Ward S, Rocke DA. Hemodynamic variability at emergent cesarean section in hypertensive patients—spinal versus general anesthesia. Anesthesiology, 1998; supple: A50.

89. Ramanathan J, Coleman P, Sibai BM. Anesthetic modification of hemodynamic and neuroendocrine stress responses to cesarean delivery in women with severe preeclampsia. Anesth Analg 1991; 73(6):772–779.

90. Alexander JM, Bloom SL, McIntire DD, Leveno KJ. Severe preeclampsia and the very low birth weight infant: is induction of labor harmful. Obstet Gynecol 1999; 93(4):485–488.

91. Chadwick HS, Easterling T. Anesthetic concerns in the patient with preeclampsia. Semin Perinatol 1991;15(5):397–409.

92. Howell P. Spinal anaesthesia in severe preeclampsia. Int J Obstet Anesth 1998; 7(4):217–219.

93. Gutsche BB, Cheek TG. Anesthesia considerations in preeclampsia-eclampsia. In: Shnider SM, Levinson G, eds. Anesthesia for Obstetrics, 3rd ed. Baltimore: Williams & Wilkins, 1993: 321.

94. Montau S, Ingermarsson I. Intrapartum fetal heart rate patterns in pregnancies complicated by hypertension. Am J Obstet Gynecol 1989; 160:283–288.

95. American College of Obstetricians and Gynecologists: Obstetric analgesia and anesthesia. Washington D.C.: ACOG Technical Bulletin No. 112, 1988.

96. Ramanathan J, Bottorff M, Jeter JN et al. The pharmacokinetics and maternal and neonatal effects of epidural lidocaine in preeclampsia. Anesth Analg 1986; 65: 120–126.

97. Hood DD, Curry R. Spinal versus epidural anesthesia for cesarean section in severely preeclamptic patients: a retrospective survey. Anesthesia 1999; 90(5):1276–1282.

98. Karinen J, Rasanen J, Alahuhta S et al. Maternal and uteroplacental state in preeclamptic patients during spinal anesthesia for caesarean section. Br J Anaesth 1996; 76(5):616–620.

99. Yudkin PL, Johnson P, Redman CWG. Obstetric factors associated with cord blood gas values at birth. Eur J Obstet Gynecol Reprod Biol 1987; 24:167–176.

100. Overdyk FJ, Harvey SC. Continuous spinal anesthesia for cesarean section in a parturient with severe preeclampsia. J Clin Anesth 1998; 10(6):510–513.

101. Hawkins JL. Anesthesia and preeclampsia/eclampsia. In: Norris MC, ed. Obstetric Anesthesia. Philadelphia: JB Lippincott, 1993: 501–527.

102. Ramanathan J, Angel JJ, Bush AJ, et al. Changes in maternal middle cerebral artery blood flow velocity associated with general anesthesia in severe preeclampsia. Anesth Analg 1999; 88:357–361.

103. Morris CM, Twickler DM, Hatab MR, et al. Cerebral blood flow and cranial magnetic resonance imaging in eclampsia and severe preeclampsia. Obstet Gynecol 1997; 89:561–568.

104. Ramanathan J, Sibai BM, Mabie MC et al. The use of labetalol for attenuation of the hypertensive response to end tracheal intubation in preeclampsia. Am J Obstet Gynecol 1988; 159:650–654.

105. Hood DD, Dewan DM, James MFM III et al. The use of nitroglycerine in preventing the hypertensive response to tracheal intubation in severe preeclampsia. Anesthesia 1985; 63:329.

106. Losasso TJ, Muzzi DA, Cucchiara RF. Response of fetal heart rate to maternal administration of esmolol. Anesthesia 1991; 74(4):782–784.

107. Ducey JP, Knape KG. Maternal esmolol administration resulting in fetal distress and cesarean section in a term pregnancy. Anesthesia 1992; 77(4):829–832.

108. Allen RW, James MFM, Uys PC. Attenuation of the pressor response to tracheal intubation in hypertensive proteinuric pregnant patients by lignocaine, alfentanil and magnesium sulphate. Br J Anaesth 1991; 66:216–223.

109. Rocke DA, Schoones GP. Rapidly progressive laryngeal oedema associated with pregnancy-aggravated hypertension. Anesthesia 1992; 47:141–143.

110. Potgieter PD, Hammond JMJ. "Cuff" test for safe extubation following laryngeal edema. Crit Care Med 1988; 16:818.

111. Vegna G, Leone S, Sorrentino M et al. New issues for nosgrafic setting of "HELLP" syndrome. Acta Eur Fertil 1989; 20:99.

112. Sibai BM. The HELLP syndrome (hemolysis, elevated liver enzymes and low platelets): much ado about nothing? Am J Obstet Gynecol 1990; 162:311–316.

113. Duffy BL. HELLP syndrome and the anesthetist. Anesthesia 1988; 43:223.

114. Chandran R, Serra-Serra V, Redman CW. Spontaneous resolution of preeclampsia-related thrombocytopenia. Br J Obstet Gynaecol 1992; 99:887–890.

115. James MFM, Anthony J. Critical care management of the pregnant patient. In:

Birnbach DJ, Gatt SP, Datta S, eds. Textbook of Obstetric Anesthesia. Philadelphia: Churchill-Livingstone, 2000: 716–732.

116. Lindheimer MD. Pre-eclampsia-eclampsia 1996: preventable? Have disputes on its treatment been resolved? (Review). Curr Opin Nephrol Hypertens 1996; 5:452–458.

117. Unal M, Senakayli OC, Serce K. Brain. MRI findings in cases with eclampsia (Review). Australas Radiol 1996; 40:348–350.

118. Sibai BM, McCubbin JH, Anderson GD et al. Eclampsia. I. Observations from 67 recent cases. Obstet Gynecol 1981; 58:609.

119. Gatt SP. Hypertensive disorders and renal disease in pregnancy and labor. In Birnbach DJ, Gatt SP, Datta S, eds. Textbook of Obstetric Anesthesia. Philadelphia: Churchill-Livingstone, 2000: 541–552.

120. Moodley J. Treatment of eclampsia. Br J Obstet Gynaecol 1990; 97(1):99–101.

Appendix: Conversion Table for Some Common Laboratory Values

	Conventional to SI units (normal range)	SI to conventional units (normal range)
Albumin	× 10 g/L (33–50)	× 0.1 g/dL (3.3–5.0)
Ammonia	× 0.74 μmol/L (12–54)	× 1.4 μg/dL (17–76)
Bilirubin (total)	× 17.1 μmol/L (3.42–17.1)	× 0.0584 mg/dL (0.2–1.0)
Calcium	× 0.25 mmol/L (2.18–2.55)	× 4.0 mg/dL (8.7–10.2)
Chloride	× 1 mmol/L (95–105)	× 1 mEq/L or mg/dL (95–105)
Cholesterol	× 0.0259 mmol/L (<5.18)	× 38.61 ml/dL (<200)
Creatinine	× 88.4 μmol/L (44.2–123.76)	× 0.0113 mg/dL (0.5–1.4)
Ethanol	× 0.217 mmol/L	× 4.61 μg/dL
Ferritin	× 1 μg/L (7–223)	× 1 nm/mL (7–223)
Fibrinogen	× 0.01 g/L (1.6–3.5)	× 100 mg/dL (160–350)
Folate	× 2.266 nmol/L	× 1 ng/mL
Glucose	× 0.0555 mmol/L (3.89–6.11)	× 18.02 mg/dL (70–110)

	Conventional to SI units (normal range)	SI to conventional units (normal range)
Haptoglobin	× 10 mg/L (500–3200)	× 0.1 mg/dL (50–320)
Hematocrit (packed cell volume [PCV])	× 0.01% (0.35–0.47)	× 100 (volume fraction) (35–47%)
Hemoglobin	× 10 g/L (117–157)	× 0.1 g/dL (11.7–15.7)
Iron	× 0.179 μmol/L (12.53–32.22)	× 5.587 μg/dL (70–180)
Iron-binding capacity	× 0.179 μmol/L	× 5.587 μg/dL
Mg^{2+}	× 0.418 mmol/L (0.63–0.84)	× 2.4 mg/dL (1.5–2.0)
Mg^{2+}	× 0.83 mEq/L (1.25–1.66)	× 1.2 mg/dL (1.5–2.0)
Osmolality	× 1 mmol/kg (285–310)	× mOsm/kg (285–310)
Platelet count	× 10^9/L (150–400)	× 10^3/mm^3 (140–400)
Potassium	× 1 mmol/L (3.5–5.3)	× 1 mEq/L (3.5–5.3)
RBC count (erythrocytes)	× 10^{12}/L (3.8–5.2)	× 10^6/μL or /mm^3 (3.8–5.2)
Sodium	× 1 mmol/L (135–148)	× 1 mEq/L (135–148)
Urea nitrogen	× 0.357 mmol/L (1.79–8.93)	× 2.8 mg/dL (5–25)
Uric acid	× 59.8 mmol/L (149.5–448.5)	× 0.0167 mg/dL (2.5–7.5)
WBC count (leukocytes)	× 0.001 cell × 10^9/L (.004–.011)	× 1000/μL or /mm^3 (4.0–11.0)

dL, deciliter; fL, femtoliter; hr, hour; kg, kilogram; L, liter; μ, micron; mEq, milliequivalent; mg, milligram; mL, milliliter; μmol, micromole; mmol, millimole; mOsm, milliosmole; mU, milliunit; ng, nanogram; nml, nanomole.

Index

About the Editors

MICHAEL A. BELFORT is Professor of Obstetrics and Gynecology at the University of Utah Health Sciences Center, Salt Lake City, and Director of the Department of Maternal-Fetal Medicine at Utah Valley Regional Medical Center, Provo, Utah. He is the author or coauthor of more than 300 articles, abstracts, book chapters, and presentations and editor of the journal *Hypertension in Pregnancy* (Marcel Dekker, Inc.). A Diplomate of the South African College of Medicine in both Anaesthesia and Obstetrics, he is a Fellow of the Royal College of Surgeons of Canada and the American College of Obstetrics and Gynecology and a Member of the Royal College of Obstetricians and Gynaecologists, the Society for Gynecologic Investigation, and the Society of Maternal-Fetal Medicine. Dr. Belfort received an M.B.B.C.H. (1981) from the University of Witwatersrand, Johannesburg, South Africa, an M.D. (1990) from the University of Cape Town, South Africa, and a Ph.D. (2001) from the Karolinska Institute in Stockholm, Sweden.

STEVEN THORNTON is Professor of Obstetrics and Gynaecology, University of Warwick, Coventry, England. The author of numerous professional publications, he is a member of the Royal College of Obstetricians & Gynaecologists, the Society for Gynaecologic Investigation, and the Society for Endocrinology. He received the B.M. (1983) and D.M. (1989) degrees from the University of Southampton, England.

GEORGE R. SAADE is Professor of Obstetrics and Gynecology and Director of the Maternal-Fetal Fellowship Training Program, University of Texas Medical Branch, Galveston. The author, coauthor, editor, or coeditor of more than 400 journal articles, book chapters, abstracts, and books, he is a Fellow of the Ameri-

can College of Obstetricians and Gynecologists and a member of the International
Society for the Study of Hypertension in Pregnancy, the American Heart Association, the Society for Gynecologic Investigation, and the Society of Maternal-Fetal
Medicine, among many other organizations. He received the M.D. degree (1985)
from the American University of Beirut Medical School, Beirut, Lebanon, and
completed residency training in Obstetrics and Gynecology at Union Memorial
Hospital, Baltimore, Maryland, as well as a Maternal-Fetal Medicine Fellowship
at Baylor College of Medicine, Houston, Texas.

ISBN 0-8247-0827-X

90000

9 780824 708276

T - #0162 - 101024 - C0 - 229/152/22 [24] - CB - 9780824708276 - Gloss Lamination